Molecular and Multimodality Imaging in Cardiovascular Disease

Thomas H. Schindler • Richard T. George
Joao A.C. Lima
Editors

Molecular and Multimodality Imaging in Cardiovascular Disease

Springer

Editors
Thomas H. Schindler
Johns Hopkins University
Radiology School of Medicine
Cardiovascular Nuclear Medicine
Baltimore, MD
USA

Joao A.C. Lima
Radiology and Epidemiology
Johns Hopkins University
School of Medicine, Cardiology
Baltimore, MD
USA

Richard T. George
Johns Hopkins University
School of Medicine, Cardiology
Baltimore, MD
USA

ISBN 978-3-319-19610-7 ISBN 978-3-319-19611-4 (eBook)
DOI 10.1007/978-3-319-19611-4

Library of Congress Control Number: 2015945382

Springer Cham Heidelberg New York Dordrecht London

Printed on acid-free paper

Springer International Publishing AG Switzerland is part of Springer Science+Business Media (www.springer.com)

Preface

Within the last decade of technical advancements, the field in cardiovascular imaging has rapidly expanded to a variety of modalities to image morphology and function with cardiac PET/MRI, CT, PET/CT, and SPECT/CT. These advanced imaging techniques now provide noninvasive coronary angiograms, unique and detailed information into the coronary arterial wall, description of cardiac structure and function, and complementary functional information as regards myocardial blood flow and perfusion, viability, and "vulnerable" arterial plaque burden. These cardiovascular imaging modalities may alter current paradigms for diagnosis and cardiovascular risk stratification while raising new questions and discussions for the researcher and clinician in this field. In view of this rapid evolution of molecular and multimodality imaging, the editors have strived to provide a comprehensive textbook that captures the full scope, potential, and promise of cardiac PET/MRI, CT, PET/CT, and SPECT/CT in imaging cardiovascular disease.

The editors have succeeded to recruit internationally renowned panel of expert authors, who are leading authorities in their respective disciplines. This book edition of *Molecular and Multimodality Imaging in Cardiovascular Disease* provides in-depth, comprehensive discussion of technical characteristics and clinical applications of each advanced imaging modality, implying their comparative strengths and weaknesses.

The first three chapters focus on physics; instrumentation, and systems of the PET/MRI; potential cardiac application; and initial experience. This is followed by chapters describing the evolving role of PET/CT in the detection and characterization of cardiac sarcoid disease and different imaging modalities to signify cardiac amyloidosis. There is also an in-depth discussion of the clinical significance in identifying hibernating-stunning myocardium in ischemic cardiomyopathy with different imaging modalities such as PET/CT, SPECT/CT, MRI, and echocardiography and how these imaging modalities may complement each other for a further refinement of viability assessment. Principles of cardiac MRI in conjunction with T1 mapping to determine extracellular volume fraction as surrogate marker of interstitial fibrosis and potential clinical value are excellently addressed. The second part of chapters focus on the exciting role of multimodality imaging in the detection of the "vulnerable" arterial plaque, the concurrent assessment of coronary morphology and myocardial perfusion or myocardial blood flow with a fused three-dimensional display, and, finally, the added prognostic value of coronary artery calcification measurements to myocardial perfusion imaging.

Noninvasive imaging modalities have become important tools for all physicians involved in the diagnosis and treatment of cardiovascular disease. PET/MRI, CT, PET/CT, and SPECT/CT confer a great potential to shed more light on cardiovascular pathophysiology, providing a framework for early diagnosis and treatment effectiveness of novel therapeutic treatment options. The current book edition is anticipated to contribute importantly to an understanding of the potential of noninvasive, molecular, and multimodality imaging in cardiovascular disease.

Baltimore, MD, USA Thomas H. Schindler, MD

Contents

Contributors

Mouaz H. Al-Mallah, MD, MSc, FACC, FAHA, FESC Cardiac Imaging, King Abdul-Aziz Cardiac Center, King Abdul-Aziz Medical City (Riyadh), National Guard Health Affairs, Riyadh, Kingdom of Saudi Arabia

Brian Mc Ardle, MD Division of Cardiology, University of Ottawa Heart Institute, Canadian Molecular Imaging Center of Excellence (CMICE), Ottawa, ON, Canada

Sharmila Dorbala, MD, MPH, FACC Noninvasive Cardiovascular Imaging Program, Departments of Radiology and Medicine (Cardiology), Heart and Vascular Center, Boston, MA, USA

Cardiac Amyloidosis Program, Department of Medicine, Boston, MA, USA

Brigham and Women's Hospital, Harvard Medical School, Boston, MA, USA

Marc R. Dweck, MD, PhD Centre for Cardiovascular Science, University of Edinburgh, Edinburgh, UK

Clinical Research Imaging Centre, University of Edinburgh, Edinburgh, UK

Heart Centre, Edinburgh, UK

Oliver Gaemperli, MD Department of Nuclear Medicine, University Hospital Zurich, Zurich, Switzerland

University Heart Center, Zuerich, Switzerland

Richard T. George, MD Johns Hopkins University, School of Medicine, Cardiology, Baltimore, MD, USA

Nikhil V. Joshi, MD Centre for Cardiovascular Science, University of Edinburgh, Edinburgh, UK

Clinical Research Imaging Centre, University of Edinburgh, Edinburgh, UK

Heart Centre, Edinburgh, UK

Philipp A. Kaufmann, MD Department of Nuclear Medicine, University Hospital Zurich, Zurich, Switzerland

University Heart Center, Zuerich, Switzerland

Paul Knaapen, MD Department of Cardiology, VU University Medical Center of Amsterdam, Amsterdam, The Netherlands

Karl P. Kunze, MSc Nuklearmedizinische Klinik und Poliklinik, Klinikum rechts der Isar, Technische Universität München, Munich, Germany

Eugene Leung, MD, FRCPC Division of Cardiology, University of Ottawa Heart Institute, Canadian Molecular Imaging Center of Excellence (CMICE), Ottawa, ON, Canada

Joao A.C. Lima, MD Radiology and Epidemiology, Johns Hopkins University, School of Medicine, Cardiology, Baltimore, MD, USA

Stephan G. Nekolla, PhD Nuklearmedizinische Klinik und Poliklinik, Klinikum rechts der Isar, Technische Universität München, Munich, Germany

Felix Nensa, MD Department of Diagnostic and Interventional Radiology, University Hospital of Essen, University of Duisburg-Essen, Essen, Germany

David E. Newby, MD, PhD Centre for Cardiovascular Science, University of Edinburgh, Edinburgh, UK

Clinical Research Imaging Centre, University of Edinburgh, Edinburgh, UK

Heart Centre, Edinburgh, UK

Hiroshi Ohira, MD Division of Cardiology, University of Ottawa Heart Institute, Canadian Molecular Imaging Center of Excellence (CMICE), Ottawa, ON, Canada

Aju P. Pazhenkottil, MD Department of Nuclear Medicine, University Hospital Zurich, Zurich, Switzerland

University Heart Center, Zurich, Switzerland

Matthieu Pelletier-Galarneau, MD, MSc Division of Cardiology, University of Ottawa Heart Institute, Canadian Molecular Imaging Center of Excellence (CMICE), Ottawa, ON, Canada

Thorsten D. Poeppel, MD Department of Diagnostic and Interventional Radiology, University Hospital of Essen, University of Duisburg-Essen, Essen, Germany

Harald H. Quick, PhD Department of Diagnostic and Interventional Radiology, High Field and Hybrid MR Imaging, University Hospital Essen, Essen, Germany

Erwin L. Hahn Institute for MR Imaging, University of Duisburg-Essen, Essen, Germany

Christoph Rischpler, MD Nuklearmedizinische Klinik und Poliklinik, Klinikum rechts der Isar, Technische Universität München, Munich, Germany

Terrence D. Ruddy, MD, FRCPC, FACC Division of Cardiology, University of Ottawa Heart Institute, Canadian Molecular Imaging Center of Excellence (CMICE), Ottawa, ON, Canada

Erik B. Schelbert, MD, MS Division of Cardiology, Department of Medicine, University of Pittsburgh, Pittsburg, PA, USA

Thomas H. Schindler, MD Johns Hopkins University, Radiology School of Medicine, Cardiovascular Nuclear Medicine, Baltimore, MD, USA

Thomas Schlosser, MD Department of Diagnostic and Interventional Radiology, University Hospital of Essen, University of Duisburg-Essen, Essen, Germany

Ravi K. Sharma, MD Division of Cardiology, Department of Medicine, Johns Hopkins University, Baltimore, MA, USA

Ines Valenta, MD Department of Radiology SOM, Nuclear Medicine, Johns Hopkins University, Baltimore, MA, USA

Timothy C. Wong, MD, MS Division of Cardiology, Department of Medicine, University of Pittsburgh, Pittsburg, PA, USA

Xiaoli Zhang, MD, PhD Department of Nuclear Medicine, State Key Laboratory of Cardiovascular Disease, Fuwai Hospital, National Center for Cardiovascular Diseases, Chinese Academy of Medical Sciences and Peking Union Medical College, Beijing, People's Republic of China

PET/MRI: Physics, Instrumentation, and Systems

1

Harald H. Quick

1.1 Introduction

Hybrid imaging with combined positron emission tomography/magnetic resonance imaging (PET/MRI) is the most recent addition to the palette of hybrid imaging modalities [1, 2]. PET/MRI synergistically combines the excellent soft tissue contrast and detailed image resolution of MR imaging with metabolic information provided by PET. Integrated PET/MRI systems furthermore offer the ability to acquire hybrid imaging data simultaneously [1, 3]. Beyond exact co-registration of PET and MR imaging data, this can be applied for MR-based motion correction of PET data. Especially in the context of diagnostic cardiac imaging, these features open up several applications, e.g., evaluation of cardiac function and viability and diagnosis of cardiac inflammatory diseases and tumorous diseases [4–7]. To fully assess the diagnostic potential of PET/MR, however, several physical and technical challenges had to be overcome and are still subject to ongoing research. Due to the absence of CT information, attenuation correction (AC) of the patient tissues in PET/MRI has to be based on MR images which are currently limited in the number of tissue classes available [8] and by undercorrection of the bone tissue [9]. Dedicated cardiac radiofrequency (RF) coils, necessary for reception of the MR signal, and ECG gating equipment are currently not considered in AC. Consequently quantification of cardiac PET data in PET/MRI, therefore, might be biased. Furthermore, the clinical workflow is rather complex and needs to be tailored to cardiac examinations.

H.H. Quick, PhD
Erwin L. Hahn Institute for MR Imaging, University of Duisburg-Essen, Essen, Germany

Department of High Field and Hybrid MR Imaging,
University Hospital Essen, Essen, Germany
e-mail: harald.quick@uni-due.de

T.H. Schindler et al. (eds.), *Molecular and Multimodality Imaging in Cardiovascular Disease*, DOI 10.1007/978-3-319-19611-4_1

In this chapter, current PET/MRI system designs are presented, physical challenges and methodological solutions for attenuation and motion correction are discussed, and furthermore, specific challenges of cardiac PET/MR hybrid imaging will be highlighted.

1.2 PET/MRI System Design

The combination of separate PET and MRI systems into a single multimodality system needed a careful design of several hardware components [1, 3]. MR imaging requires well-controlled and uniform static magnetic fields for spin polarization, linear gradient fields for spatial signal encoding, and radiofrequency fields for spin excitation and signal readout. Therefore, any unshielded additional electronic hardware can affect the accuracy and quality of MR images. On the other hand, conventional PET detectors and associated hardware and electronics are not designed for the use inside strong electromagnetic fields. In particular, PET detectors based on photomultiplier tubes (PMTs), which are needed to convert and amplify signal from scintillation crystals into electronic signal, do not function properly in or near strong magnetic fields [10, 11].

Integrating PET detectors based on PMT within an MR system has proven to be a difficult task, requiring vendors to either opt for avalanche photodiodes (APDs) [10, 11] or physically separate the PET and MR imaging units [2]. The performance of APD detectors, used to replace PMT, is not affected by strong magnetic fields [10, 11]. In the context of PET/MR hybrid imaging, conventional PMT detectors can only be used if the PET unit is placed sufficiently far away from the MR imaging unit such that the magnetic field strength at the position of the PET unit is very low [2]. A recently available integrated PET/MRI system contains new semiconductor detectors, e.g., silicon photon multipliers (SiPMs) [12, 13]. Like APD detectors, SiPM detectors are not sensitive to the magnetic field and, consequently, can be integrated inside an MR system. Four current PET/MR hybrid imaging systems are shown in Fig. 1.1. A schematic drawing of an integrated PET/MRI system and MR-compatible APD-based PET detectors are displayed in Fig. 1.2.

1.3 Attenuation Correction

1.3.1 Attenuation Correction in PET/CT

A technical challenge in PET/MR hybrid imaging is the attenuation correction of PET emission images based on MR information, necessary for an accurate quantitative measurement of the tracer activity concentration. In PET/CT hybrid imaging, the CT image providing spatial representation of Hounsfield units (HU) of the patient tissues and hardware components, such as patient table, can be used to calculate attenuation maps (μ-maps) by applying an appropriate energy scaling (Fig. 1.3). This is achieved by using the inherent 3D CT data of the patient tissues and patient table. The CT data (in HU) is then directly

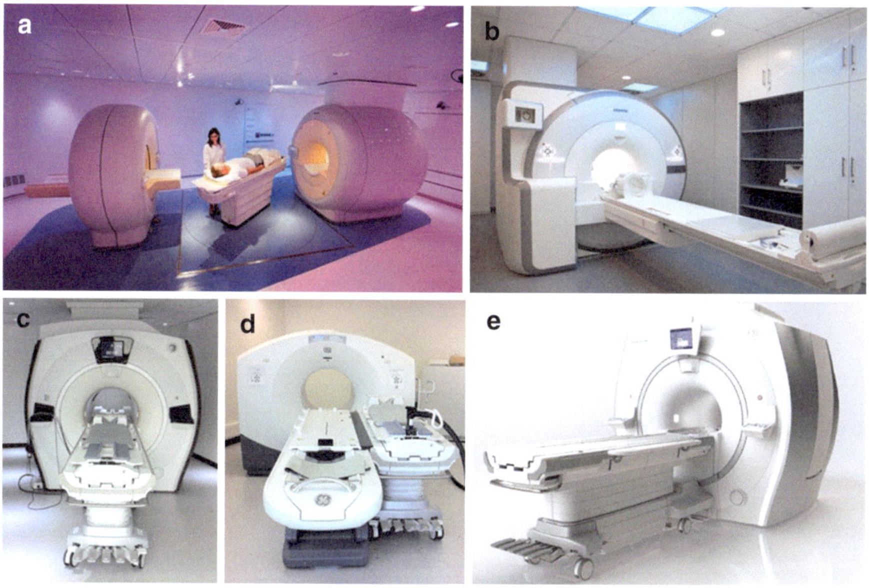

Fig. 1.1 Four current systems for PET/MR hybrid imaging: (**a**) Philips Ingenuity TF, (**b**) Siemens Biograph mMR, (**c**, **d**) GE Tri-modality MR (**c**) and PET/CT (**d**) connected via a patient table shuttle system, (**e**) GE Signa PET/MR. All four systems perform at 3 Tesla field strength. Systems (**a**) and (**c**, **d**) provide sequential PET/MR examinations while systems (**b**) and (**e**) allow for simultaneous PET and MR data acquisition

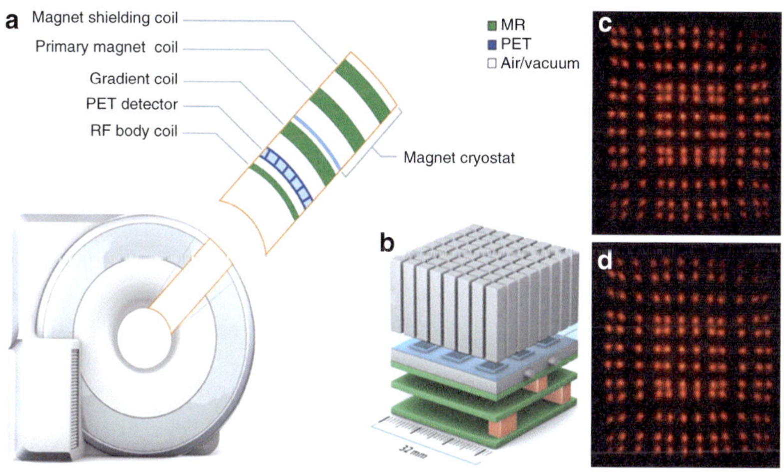

Fig. 1.2 (**a**) Schematic drawing of an integrated PET/MR system (Biograph mMR, Siemens AG, Healthcare Sector). The drawing shows the integration of the PET detectors in the MR system structure. From the inside to the outside: radiofrequency body coil, PET detector, gradient coil assembly, primary magnet coil, and magnet shielding coil. (**b**) PET detector block assembly where 64 lutetium oxyorthosilicate (LSO) crystals form one detector block that are read out by MR-compatible avalanche photodiode (APD) detectors. (**c**, **d**) Demonstration of the MR compatibility of an LSO crystal with APD-based PET detector. The PET signal footprint in (**c**) was acquired without magnetic field, while the signal footprint in (**d**) was acquired at 7.0 Tesla magnetic field strength. No magnetic field-related signal distortions can be seen in (**d**) (**c**, **d** from Lecomte et al. [11])

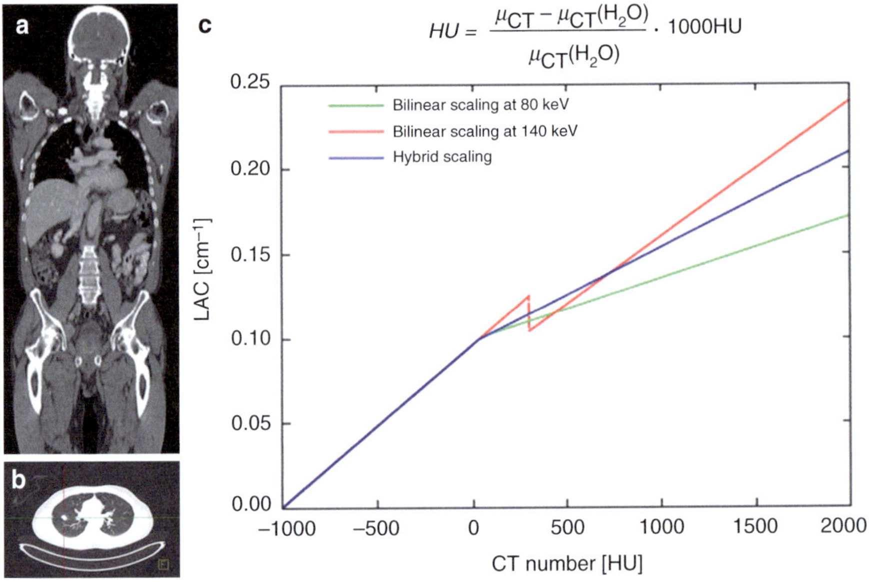

Fig. 1.3 Attenuation correction of PET data in PET/CT hybrid imaging. In PET/CT, attenuation correction is achieved by synergistically using the inherent three-dimensional CT data of the patient tissues (**a**) and patient table (**b**). The CT data (Hounsfield Units, HU) is then directly converted from its energy level (e.g., 80–140 keV) by bilinear conversion models (From Carney et al. [14]) to linear attenuation coefficients (LAC) of PET at 511 keV energy level (**c**)

converted from its energy level (e.g., 80–140 keV) by bilinear conversion models to linear attenuation coefficients (LAC) of PET at 511 keV energy level (Fig. 1.3) [14].

1.3.2 Attenuation Correction in PET/MRI

PET data needs to be attenuation corrected in the reconstruction process in order to provide a valid quantification of tracer activity distribution in the human body. Scanner hardware components (e.g., tabletop, RF coils) as well as patient tissues within the FOV of the PET detector during data acquisition attenuate the number of true annihilation events and consequently may lead to false results without providing AC. Depending on the position of the heart in the thorax, photons emitted from the myocardium may experience different attenuations on their way through different body tissues to the PET detector. Non-AC PET data generally shows underestimation of the real tracer activity deep in the patient's body and also in the heart. Since the PET/MRI system cannot measure linear attenuation directly as in PET/CT hybrid imaging, AC here needs to be performed differently (Fig. 1.4).

1.3.2.1 Attenuation Correction of Patient Tissues

Attenuation correction of human soft tissue is necessary to correct for the individual patient anatomy. Since no linear attenuation coefficient-based CT information is

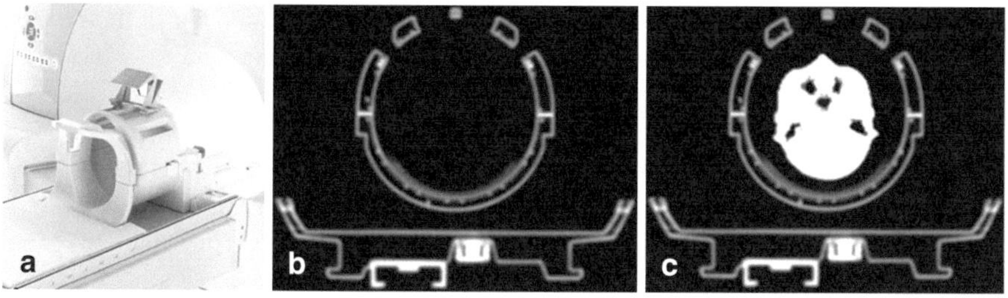

Fig. 1.4 Attenuation correction PET/MR hybrid imaging. Photograph (**a**) shows a head/neck radiofrequency coil that was optimized for PET transparency for use in an integrated PET/MR hybrid system. Image (**b**) shows a transversal view through the CT-based hardware attenuation map of a PET/MR system's patient table with a radiofrequency head coil in place. In image (**c**) the MR-based attenuation correction map of the patient tissues (head) has been added. Thus (**c**) shows the completed attenuation map that represents the geometric distribution of attenuating hardware and soft tissue structures in the PET field of view

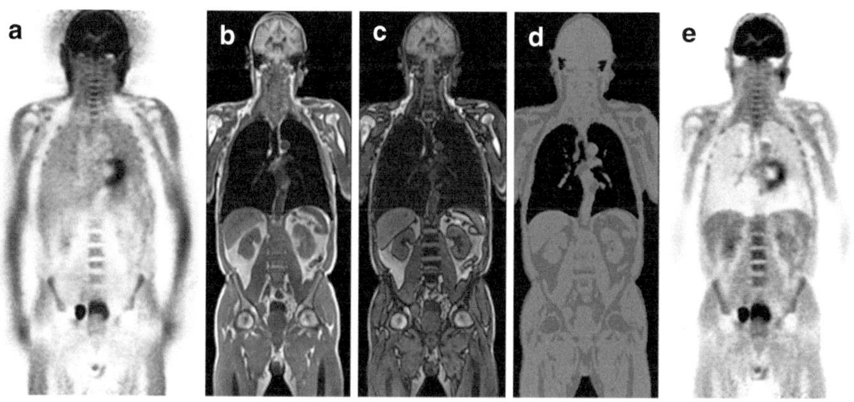

Fig. 1.5 Patient-tissue attenuation correction based on MR imaging. (**a**) Uncorrected whole-body PET scan showing relative activity enhancement in the lungs and along the outer contours of the patient. (**b**, **c**) Dixon-based MR sequence providing separate water/fat "in-phase" and "opposed-phase" images that serve as basis for soft tissue segmentation. (**d**) Segmented soft tissue groups (air, fat, muscle, lungs) that can be assigned to a PET attenuation map of the patient tissues. (**e**) Resulting attenuation-corrected PET scan of the initial data set (**a**). *Note*: Bone signal is assigned as soft tissue values in this MR-based approach for AC

available in integrated PET/MRI, tissue-specific AC has to be based on MR information which is based on proton density and relaxation properties (e.g., T1 and T2 relaxation times), rather than on the attenuation of X-rays in tissue. Both air and solid bones lack signal in MRI; thus these fundamentally different tissue classes are difficult to separate. In the current implementation of integrated PET/MRI systems, tissue attenuation and scatter correction is performed using a three-dimensional (3D) Dixon-based MR imaging technique, providing two sets of images where water and fat are "in phase" and "out of phase" (Fig. 1.5) [8]. This allows reconstruction of fat-only, water-only, and fat-water images and results in tissue segmentation of air, fat, muscle, and lungs in the reconstructed and displayed μ-maps

(Fig. 1.5) [8]. The cortical bone is currently not being accounted for in the Dixon-based AC approach. The bone is here classified as soft tissue, and thus the exact magnitude of PET signal attenuation of the bone might be underestimated [9].

1.3.2.2 Attenuation Correction of System Hardware Components

Radiofrequency surface receiver coils are a technical precondition for high-resolution MR imaging and are well established in clinical MRI. In a standard setup of integrated PET/MR cardiac imaging, the patient is placed on top of a rigid phased-array spine RF coil. For anterior signal detection, a second multichannel phased-array RF surface coil is placed on the thorax of the patient during simultaneous MR and PET data acquisition (Fig. 1.6). Thus, all RF surface coils used in the PET field of view during simultaneous PET data acquisition have to be optimized for PET transparency, i.e., such coils should attenuate the photons only minimally [15–18].

The PET signal attenuation of rigid and stationary equipment such as the RF spine array and the RF head/neck coil can be compensated for by straightforward AC methods. After scanning this equipment by using CT, a 3D map of attenuation values can be generated. This data can then be converted into a 3D representation of the 511 keV attenuation values, the so-called μ-map. By linking the RF spine or RF head coil's position to the patient's table position, the corresponding AC μ-map for each table position is automatically selected by the system for PET image reconstruction [17].

For flexible surface RF coils like the 6-channel RF body phased array (Fig. 1.6) which may be used in the context of cardiac PET/MR, the AC is performed differently. Because the design of such surface RF coils is flexible, the individual position and shape of this RF coil during a patient examination is not known. Thus a

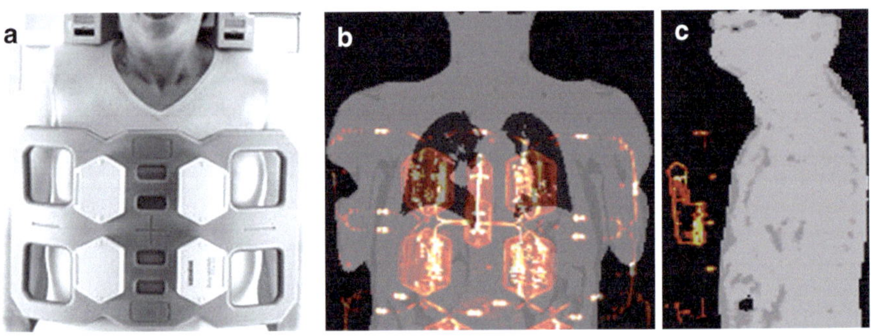

Fig. 1.6 (**a**) Six-channel thorax radiofrequency coil for MR signal reception during simultaneous cardiac PET/MR data acquisition. Images (**b**, **c**) show MR-based attenuation maps of the patient tissues that were acquired with a 3D Dixon-based sequence. The hardware attenuation correction map of the flexible RF coil (*orange/red color*) here was co-registered with nonrigid registration on the patient tissue attenuation correction map. Such attenuation maps represent the geometric distribution of PET signal-attenuating hardware and soft tissue structures in the PET field of view

pre-acquired rigid 3D CT template cannot directly be co-registered [17]. As alternative strategy for AC of flexible RF coils, visible markers have been proposed to perform an automatic nonrigid co-registration of the pre-acquired 3D CT attenuation template to the individual position and shape of the flexible RF coil during the cardiac PET/MR examination (Fig. 1.6) [17, 19].

1.4 Motion Correction (MC)

Integrated PET/MRI systems provide the inherent advantage of simultaneous PET and MR data acquisition. In view of motion correction (MC), this is an inherent advantage over PET/CT that is currently being further explored [20–27]. While in PET/CT the CT data is static and for dose considerations is acquired only once at the beginning at a typical hybrid examination, the MR data in PET/MRI is acquired simultaneously to PET data acquisition, and this applies to data acquisition in each bed position. This inherently leads to less deviation and less gross motion between both imaging modalities when compared to PET/CT imaging. Furthermore, real-time MRI data and 4D MR data of breathing motion can be used to retrospectively motion correct PET data to provide improved fusion of PET and MR data sets [20–27]. This may potentially lead to improved lesion visibility in the lungs, upper abdomen, and liver and may also result in better quantification of activity in the myocardium since all structures are depicted with sharper contours and less smeared over a larger volume which otherwise leads to reduced standardized uptake values (SUV) of regions subject to motion [25].

With the heart being subject to cardiac and breathing motion during PET and MR data acquisition, it is expected that the further development and application of advanced triggering, nonrigid motion correction, and attenuation correction methods will have a substantial impact on PET/MR cardiac imaging in general and more specific in myocardial tissue quantification [26].

1.4.1 Cardiac Gating

Most MRI sequences as well as reconstruction of cardiac PET data recorded in list mode require a sufficiently good ECG signal in order to control or selectively use data from an acquired image of a specific cardiac phase. In contrast to PET examinations in PET/CT procedures, during integrated PET/MRI, it must be considered that ECG signals can be significantly influenced by the magnetic field and radiofrequency pulses, thus requiring special care when applying the electrodes and monitoring the ECG signal. The relatively long duration of the simultaneous MRI examination can be used almost in its entirety for the parallel acquisition of PET data; this compensates for the loss of PET acquisition time caused by ECG gating and results in high PET image quality (Fig. 1.7) [4, 27, 28].

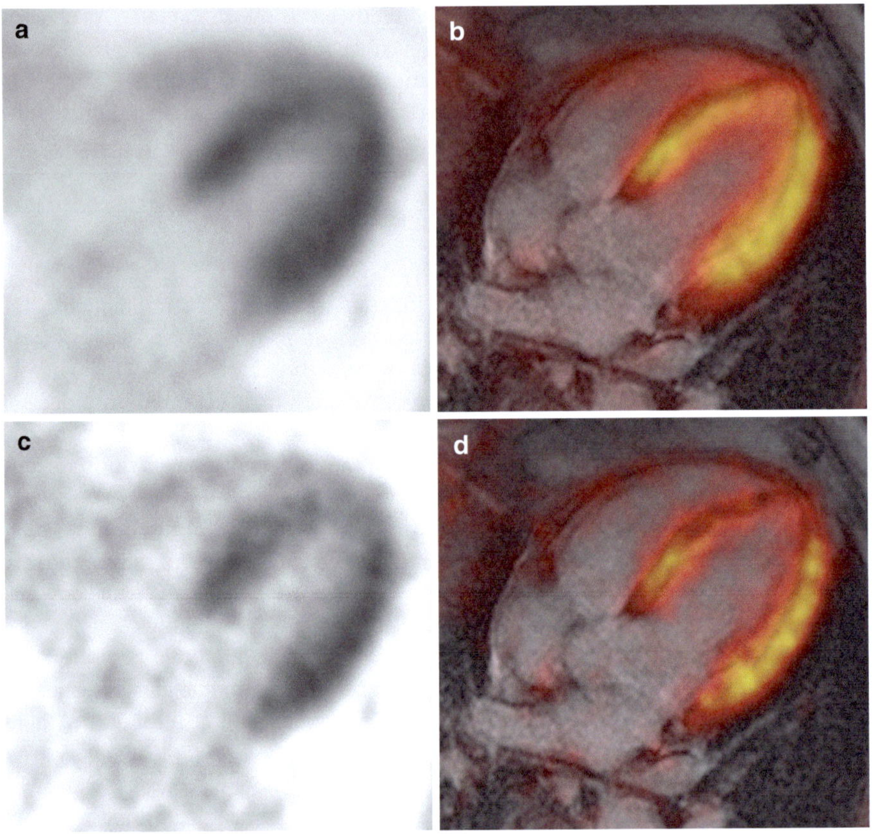

Fig. 1.7 Impact of ECG gating on cardiac PET imaging. The images show an end-diastolic four-chamber view of PET (**a**, **c**) and PET/MR fused with late gadolinium-enhanced ECG-gated MRI (**b**, **d**). The PET data in (**a**, **b**) was non-ECG gated; the PET data in (**c**, **d**) was ECG gated. While the non-ECG gated PET data (**a**, **b**) here shows better signal-to-noise ratio due to longer data acquisition, the ECG-gated PET data showing one out of eight cardiac motion phases (**c**, **d**) provides sharper depiction of the activity distribution constrained to the myocardial wall

1.5 Hybrid Imaging Workflow

Simultaneous and independent PET and MR data acquisition provides the basis for cardiac PET/MRI studies. In view of data synchronization, this acquisition scheme also provides an inherent advantage of cardiac PET/MR when compared to PET/CT since the acquisition times of both imaging modalities are closely matched in PET/MR, while in PET/CT the CT data acquisition is to be finished within few seconds. Thus, the rather long acquisition times of a cardiac MR exam encompassing evaluation of anatomy, function, and perfusion can be used synergistically to extend the acquisition time of PET. This, in combination with PET data acquisition in list

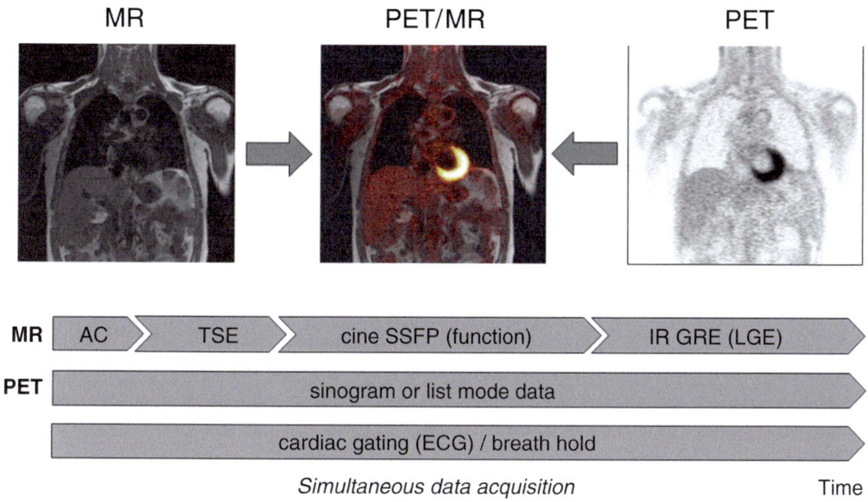

Fig. 1.8 PET/MR simultaneous imaging workflow. MR (*left*) and PET (*right*) data acquisition is performed simultaneously. The standard cardiac MR examination encompasses sequences for attenuation correction, e.g., turbo spin echo (*TSE*) for anatomic reference and cardiac-gated cine-cine steady-state free precession (*SSFP*) sequences for assessment of cardiac function. Late gadolinium enhancement (*LGE*) using an inversion recovery (*IR*) gradient echo (*GRE*) sequence reveals cardiac infarction that then can be correlated to the metabolic information of simultaneously acquired F18-FDG-PET

Table 1.1 Challenges and current correction methods relevant for cardiac PET/MRI

Challenge	Correction method	Reference #
Attenuation correction of patient tissues	MR-based tissue segmentation into tissue classes (e.g., background air, soft tissues, fat, lung) with Dixon-based MR sequences	[8, 9]
Attenuation correction of hardware components	CT-based and energy-converted templates of hardware components (e.g., patient table, RF coils)	[14–19]
Motion during MR and/or PET data acquisition	MR-derived motion fields applied to PET reconstruction	[20–27]
Motion between MR-based attenuation map and PET data acquisition	Acquisition of multiphase MR-based AC maps during breathing and co-reconstruction of list-mode PET-data to matching AC phase	[24, 25]

mode, allows for ECG gating or even double gating of cardiac and breathing motion while enough PET data is acquired to support retrospective data reconstruction with good image quality of gated and time-resolved PET studies (Fig. 1.8). All challenges and current correction methods associated with cardiac PET/MRI are listed in Table 1.1.

1.6 Summary

Whole-body PET/MR hybrid imaging has entered the clinical arena. On the technical and hardware development level, several challenges had to be overcome that ultimately have led to the availability of integrated whole-body PET/MR systems. Innovative methods have been developed to provide viable solutions for MR-based attenuation correction and motion correction of PET data and are still subject to ongoing research. Unlike any other clinical PET/MR imaging application, cardiac PET/MRI will benefit from further evolution and application of attenuation correction and motion correction algorithms to unveil its full diagnostic potential.

References

1. Delso G, Furst S, Jakoby B, et al. Performance measurements of the Siemens mMR integrated whole-body PET/MR scanner. J Nucl Med. 2011;52:1914–22.
2. Zaidi H, Ojha N, Morich M, et al. Design and performance evaluation of a whole-body Ingenuity TF PET-MRI system. Phys Med Biol. 2011;56:3091–106.
3. Quick HH. Integrated PET/MR. J Magn Reson Imaging. 2014;39:243–58.
4. Nensa F, Poeppel TD, Beiderwellen K, et al. Hybrid PET/MR imaging of the heart: feasibility and initial results. Radiology. 2013;268:366–73.
5. Rischpler C, Nekolla SG, Dregely I, Schwaiger M. Hybrid PET/MR imaging of the heart: potential, initial experiences, and future prospects. J Nucl Med. 2013;54:402–15.
6. Schlosser T, Nensa F, Mahabadi AA, Poeppel TD. Hybrid MRI/PET of the heart: a new complementary imaging technique for simultaneous acquisition of MRI and PET data. Heart. 2013;99:351–2.
7. Lee WW, Marinelli B, Van der Laan AM, et al. PET/MRI of inflammation in myocardial infarction. J Am Coll Cardiol. 2013;59:153–63.
8. Martinez-Moller A, Souvatzoglou M, Delso G, et al. Tissue classification as a potential approach for attenuation correction in whole-body PET/MRI: evaluation with PET/CT data. J Nucl Med. 2009;50:520–6.
9. Samarin A, Burger C, Wollenweber SD, et al. PET/MR imaging of bone lesions – implications for PET quantification from imperfect attenuation correction. Eur J Nucl Med Mol Imaging. 2012;39:1154–60.
10. Pichler BJ, Judenhofer MS, Catana C, et al. Performance test of an LSO-APD detector in a 7-T MRI scanner for simultaneous PET/MRI. J Nucl Med. 2006;47:639–47.
11. Lecomte R. Novel detector technology for clinical PET. Eur J Nucl Med Mol Imaging. 2009;32:S69–85.
12. Schaart DR, van Dam HT, Seifert S, et al. A novel, SiPM-array-based, monolithic scintillator detector for PET. Phys Med Biol. 2009;54:3501–12.
13. Levin C, Glover G, Deller T, et al. Prototype time-of-flight PET ring integrated with a 3T MRI system for simultaneous whole-body PET/MR imaging [abstract]. J Nucl Med. 2013;54 Suppl 2:148.
14. Carney JPJ, Townsend DW, Rappoport V, Bendriem B. Method for transforming CT images for attenuation correction in PET/CT imaging. Med Phys. 2006;33:976–83.
15. Delso G, Martinez-Möller A, Bundschuh RA, et al. Evaluation of the attenuation properties of MR equipment for its use in a whole-body PET/MR scanner. Phys Med Biol. 2010;55:4361–74.
16. Tellmann L, Quick HH, Bockisch A, Herzog H, Beyer T. The effect of MR surface coils on PET quantification in whole-body PET/MR. Med Phys. 2011;38:2795–805.
17. Paulus DH, Braun H, Aklan, Quick HH. Simultaneous PET/MR imaging: MR-based attenuation correction of local radiofrequency surface coils. Med Phys. 2012;39:4306–15.

18. Paulus DH, Tellmann L, Quick HH. Towards improved hardware component attenuation correction in PET/MR hybrid imaging. Phys Med Biol. 2013;58:8021–40.
19. Kartmann R, Paulus DH, Braun H, et al. Integrated PET/MR imaging: automatic attenuation correction of flexible RF coils. Med Phys. 2013;40(8):082301. doi:10.1118/1.4812685.
20. Tsoumpas C, Mackewn JE, Halsted P. Simultaneous PET-MR acquisition and MR-derived motion fields for correction of non-rigid motion in PET. Ann Nucl Med. 2010;24:745–50.
21. Tsoumpas C, Buerger C, King AP, et al. Fast generation of 4D PET-MR data from real dynamic MR acquisitions. Phys Med Biol. 2011;56:6597–613.
22. Catana C, Benner T, van der Kouwe A, et al. MRI-assisted PET motion correction for neurologic studies in an integrated MR/PET scanner. J Nucl Med. 2011;52:154–61.
23. Brendle CB, Schmidt H, Fleischer S, Braeuning UH, Pfannenberg CA, Schwenzer NF. Simultaneously acquired MR/PET images compared with sequential MR/PET and PET/CT: alignment quality. Radiology. 2013;268:190–9.
24. Wuerslin C, Schmidt H, Martirosian P, et al. Respiratory motion correction in oncologic PET using T1-weighted MR imaging on a simultaneous whole-body PET/MR system. J Nucl Med. 2013;54:464–71.
25. Grimm R, Fürst S, Dregely I, et al. Self-gated radial MRI for respiratory motion compensation on hybrid PET/MR systems. Med Image Comput Comput Assist Interv. 2013;16:17–24.
26. Fieseler M, Kugel H, Gigengack F, et al. A dynamic thorax phantom for the assessment of cardiac and respiratory motion correction in PET/MRI: a preliminary evaluation. Nuc Instr Meth Phys Res A. 2013;702:59–63.
27. Baumgartner CF, Kolbitsch C, Balfour DR, et al. High-resolution dynamic MR imaging of the thorax for respiratory motion correction of PET using groupwise manifold alignment. Med Image Anal. 2014;18:939–52.
28. Nensa F, Schlosser T. Cardiovascular hybrid imaging using PET/MRI. Rofo. 2014;186:1094–101.

Potential Role of Cardiac PET/MRI in Cardiovascular Disease: Initial Experience

2

Felix Nensa, Thorsten D. Poeppel, and Thomas Schlosser

2.1 Introduction

Hybrid PET/MR imaging using sequential and integrated scanner platforms has been available for several years, and from the beginning, expectations toward cardiovascular applications have been high. Both PET and MRI have been used in cardiovascular imaging for decades, and in recent years, MRI became a standard of reference with respect to a variety of cardiovascular diseases. Cardiac MRI allows for the detailed anatomical assessment of the cardiovascular system, quantification of cardiovascular function, and multiparametric tissue classification. PET imaging allows for the precise quantification of myocardial perfusion and coronary blood flow reserve, visualization of specific metabolic processes, as well as quantification on the molecular level. Despite a certain overlap between modalities, the excellent morphologic and functional imaging capabilities of MRI in combination with the high sensitivity and quantification capabilities of PET are poised to provide added value in a variety of cardiac diseases. The following chapter provides a summary of the current state of scientific research in cardiovascular PET/MRI.

F. Nensa, MD (✉) • T. Schlosser, MD
Department of Diagnostic and Interventional Radiology and Neuroradiology, University Hospital of Essen, University of Duisburg-Essen, Essen, Germany
e-mail: felix.nensa@gmail.com; thomas.schlosser@uni-due.de

T.D. Poeppel, MD
Clinic for Nuclear Medicine, University Hospital of Essen, University of Duisburg-Essen, Essen, Germany
e-mail: thorsten.poeppel@uni-due.de

T.H. Schindler et al. (eds.), *Molecular and Multimodality Imaging in Cardiovascular Disease*, DOI 10.1007/978-3-319-19611-4_2

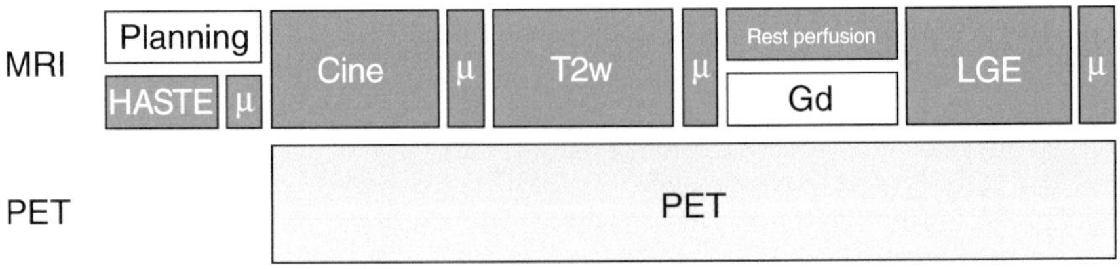

Fig. 2.1 Basic protocol for simultaneous cardiac PET/MR imaging. *HASTE* axial 2D half Fourier acquisition single-shot turbo spin echo sequence, *μ* attenuation map (μ-map) using 2-point Dixon sequences, *Cine* Cine imaging using balanced SSFP sequence, *T2w* T2-weighted imaging using turbo inversion recovery magnitude sequence, *Rest Perfusion* rest perfusion imaging using saturation recovery fast low-angle shot sequence, *Gd* ~10 min waiting for late gadolinium enhancement, *LGE* late gadolinium enhancement imaging using segmented 2D inversion recovery turbo FLASH sequence

2.2 Feasibility

Being clinically well established, cardiac MRI still remains a challenge. Several sources of motion originating from cardiac movement, from breathing, and from multidirectional blood flow require fast and robust imaging, while the involvement of small anatomical structures like papillary muscles or heart valves demands high spatial image resolution. To meet these requirements, cardiac MRI employs highly optimized and complex acquisition techniques, which potentially could be more susceptible to inhomogeneity of the magnetic field. However, despite the presence of PET detectors in the magnetic field of the MR imaging unit, being a potential source of field inhomogeneities, eddy currents, and electromagnetic interference, several reports have demonstrated the technical feasibility and high image quality of cardiac PET/MR imaging on an integrated scanner (Fig. 2.1) [1–5]. Using standard MR sequences for cardiac imaging and dedicated low-attenuation body surface coils, no negative side effects from the integrated imaging system design have been observed [5].

Myocardial PET imaging with FDG usually requires a special dietary preparation [3, 6], which is known to be a source of patient discomfort and potential incompliance. In addition, the relatively long duration of cardiac MRI examinations associated with noise, narrowness, and immobility can result in premature cancellation of examinations by the patient. Indeed, a cardiac PET/MRI study revealed long examination times, the PET/MR imaging examination itself, and fasting to be the main sources of discomfort, resulting in only moderate patient compliance [5]. Thus, it seems mandatory to further optimize patient preparation and implement compact imaging protocols to pave the way for the clinical establishment of cardiac PET/MRI.

2.3 MRI-Based Attenuation Correction

Since there is no direct translation of MR-acquired image contrasts into gamma ray attenuation coefficients of tissue, alternative techniques for attenuation correction of PET data had to be developed. While in principle several methods are available [7], currently an MR-based image segmentation approach is typically used in

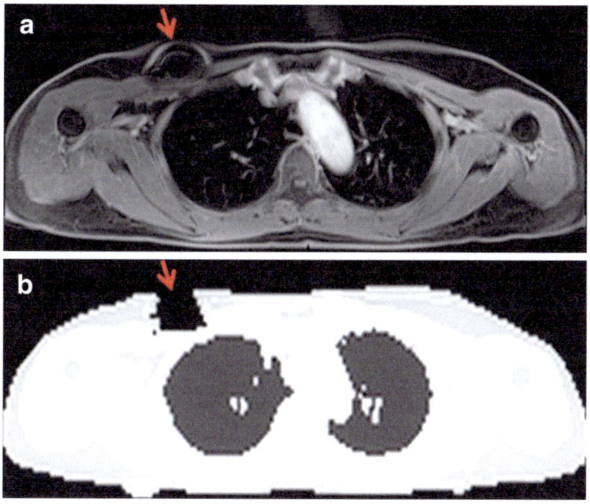

Fig. 2.2 Source of imaging artifacts. Implanted port system causing MR imaging artifacts (**a**, *arrow*) resulting in erroneous attenuation coefficients in μ-maps (**b**, *arrow*)

integrated cardiac PET/MR imaging [8]. This method usually segments tissue into four compartments (background, lung, fat, and soft tissue) with fixed attenuation coefficients assigned to each compartment. Consequently, the resulting attenuation maps are relatively coarse as finer nuances between tissue attenuations are not represented; e.g., the myocardium vs. the blood, which are both classified as soft tissue. Moreover, the bone is also classified as soft tissue and thus severely misclassified regarding its attenuation for gamma rays. Therefore, in the bone tissue and in its vicinity, standardized uptake values (SUVs) derived from PET/MRI systems might be significantly underestimated when compared to standardized uptake values derived from PET/CT [9]. Using ultrashort echo time (UTE) sequences, the segmentation of tissue with very short T2* (such as the bone) has been demonstrated to be feasible [10]. However, this technique is still limited to a rather small field of view and thus not yet available in cardiac PET/MR imaging.

The segmentation-based approach is dependent on the accuracy of the tissue segmentation algorithm, which can be significantly wrong in the presence of artifacts in the underlying MR images. Artifacts that are frequently found in cardiac imaging often originate from foreign objects like implantable port systems, sternal wire cerclages, artificial heart valves, or artificial joint replacement of the humerus (Fig. 2.2).

Also, cardiac MR imaging is usually performed with the patient's arms aligned along the body axis. In larger patients, this can result in parts of the arms being placed outside the MR field of view, causing so-called truncation artifacts at the edges of the attenuation maps. This can at least partially be avoided by imaging in the arms-up position, extension of the MR field of view [11], or partial correction with PET emission data using maximum-likelihood reconstruction of attenuation and activity (MLAA) [12].

Nevertheless, segmentation-based attenuation correction has been demonstrated to be a reasonably reliable procedure with regard to visual assessment of PET data by the experienced observer [8]. Regarding cardiac PET/MR imaging, it has been shown to provide excellent visual PET image quality that was in good concordance

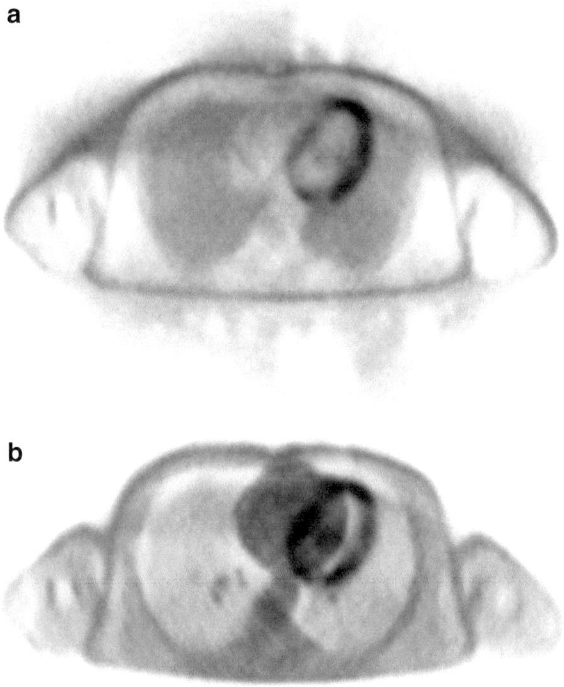

Fig. 2.3 Source of imaging artifacts. PET image artifacts due to patient movement (primarily in z-axis direction) during PET acquisition (**a**) (PET image without attenuation correction). The artifacts are even more pronounced using the wrong (no longer correctly co-registered) μ-map for attenuation correction (**b**)

with corresponding PET images from PET/CT [5]. In a study comparing standardized uptake values for FDG using PET/MR and PET/CT in normal organ tissues of oncologic patients, excellent correlations between both modalities were found in the myocardium [13]. In another study in oncologic patients, an excellent correlation of myocardial standardized uptake values between non-ECG-gated PET/MRI and PET/CT has been reported. Furthermore, a variation over the cardiac cycle with higher standardized uptake values at end-systole and lower standardized uptake values at end-diastole was observed using ECG-gated PET/MRI [14]. In a dedicated cardiac PET/MRI study in patients with myocardial infarction, analysis of maximum standardized uptake values in the myocardium showed considerable variation between PET/MRI- and PET/CT-acquired data, while pairwise comparison did not show a significant difference between both modalities [5]. In summary, quantitative PET data acquired on an integrated PET/MR scanner should still be treated with caution, and visual assessment of attenuation maps and PET images for technical errors is mandatory (Fig. 2.3).

2.4 Acute Myocardial Infarction

An initial report of integrated PET/MRI in a patient with a large transmural infarction after occlusion of the left circumflex artery and symptom-to-reperfusion time of 6 h demonstrated a nearly perfect match between the myocardium showing late

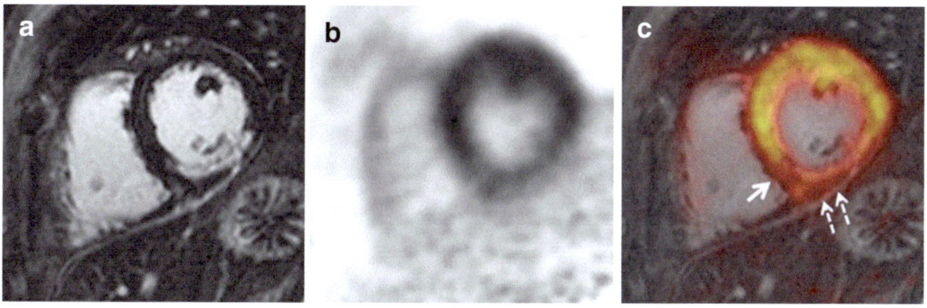

Fig. 2.4 FDG PET/MRI in a patient with reperfused acute myocardial infarction. Late gadolinium-enhanced MRI demonstrated 50–90 % transmural myocardial infarction in the perfusion territory of the right coronary artery (**a**). FDG uptake (**b**) was significantly reduced in the infarct area. Closer inspection of fused images (**c**) and comparison between late gadolinium enhancement and FDG uptake reveals lateral (**c**, *solid arrow*) and epicardial (**c**, *dashed arrows*) extent of reduced FDG uptake. Overall, the area of reduced FDG uptake was significantly larger than the infarct area and thus could rather correspond to the total area at risk than myocardial necrosis alone

gadolinium enhancement and the myocardium showing reduced FDG uptake [1]. In a feasibility study in patients with acute and chronic myocardial infarction, a good agreement between myocardial segments showing late gadolinium enhancement (LGE) and reduced FDG uptake was found. However, that feasibility study was based on visual evaluation of PET and LGE images by reference to the 17-segment model of the left ventricle, and no subgroup analyses between acute and chronic myocardial infarction were performed. Slightly more segments with reduced FDG uptake were found; however, particularly the findings in one patient with acute occlusion of the left anterior descending artery with ST-elevation myocardial infarction and symptom-to-reperfusion time of 3 h were unexpected. While no infarction was found on LGE images, PET images showed a reduced tracer uptake in the anterior wall that closely matched myocardial edema found on T2-weighted images [5]. Therefore it was hypothesized that reduced FDG uptake could be related to the area at risk in patients with reperfused acute myocardial infarction. In a follow-up study in patients with reperfused acute myocardial infarction, PET and MRI were compared by quantitative assessment of the myocardium showing late gadolinium enhancement and reduced FDG uptake. Also, the endocardial surface area (ESA) was calculated from LGE images and used as a reference standard for the area at risk. It was found that the area showing reduced FDG uptake was significantly larger than the area showing late gadolinium enhancement (Fig. 2.4). Furthermore, in six patients with complete salvage after reperfusion (in terms of showing no late gadolinium enhancement), an area of reduced FDG uptake was found in the perfusion territory of the culprit artery. And finally in patients with both late gadolinium enhancement and reduced FDG uptake, a good correlation between the area of reduced FDG uptake and the endocardial surface area was found [15]. However, the ESA method for the assessment of the area at risk is technically limited in that it cannot detect the area at risk in the absence of LGE or its extent lateral to the myocardium showing LGE. Thus, further validation using an alternative standard of reference such as the assessment of myocardial edema by T2-weighted MR imaging is needed. If reduced FDG uptake can be confirmed to reflect the area at risk in terms of a metabolic imprint of ischemia, PET/MRI could allow for the retrospective assessment of myocardial salvage in patients with reperfused acute myocardial infarction. This could be used for the prediction of left ventricular functional recovery in these patients or as a surrogate parameter for the evaluation of strategies to reduce infarct size, such as pre- and post-conditioning or remote conditioning.

2.5 Chronic Myocardial Infarction and Ischemic Cardiomyopathy

Data on simultaneous PET/MR imaging of coronary artery disease is still sparse. The available data from PET/CT and MR studies indicates that simultaneous PET/MRI with tracers for PET perfusion imaging could be a powerful modality for the assessment of coronary artery disease and myocardial viability. In such imaging protocols, viability imaging could be performed using LGE MRI, which seems not only to be the most accurate method but would also allow omitting FDG imaging. This could greatly simplify the PET examination as the complex task of a dual-tracer study would become obsolete. On the other hand, PET myocardial perfusion imaging has been demonstrated to yield the highest sensitivity and specificity for the noninvasive detection of coronary stenosis and to allow for the absolute quantification of myocardial blood flow, which thus could be an improvement over MR perfusion imaging [16]. In an older side-by-side comparison of sequentially performed FDG PET/CT and LGE MRI of the heart in patients with known coronary artery disease, a close agreement between PET and MRI in detecting transmural myocardial scars was found. However, a significant number of segments with subendocardial late gadolinium enhancement showed normal FDG uptake in the PET study, thus indicating a higher sensitivity of LGE imaging for the detection of subendocardial scars. These findings have not yet been confirmed using simultaneous PET/MRI. Preliminary data shows the feasibility of simultaneous PET/MR perfusion imaging using ^{13}N-ammonia. In this context, a protocol for the parallel acquisition and comparison of simultaneous PET and MR measurements of myocardial perfusion at rest and during pharmacologic stress has been demonstrated [17]. A more recent study compared 13 N-ammonia PET/MR to SPECT perfusion imaging and reported superior specificity and diagnostic accuracy of PET/MR in patients with reversible ischemia [18].

2.6 Myocarditis and Cardiac Sarcoidosis

FDG PET/MRI represents a promising noninvasive imaging technique to identify and monitor inflammatory condition of the heart. Cardiac MRI has become the reference standard for the imaging assessment of myocardial inflammation, as it allows a multiparametric evaluation of cardiac function, myocardial edema, and necrosis as well as myocardial hyperemia and pericardial effusion [19]. With cardiac MRI, one can rapidly detect the disease, evaluate its extent, and quantify the impairment of cardiac function. FDG PET, however, is increasingly recognized as a valuable tool for the assessment of various inflammatory conditions including those of the heart [20]. FDG uptake is not only a sensitive marker of inflammation but also a quantifiably parameter for disease activity that could complement cardiac MRI in the detection, differential diagnosis, and monitoring of cardiac inflammation.

PET imaging of myocardial inflammation using FDG is complicated by the fact that cardiomyocytes metabolize a variable mixture of glucose and fatty acids under uncontrolled conditions, with a preference for fatty acid metabolism. To differentiate FDG uptake of intramyocardial inflammatory infiltrates from normal myocardial FDG uptake, the latter needs to be shifted to a more or less exclusive utilization of fatty acids. However, several techniques including long fasting, high-fat low-carbohydrate diet, and heparin loading have been demonstrated to successfully suppress myocardial FDG uptake [21–23].

To date, no studies have been published that evaluate PET/MR for the imaging of myocarditis. However, several case reports indicate the potential of PET/MRI in that context. One report has demonstrated the use of FDG PET/MRI in a case of myocarditis caused by parvovirus B19 and highlights the multiparametric imaging features available for diagnostic workup [24]. While neither an impairment of cardiac function nor a pericardial effusion was found, T2 and LGE imaging revealed focal edema and necrosis in the anterior left ventricular wall, matched by significant hyperemia as assessed by dynamic MR perfusion imaging. These findings were in excellent agreement with increased FDG uptake in the anterior wall.

In addition, another case report demonstrated the feasibility of FDG PET/MRI in a case of diffuse myocarditis of the lateral wall caused by an Epstein-Barr virus infection [25]. In this case, T2-weighted MRI only revealed very subtle signs of myocardial edema, while LGE imaging demonstrated focal intramyocardial nodules and diffuse subepicardial enhancement of the lateral wall. Therefore, these MR imaging findings were compatible with either acute myocarditis or chronic myocarditis or myocardial scarring. However, intense FDG uptake in the lateral wall allowed for the diagnosis of acute myocarditis.

Several case reports have already demonstrated the feasibility of FDG PET/MRI in cardiac sarcoidosis [4, 26, 27]. A study in 51 consecutive patients with cardiac sarcoidosis has found an improved diagnostic accuracy of combined FDG PET/MRI over PET and MRI alone [28]. Cardiac involvement is the major risk factor for fatal outcome in sarcoidosis, often manifesting in arrhythmia and heart failure. Besides direct treatment of cardiac symptoms, in many cases therapy comprises also immunosuppression, which needs to be carefully balanced regarding side effects. Thus, not only methods for the accurate diagnosis but also for monitoring of disease activity with the objective of drug titration are needed (Figs. 2.5 and 2.6).

While LGE imaging has a high sensitivity for the detection of myocardial necrosis and scarring and thus can detect cardiac sarcoidosis well [29], it will more likely reflect the integral of myocardial damage than the current activity of disease. T2-weighted imaging of myocardial edema may in principle differentiate between active and chronic disease, because the presence of edema is associated with more

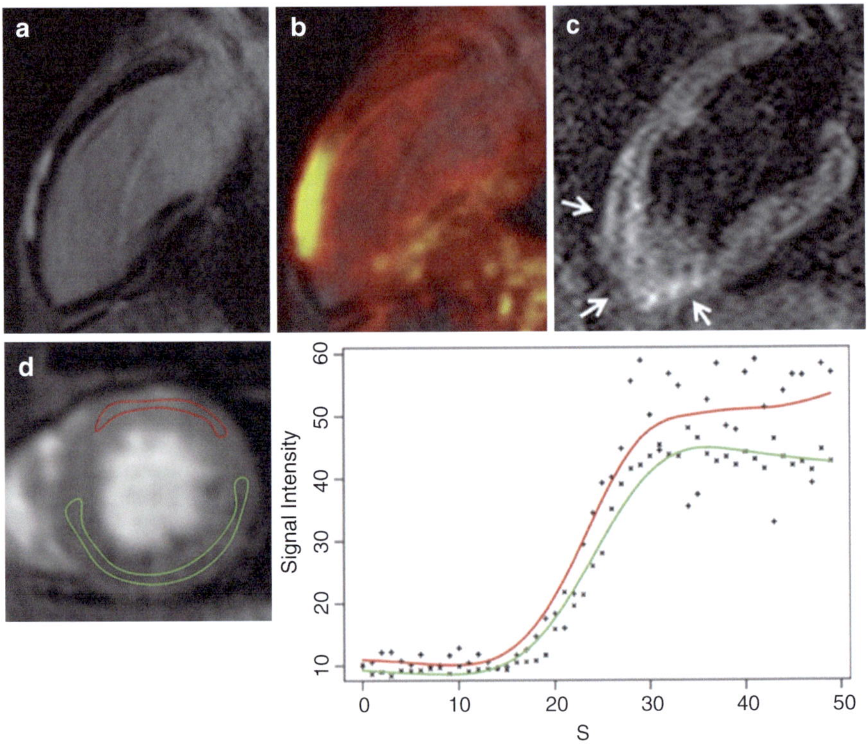

Fig. 2.5 Multiparametric assessment of myocarditis using simultaneous positron emission tomography/magnetic resonance imaging. FDG PET/MRI in a patient with acute viral myocarditis caused by parvovirus B19. Subepicardial late gadolinium enhancement (**a**) was found in the LV anterior wall that was in excellent agreement with increased FDG uptake (**b**). T2-weighted images revealed an edema in the LV anterior wall (**c**). Dynamic perfusion imaging revealed hyperemia in the LV anterior wall (**d**) (With kind permission from Ref. [24])

active inflammation. However, edema is generally less intense in granulomatous inflammation, and it is questionable if that will allow for the accurate monitoring of disease activity under treatment. Also, T2-weighted MR imaging is vulnerable to artifacts and often does not yield a consistent image quality in patients with arrhythmia [30]. FDG-PET on the other hand is not particularly susceptible to motion artifacts and already known for its ability to quantitatively monitor the activity of inflammatory disease and to visualize therapy response [4, 31]. A recent case report has demonstrated the ability of FDG PET/MRI to monitor inflammatory activity of cardiac sarcoidosis that correlated with the improvement of clinical symptoms (Fig. 2.5). Thus, FDG PET/MRI seems to be well suited to diagnose and accurately monitor cardiac sarcoidosis under treatment [32].

Another case report has demonstrated the utility of FDG PET/MRI in the assessment of Loeffler endocarditis [33]. In this report, the confirmation of diagnosis and graduation of inflammatory activity was performed noninvasively using PET/MRI,

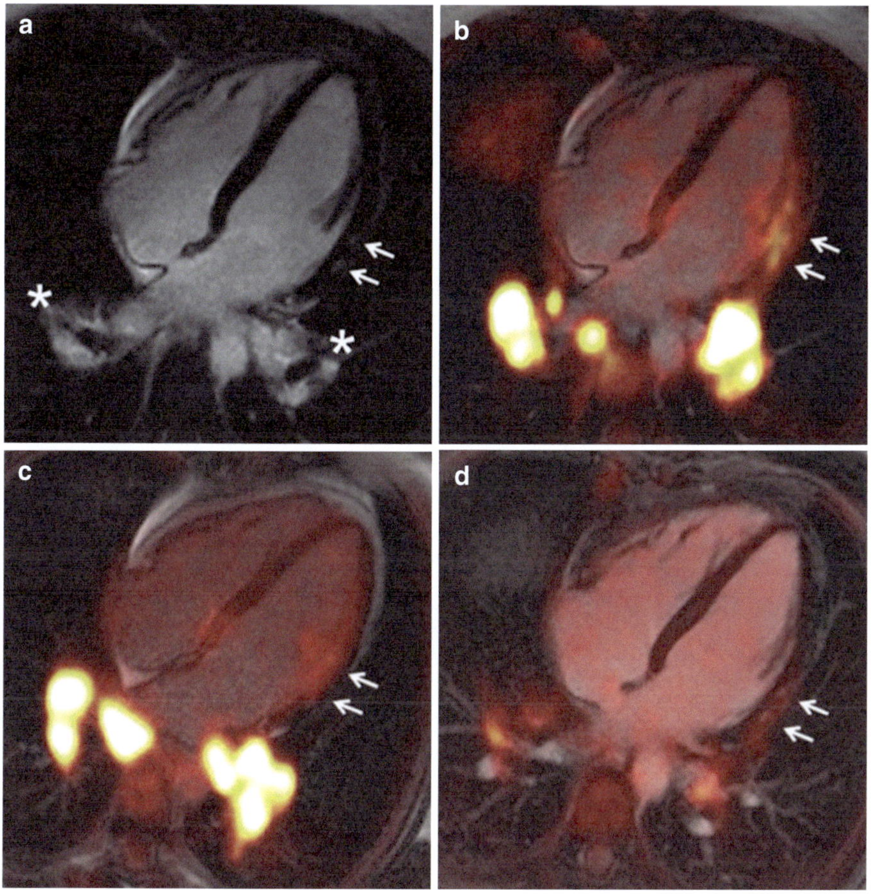

Fig. 2.6 Diagnosis and treatment response evaluation of cardiac sarcoidosis using PET/MRI. FDG PET/MRI in a patient with general malaise, acute retrosternal chest pain, and palpitations. Baseline examination (B + B) showed bihilär lymphadenopathy (**a**, *stars*) and focal late gadolinium enhancement in the lateral left ventricular wall (**a**, *arrows*). Both lymph nodes and myocardial lesions showed intense FDG uptake (**b**), and sarcoidosis with myocardial involvement was diagnosed. After 4 weeks of treatment, PET images (**c**) still demonstrated increased lymphonodular and myocardial (**c**, *arrows*) FDG uptake, whereas FDG uptake was significantly reduced after 4 months of treatment (**d**). In contrast to FDG uptake, myocardial late gadolinium enhancement remained constant in all three examinations and thus was not an indicator of treatment response (With kind permission from Ref. [32])

which was preferred over biopsy because of the increased risk of embolism associated with Loeffler endocarditis. While LGE MR imaging can also detect this disease as circumferential enhancement of the endocardium, the assessment of inflammatory activity via FDG PEt allows for the differentiation between clinically silent acute necrotic, symptomatic thrombotic, and late fibrotic stage of disease. And similar to other inflammatory diseases, the graduation of inflammatory activity using FDG PET could also allow for the monitoring of the effect of anti-inflammatory therapy.

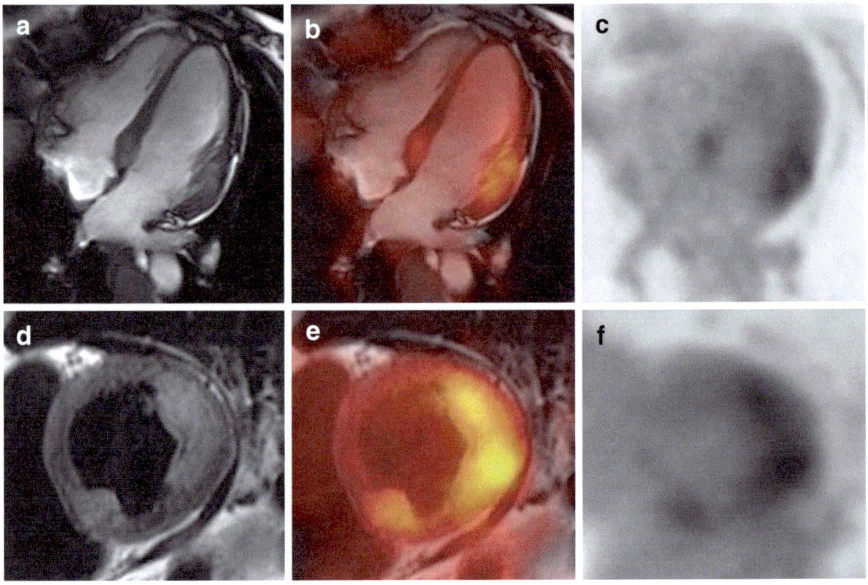

Fig. 2.7 Cardiac tumors. FDG PET/MRI in a patient with angiosarcoma of the limb. Myocardial metastases are visible as hyperintense lesions in the basal septum and the basolateral wall in a 4-chamber SSFP image (**a**) and a T2-weighted short-axis image (**d**). Malignancy of the lesions was confirmed by intense FDG uptake in PET images (**c** and **f**, fusion **b** and **e**)

2.7 Cardiac Tumors

Cardiac MRI plays an essential role in the diagnosis of cardiac tumors, and one of the biggest strength of PET is oncologic imaging. Thus, a combination of both seems to be an interesting combination for the diagnostic workup of cardiac tumors. However, published work on PET/MRI for the assessment of cardiac tumors is scarce. An older case report of cardiac metastasis in a patient with squamous epithelial cancer of the lung demonstrated the feasibility of post hoc fused PET/MRI [34]. A more recent pilot study in 20 patients with cardiac masses of unknown identity evaluated if integrated FDG PET/MRI provides significant benefit over FDG PET or MRI alone [35]. The study found both FDG PET and MRI to yield 100 % sensitivity and 92 % specificity in determining tumor malignancy when interpreted independently, while a combined interpretation yielded 100 % sensitivity and specificity. It was concluded that simultaneous PET/MRI might be reserved for selected cases of cardiac tumors where true benefit can be expected, as competitive and more available methods like PET/CT and MRI already demonstrate strong diagnostic performance [36, 37]. Such cases could include the planning of surgery in patients with complex cardiac infiltration or the differentiation of scar tissue vs. relapse in follow-up examinations after surgery (Fig. 2.7).

2.8 Rare Cardiomyopathies

A case report has demonstrated the use of FDG PET/MRI in a patient with stress-induced transient midventricular ballooning syndrome, a variant of Takotsubo cardiomyopathy [2]. The patient was prepared with a high-fat, low-carbohydrate diet before the examination, and increased glucose metabolism within the dysfunctional midventricular segments was found, while FDG uptake within normal myocardium was suppressed. Cine MRI demonstrated left ventricular midventricular dysfunction, and late gadolinium enhancement MRI did not depict any myocardial hyperenhancement. The combined information allowed for the delineation of neurogenic myocardial stunning. The authors concluded that cardiac PET/MRI may provide further insight into the underlying pathophysiology of stress-induced cardiomyopathy. Another case report demonstrated the use of FDG PET/MRI in a patient with nonobstructive hypertrophic cardiomyopathy (HCM) [38]. The FDG PET/MR scan was performed after oral glucose loading. First-pass MR perfusion imaging showed reduced myocardial blood flow in the hypertrophic septum that corresponded with contrast enhancement in LGE images and patchy FDG uptake defects in PET images and thus was interpreted as myocardial fibrosis. Based on the results of an animal study, the authors speculate that the reduction of glucose uptake in progressive HCM over time could precede its progression to heart failure [39]. They conclude that cardiac FDG PET/MRI could be helpful in the differential diagnosis of LGE and risk stratification of HCM.

2.9 Atherosclerosis and Vasculitis

The risk assessment of cardiovascular events based on the detection of macroscopic calcification in the coronary arteries using computed tomography is well established. However, the amount of coronary calcification is not necessarily correlated with the likelihood of plaque rupture and subsequent coronary thrombosis. Thus, additional techniques that can detect vulnerable (unstable) plaques are of great scientific and clinical interest. FDG PET is well known to demonstrate macrophage activity within atherosclerotic plaques [40] and has been shown to monitor plaque inflammation under lipid-lowering therapy [41]. Recently, a PET/CT study demonstrated ^{18}F-sodium fluoride (NaF) uptake to be elevated in ruptured coronary plaques in patients with acute myocardial infarction [42]. This study also found increased NaF uptake at the site of all carotid plaque ruptures that was associated with histological evidence of active calcification, macrophage infiltration, apoptosis, and necrosis. Newer tracers like those targeted against matrix metalloproteinases have been demonstrated to be markers of plaque vulnerability in preclinical studies [43].

MRI is known to be particularly suitable for the morphologic assessment of plaque features and plaque vulnerability [44, 45]. In combination with PET, which is able to visualize and quantify plaque metabolism on the molecular level, integrated PET/MRI allows for multiparametric plaque imaging and eventually could improve the detection of plaque vulnerability. The feasibility of plaque imaging using integrated FDG PET/MR has been demonstrated in a small group of six HIV-positive men on stable antiviral therapy and increased risk of atherosclerosis [46]. Using a dedicated head and neck coil, the MRI protocol included 3D time-of-flight (TOF) angiography to obtain lumen contours and axial 2D turbo spin echo dark blood images with fat suppression in proton density, T1 and T2 weightings. PET/MR examinations were feasible in all patients and all slices were analyzable. The study also compared PET/MR with PET/CT and found FDG quantification to be comparable between both modalities; however, PET/MR provided superior delineation of the vessel wall. Another study from the same group successfully evaluated integrated FDG PET/MRI in a preclinical model of diet-induced atherosclerosis in mini pigs, which paves the way for translational PET/MRI studies of atherosclerosis in an in vivo animal model [47].

Vasculitis represents an inflammatory condition of the walls of blood vessels, including thickening, weakening, narrowing, and scarring. Using MRI, a variety of morphologic changes can be observed. Thickening of the arterial wall can be accurately assessed with sequences that provide good spatial resolution. Further tissue classification can be performed using different techniques such as T2-weighted imaging for the assessment of wall edema or susceptibility-weighted imaging for the detection of hemosiderin and calcification (Fig. 2.8).

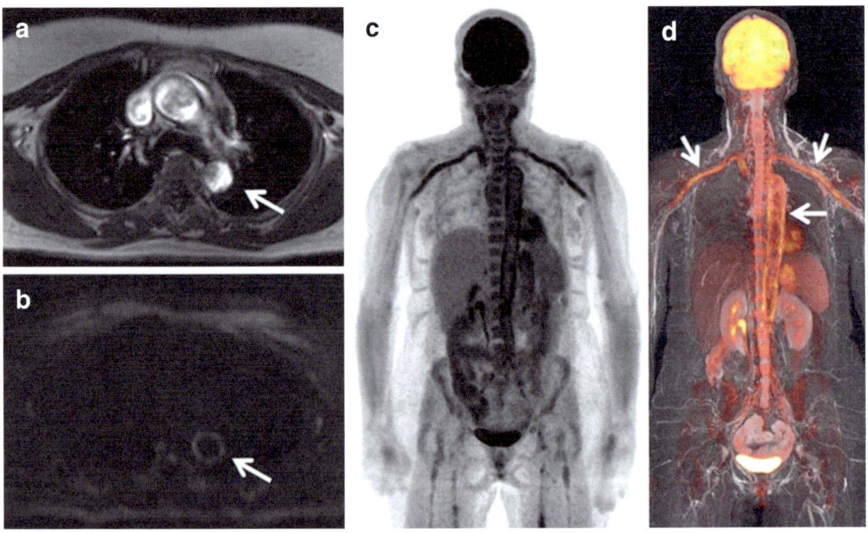

Fig. 2.8 FDG PET/MRI examination of a patient with a form of giant cell arteritis in which only the aorta and large arteries were affected. The axial T1-weighted MR image after contrast medium injection shows a hypointense thickening (max. 8 mm) in the aortic wall (**a**, *arrow*). The axial diffusion-weighted image (**b**) (value 500 s/mm^2) shows a hyperintense T2 shine-through signal in the aortic wall (**b**, *arrow*). The coronary maximum-intensity projection (MIP, slab: 150 mm) of PET data (**c**) and fusion with a T2-weighted MR image (**d**, *arrow*) show increased glucose utilization in the inflamed blood vessel walls (With kind permission from Ref. [6])

Increased perfusion, which is typically found in active inflammation, can be detected using i.v. contrast agents. The mechanism of late gadolinium enhancement has been successfully employed in arterial scar detection in Takayasu arteritis [48]. Furthermore, MRI provides several techniques for noninvasive angiography. These are not only useful in the diagnosis of vasculitis but also in the detection and follow-up of typical complications such as aneurysm and stenosis. In combination with the detection and monitoring of inflammatory activity using FDG PET, integrated PET/MRI seems to be a promising option in the assessment of vasculitis [6]. However, no studies on PET/MR imaging of vasculitis have been published so far.

2.10 Summary

Hybrid PET/MR scanners have been available for a few years, and several studies have demonstrated the technical feasibility and high image quality of cardiac PET/MR imaging on these platforms. Initial results indicate added value of cardiac PET/MRI – either in the clinical routine or within studies – in pathologies like acute myocardial infarction, myocarditis, cardiac sarcoidosis, and cardiac tumors. However, additional studies will first have to demonstrate such added value of PET/MRI over the current standards of care to justify the investments in this expensive technology. Also, ongoing development of scanner hard- and software is needed to improve on current technical issues like attenuation correction and to take advantage of new opportunities like MR-based motion correction for PET in cardiac imaging. Hopefully, the translation of new PET tracers from preclinical evaluation into clinical imaging will open up new fields of application for cardiac PET/MRI.

References

1. Schlosser T, Nensa F, Mahabadi AA, Poeppel TD. Hybrid MRI/PET of the heart: a new complementary imaging technique for simultaneous acquisition of MRI and PET data. Heart. 2012;5:351–2.
2. Ibrahim T, Nekolla SG, Langwieser N, et al. Simultaneous positron emission tomography/magnetic resonance imaging identifies sustained regional abnormalities in cardiac metabolism and function in stress-induced transient midventricular ballooning syndrome. Circulation. 2012;21:e324–6.
3. Rischpler C, Nekolla SG, Dregely I, Schwaiger M. Hybrid PET/MR imaging of the heart: potential, initial experiences, and future prospects. J Nucl Med. 2013;3:402–15.
4. White JA, Rajchl M, Butler J, Thompson RT, Prato FS, Wisenberg G. Active cardiac sarcoidosis: first clinical experience of simultaneous positron emission tomography-magnetic resonance imaging for the diagnosis of cardiac disease. Circulation. 2013;22:e639–41.
5. Nensa F, Poeppel TD, Beiderwellen K, et al. Hybrid PET/MR imaging of the heart: feasibility and initial results. Radiology. 2013;2:366–73.
6. Nensa F, Schlosser T. Cardiovascular hybrid imaging using PET/MRI. Rofo. 2014;12:1094–101.
7. Quick HH. Integrated PET/MR. J Magn Reson Imaging. 2013;2:243–58.

8. Martinez-Möller A, Souvatzoglou M, Delso G, et al. Tissue classification as a potential approach for attenuation correction in whole-body PET/MRI: evaluation with PET/CT data. J Nucl Med. 2009;4:520–6.
9. Kim JH, Lee JS, Song IC, Lee DS. Comparison of segmentation-based attenuation correction methods for PET/MRI: evaluation of bone and liver standardized uptake value with oncologic PET/CT data. J Nucl Med. 2012;12:1878–82.
10. Keereman V, Fierens Y, Broux T, De Deene Y, Lonneux M, Vandenberghe S. MRI-based attenuation correction for PET/MRI using ultrashort echo time sequences. J Nucl Med. 2010;5:812–8.
11. Blumhagen JO, Ladebeck R, Fenchel M, Scheffler K. MR-based field-of-view extension in MR/PET: B(0) homogenization using gradient enhancement (HUGE). Magn Reson Med. 2012;4:1047–57.
12. Nuyts J, Bal G, Kehren F, Fenchel M, Michel C, Watson C. Completion of a truncated attenuation image from the attenuated PET emission data. IEEE Trans Med Imaging. 2013;2:237–46.
13. Heusch P, Buchbender C, Beiderwellen K, et al. Standardized uptake values for [18F] FDG in normal organ tissues: comparison of whole-body PET/CT and PET/MRI. Eur J Radiol. 2013;5:870–6.
14. Lau JMC, Laforest R, Sharma S, et al. Feasibility of MRI attenuation correction in cardiac-gated FDG-PET. Paper presented at the ISMRM 21st Annual Meeting & Exhibition, Salt Lake City; 2013.
15. Nensa F, Tezgalı E, and Poeppel TD, et al. Integrated FDG-PET/MRI for the assessment of myocardial salvage in reperfused acute myocardial infarction. Radiology. 2015 Apr 3:140564. [Epub ahead of print]. See http://www.ncbi.nlm.nih.gov/pubmed/25848898.
16. Jaarsma C, Leiner T, Bekkers SC, et al. Diagnostic performance of noninvasive myocardial perfusion imaging using single-photon emission computed tomography, cardiac magnetic resonance, and positron emission tomography imaging for the detection of obstructive coronary artery disease: a meta-analysis. J Am Coll Cardiol. 2012;19:1719–28.
17. Zhang HS, Rischpler C, Langwieser N, et al. Simultaneous measurement of myocardial perfusion by dynamic contrast enhancement MR and ammonia PET. Paper presented at the ISMRM 21st Annual Meeting & Exhibition, Salt Lake City; 2013.
18. Lau JMC, Laforest R, Zheng J, et al. 13N-Ammonia PET/MR myocardial stress perfusion imaging early experience. Paper presented at the SNMMI 2014 Annual Meeting, St. Louis; 2014.
19. Friedrich MG, Sechtem U, Schulz-Menger J, et al. Cardiovascular magnetic resonance in myocarditis: a JACC White Paper. J Am Coll Cardiol. 2009;17:1475–87.
20. Erba PA, Sollini M, Lazzeri E, Mariani G. FDG-PET in cardiac infections. Semin Nucl Med. 2013;5:377–95.
21. Harisankar CN, Mittal BR, Agrawal KL, Abrar ML, Bhattacharya A. Utility of high fat and low carbohydrate diet in suppressing myocardial FDG uptake. J Nucl Cardiol. 2011;5:926–36.
22. Ito K, Morooka M, Okazaki O, Minaminoto R, Kubota K, Hiroe M. Efficacy of heparin loading during an 18F-FDG PET/CT examination to search for cardiac sarcoidosis activity. Clin Nucl Med. 2013;2:128–30.
23. Morooka M, Moroi M, Uno K, et al. Long fasting is effective in inhibiting physiological myocardial 18F-FDG uptake and for evaluating active lesions of cardiac sarcoidosis. EJNMMI Res. 2014;1:1.
24. Nensa F, Poeppel TD, Krings P, Schlosser T. Multiparametric assessment of myocarditis using simultaneous positron emission tomography/magnetic resonance imaging. Eur Heart J. 2014;35(32):2173.
25. Olshausen GV, Hyafil F, Langwieser N, Laugwitz K-L, Schwaiger M, Ibrahim T. Detection of acute inflammatory myocarditis in Epstein Barr virus infection using hybrid 18F-fluoro-deoxyglucose–positron emission tomography/magnetic resonance imaging. Circulation. 2014;11:925–6.
26. O'Meara C, Menezes LJ, White SK, Wicks E, Elliott P. Initial experience of imaging cardiac sarcoidosis using hybrid PET-MR – a technologist's case study. J Cardiovasc Magn Reson. 2013;15 Suppl 1:T1.

27. Schneider S, Batrice A, Rischpler C, Eiber M, Ibrahim T, Nekolla SG. Utility of multimodal cardiac imaging with PET/MRI in cardiac sarcoidosis: implications for diagnosis, monitoring and treatment. Eur Heart J. 2014;5:312.
28. Wicks E, Menezes L, Pantazis A, et al. Novel hybrid positron emission tomography – magnetic resonance (PET-MR) multi-modality inflammatory imaging has improved diagnostic accuracy for detecting cardiac sarcoidosis. Heart. 2014;100 Suppl 3:A80.
29. Greulich S, Deluigi CC, Gloekler S, et al. CMR imaging predicts death and other adverse events in suspected cardiac sarcoidosis. JACC Cardiovasc Imaging. 2013;4:501–11.
30. Carbone I, Friedrich MG. Myocardial edema imaging by cardiovascular magnetic resonance: current status and future potential. Curr Cardiol Rep. 2012;1:1–6.
31. Sobic-Saranovic DP, Grozdic IT, Videnovic-Ivanov J, et al. Responsiveness of FDG PET/CT to treatment of patients with active chronic sarcoidosis. Clin Nucl Med. 2013;7:516–21.
32. Nensa F, Tezgah E, Poeppel TD, Nassenstein K, Schlosser T. Diagnosis and treatment response evaluation of cardiac sarcoidosis using PET/MRI. Eur Heart J. 2015;36(9):550.
33. Langwieser N, von Olshausen G, Rischpler C, Ibrahim T. Confirmation of diagnosis and graduation of inflammatory activity of Loeffler endocarditis by hybrid positron emission tomography/magnetic resonance imaging. Eur Heart J. 2014;36:2496.
34. Probst S, Seltzer A, Spieler B, Chachoua A, Friedman K. The appearance of cardiac metastasis from squamous cell carcinoma of the lung on F-18 FDG PET/CT and post hoc PET/MRI. Clin Nucl Med. 2011;4:311–2.
35. Nensa F, Tezgah E, Poeppel TD, et al. Integrated 18F-FDG-PET/MRI in the assessment of cardiac masses: a pilot study. J Nucl Med. 2015;56(2):255–60.
36. Hoffmann U, Globits S, Schima W, et al. Usefulness of magnetic resonance imaging of cardiac and paracardiac masses. Am J Cardiol. 2003;7:890–5.
37. Rahbar K, Seifarth H, Schäfers M, et al. Differentiation of malignant and benign cardiac tumors using 18F-FDG PET/CT. J Nucl Med. 2012;6:856–63.
38. Kong E-J, Lee S-H, Cho I-H. Myocardial fibrosis in hypertrophic cardiomyopathy demonstrated by integrated cardiac F-18 FDG PET/MR. Nucl Med Mol Imaging. 2013;3:196–200.
39. Handa N, Magata Y, Mukai T, Nishina T, Konishi J, Komeda M. Quantitative FDG-uptake by positron emission tomography in progressive hypertrophy of rat hearts in vivo. Ann Nucl Med. 2007;10:569–76.
40. Rudd JH, Warburton EA, Fryer TD, et al. Imaging atherosclerotic plaque inflammation with [18F]-fluorodeoxyglucose positron emission tomography. Circulation. 2002;23:2708–11.
41. Tahara N, Kai H, Ishibashi M, et al. Simvastatin attenuates plaque inflammation: evaluation by fluorodeoxyglucose positron emission tomography. J Am Coll Cardiol. 2006;9:1825–31.
42. Joshi NV, Vesey AT, Williams MC, et al. 18F-fluoride positron emission tomography for identification of ruptured and high-risk coronary atherosclerotic plaques: a prospective clinical trial. Lancet. 2013;9918:705–13.
43. Hermann S, Starsichova A, Waschkau B, et al. Non FDG imaging of atherosclerosis: will imaging of MMPs assess plaque vulnerability? J Nucl Cardiol. 2012;3:609–17.
44. Yuan C, Mitsumori LM, Beach KW, Maravilla KR. Carotid atherosclerotic plaque: noninvasive MR characterization and identification of vulnerable lesions. Radiology. 2001;2:285–99.
45. Saam T, Hatsukami TS, Takaya N, et al. The vulnerable, or high-risk, atherosclerotic plaque: noninvasive MR imaging for characterization and assessment. Radiology. 2007;1:64–77.
46. Ripa RS, Knudsen A, Hag AM, et al. Feasibility of simultaneous PET/MR of the carotid artery: first clinical experience and comparison to PET/CT. Am J Nucl Med Mol Imaging. 2013;4:361–71.
47. Pedersen SF, Ludvigsen TP, Johannesen HH, et al. Feasibility of simultaneous PET/MR in diet-induced atherosclerotic minipig: a pilot study for translational imaging. Am J Nucl Med Mol Imaging. 2014;5:448–58.
48. Schneeweis C, Schnackenburg B, Stuber M, et al. Delayed contrast-enhanced MRI of the coronary artery wall in takayasu arteritis. PLoS One. 2012;12, e50655.

3 PET/MRI for Cardiac Imaging: Technical Considerations and Potential Applications

Stephan G. Nekolla, Christoph Rischpler, and Karl P. Kunze

3.1 Introduction

To investigate the potential role of cardiac PET/MRI, it is useful to consider the clinical and economical boundary conditions in cardiac imaging. Two factors have a large influence: Firstly, the overwhelming mainstay of nuclear cardiology is SPECT imaging. It is an easy-to-perform methodology with a high clinical utility, and considerable activities are ongoing to reduce the clinical examination times as well as exposition to ionizing radiation [1, 2].

Secondly, as published by The Task Force on Myocardial Revascularization of the European Society of Cardiology (ESC) and the European Association for Cardio-Thoracic Surgery (EACTS), the recent guidelines on myocardial revascularization consider several cardiac imaging approaches (stress echo, SPECT, PET, and MRI perfusion) *equally* suitable for the diagnosis of patients with suspected coronary artery diseases (CADs) with an intermediate pretest probability [3]. Although this strictly represents the European perspective, it is anticipated that this situation will apply worldwide as well. Fortunately, the same document introduces hybrid imaging for the first time and classifies it as IIa ("should be considered"). This primarily reflects the incremental value of adding (morphological) information derived from CT to perfusion data generated with nuclear imaging [4]. However, a common observation in hybrid imaging systems is an increased complexity of the workflow, which may result in a higher susceptibility to errors. Regarding the disproportionately higher complexity of MR compared to CT, it is clear that this is a relevant issue for integrated PET/MRI systems.

S.G. Nekolla, PhD (✉) • C. Rischpler, MD • K.P. Kunze, MSc
Nuklearmedizinische Klinik und Poliklinik, Klinikum rechts der Isar,
Technische Universität München, Munich, Germany
e-mail: stephan.nekolla@tum.de

T.H. Schindler et al. (eds.), *Molecular and Multimodality Imaging in Cardiovascular Disease*, DOI 10.1007/978-3-319-19611-4_3

So, what does this mean specifically for cardiac PET/MRI? At the time of writing this chapter, the number of review articles and book chapters outnumbers those of actual research articles (taking case studies out of the focus for the moment) and is small even if compared to the very modest number of PET/MRI systems installed since 2010 which is estimated to be slightly above 50. Still, the aspects favoring MRI such as the higher soft tissue spatial resolution, the lack of ionizing radiation, and the better tolerable contrast agents hold true. Those aspects are supplemented with the high rate of technological innovations in cardiac MRI such as perfusion imaging and T1 mapping [5, 6]. Integrating all these results in an approach where the fact that PET/MRI is not a sequential technique but allows fully parallel imaging offers a time-effective methodology with *both* modalities acquiring simultaneously what they can do in a reliable manner. Examples would be highly specific PET probes (e.g., innervation and/or inflammation) combined with MRI delineating anatomical references, perfusion, or tissue with an altered volume of distribution for contrast media in complex cardiac pathophysiologies, for which high throughput and low costs are not the limiting factors.

This chapter tries to provide insights on the technical aspects, investigate available applications, and target its potential strengths especially in nonstandard applications beyond conventional perfusion and viability imaging.

3.2 Technical Considerations

A fully integrated PET/MRI system is a complex technology as the combination of high static magnetic fields, variable gradient fields, and powerful radiofrequency in the range of several kilowatts would interact with conventional photomultiplier tubes and the PET electronics. In the other direction, PET-related components cause inhomogeneities in the magnetic fields, and electromagnetic interferences could result in a degradation of the MR image quality. To date, three different constructions of PET/MRI systems are available and regulatory approved. A sequential design aligns the PET and MR components axially and connects with the patient bed on a rail system (Ingenuity TF PET/MRI, Philips, Best, the Netherlands) [7]. The first truly integrated device with simultaneous MR and PET acquisitions was the Biograph mMR (Siemens Healthcare, Erlangen, Germany) [8]. This device uses avalanche photodiodes (APDs) which are insensitive to the magnetic field [9]. Recently, a second integrated system, the SIGNA PET/MRI (General Electric Healthcare, Milwaukee, USA) was introduced. It uses silicon photomultiplier detectors (SiPM) enabling time-of-flight PET imaging [10, 11].

3.2.1 Attenuation Correction

A correct attenuation map is the cornerstone of PET quantification. Errors in this map result in significant deviations as shown in several studies where the misalignment between PET and CT was investigated (Fig. 3.1) [12, 13].

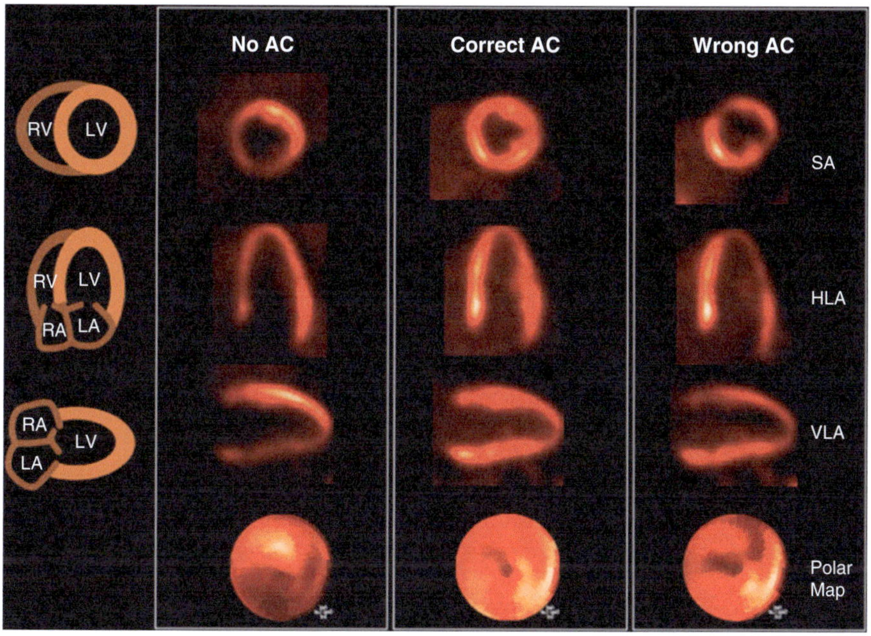

Fig. 3.1 Attenuation correction in cardiac PET. Attenuation correction is the cornerstone of quantification in PET imaging. Cardiac PET is especially prone to this as shown below. In contrast to cardiac SPECT where non-AC data are routinely used in the clinical reading, the effects in PET are much larger (*left column*). Even modest misalignment of 6 mm as shown in the right column alters the apparent tracer distribution

In stand-alone PET systems the attenuation map is generated by a rotating rod source, while in PET/CT systems the attenuation map is estimated from CT data. This adds to the total radiation exposure; however, using suitable protocols, values as low as using rotational sources can be achieved [14, 15]. Unfortunately, MRI is not able to directly retrieve the desired information as it has no access to the absorption of high-energy photons. We approached this problem by using tissue segmentation and assigning standardized, non-patient-specific attenuation values to the tissue classes (Fig. 3.2) [16].

As in stand-alone PET using rod sources, the cortical bone is ignored. The acquisition of these images requires usually about 18 s per bed position during one breath-hold. Alternatively, T1-weighted turbo spin-echo sequences are used with the advantage of a shorter acquisition time but combining fat and water into a single tissue class [17]. Obviously, the major disadvantage of the segmentation-based approach is the limited number of tissue classes especially if a significant inter-patient variability in lung structure and location could be anticipated. General disadvantages of this approach are that metal implants do not contribute to the attenuation map and that contrast agents may cause inaccuracies due to reduced T1 values (Fig. 3.3) [18]. However, this segmentation-based approach is currently used in commercially available PET/MRI scanners [16, 17], and our group has demonstrated a good correlation between PET/MRI

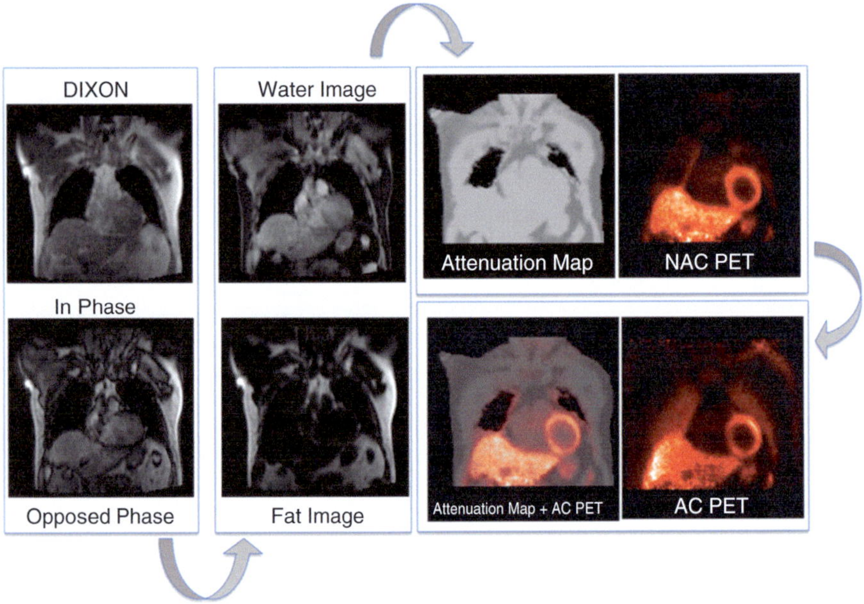

Fig. 3.2 Attenuation correction in PET/MR. The attenuation map is generated using in- and opposed-phase MR Dixon images from which fat and water images are computed. In the attenuation map air, lung, fat, and soft tissues are automatically segmented. Using this attenuation map and NAC (non-attenuation-corrected) PET data, the final AC PET images are calculated

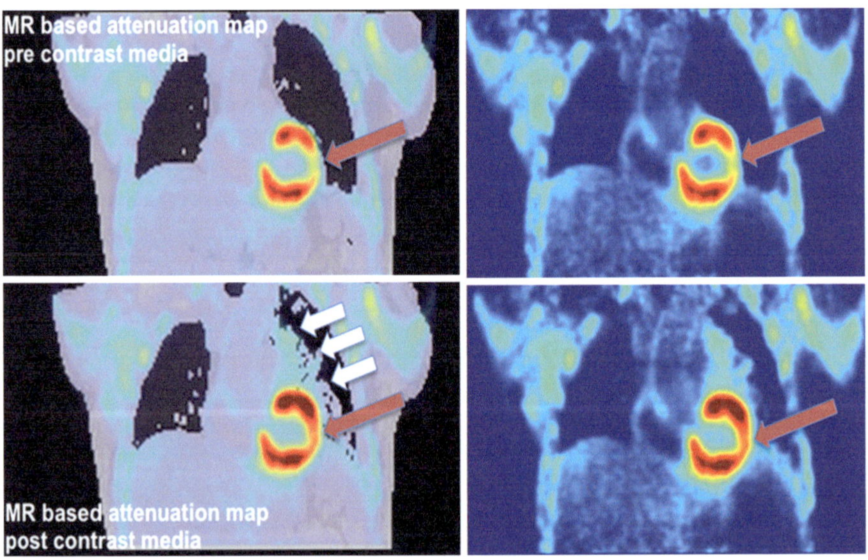

Fig. 3.3 AC pre/post KM. Dixon-based attenuation maps prior (*top left*) and after (*bottom left*) injection of contrast media shown together with reconstructions from the same PET scan but using the respective attenuation maps. Both PET data sets are scaled to the same maximum. Due to an overcorrection caused by the (apparent) larger amount of attenuating "lung" (*white arrows*) tissue, the myocardial PET values using the post-contrast attenuation maps differ (*red arrows*)

and PET/CT data in oncologic studies [19]. Initial work in cardiac patients has also shown good agreement between sequentially acquired patients with PET/CT and PET/MRI [20].

Another PET/MRI specific limitation, which affects attenuation correction, is the limited field of view (FOV) of the MR system potentially truncating the MR data. In other words, the PET scanner has a larger FOV as the MR system. This results in MR "invisible" tissue where body parts are outside the FOV introducing a bias in the attenuation correction. Thus, based on PET emission data, tissue is extrapolated and added to the map [21, 22]. A more desirable solution would be, however, the extension of the field of view, as was recently suggested and showed promising results [23].

Multiple components outside the body but inside the PET/MRI field of view, such as coils, positioning aids, monitoring devices, cables, earphones, and the – as compared to PET/CT, more massive – patient bed, are an additional source of photon scatter and attenuation. Most of these objects are MR "invisible" and are at rather random locations and thus do not necessarily contribute (although they should do) to the attenuation map. Only the patient bed and the fixed coils with known location are added to the final attenuation map [24–26]. As a result of this issue, vendors of such devices have redesigned them to reduce size and weight, but the effects are still measurable although small. If this has a relevant impact on the diagnostic performance, however, is not known yet. It might be anticipated that the effects are in the same order of objects overestimated in PET/CT imaging due to CT reconstruction artifacts or non-ferromagnetic signal voids in non-hybrid MR imaging.

A special group of artifacts in cardiac imaging arises from implantable devices. In difference to cardiac PET/CT and SPECT/CT, implantable cardiac devices (ICDs, CRT devices, or pacemakers) are of significant concern in MR imaging. As mentioned before, the devices cause CT artifacts, which potentially result in a biased attenuation correction, although initial work in PET/CT showed only little effects [27]. But in MRI, the effects are twofold. Nonmagnetic metals disturb the homogeneity of the magnetic field and cause signal voids, which clearly exceed the actual size of the object and thus underestimate the true attenuation. The second, more critical effect stems from an interaction with the radiofrequency and could cause life-threatening malfunction or local heating. Thus, many patients are excluded from MRI (including PET/MRI) which represents an increasing problem as the number of patients with diseases qualifying for the implantation of those devices is growing [28, 29]. Although newer generations of these devices are MR compatible, the logistical hurdles are significant and the procedures can be time-consuming. In general, it is advisable that the clinical reader is informed about potential sources of artifacts and a strict quality control with a special emphasis on correct alignment of MR-derived attenuation correction maps and PET data should be performed.

3.2.2 Imaging Workflow

We mentioned already that proper attenuation correction and exact alignment of the attenuation map is mandatory for correct diagnostic performance. Regarding this point, one major advantage of MR compared to CT is that the AC scan may be repeated as often as necessary without any ionizing radiation. The subsequent choice of the optimal attenuation map, however, is rather time-consuming and thus inefficient and inconvenient. Recent developments in PET/CT, however, indicate that software-assisted solutions will become available soon [30, 31].

It is relevant to remember that considerations on PET/MRI workflows include the fact that most data are acquired in "parallel" and not "simultaneously." PET measures in volume rather than slice modes with variable frame lengths between seconds and up to 20–30 min (or more) depending on the chosen tracer, the uptake pattern and its half-life, the injected activity, and the patience of the patient. Thus, PET data integrates always the voluntary and involuntary patient motion (respiration, contractile motion, and "true" patient motion). This is in quite some difference to the MR acquisitions. As MR is so motion sensitive due to its image generation physics, MR data is usually acquired sequentially, with slice acquisition durations ranging from milliseconds for dynamic scans to several breath-holds for high-resolution images. It is inherent to sequential imaging that if data is acquired over several breath-holds, the limited reproducibility of the patient's breath-holding creates spatially somewhat inconstant images. This has an underestimated limitation that ungated (regarding the cardiac cycle and the ventilation) PET images are fused with spatiotemporal consistent MR images (e.g., end-diastole in expiration). Related to this, the reading process of PET/MRI data is more complex than typically found in PET/CT or SPECT/CT as PET volume data ultimately is mapped on various (partly overlapping) MR slices acquired in various positions and orientations (e.g., short axes; two-, three-, and four-chamber view). This is tedious, and the future will hopefully bring motion-triggered acquisition [32] or software corrections [33] in order to allow free-breathing imaging.

However, there are also applications that might benefit from truly simultaneous acquisition of PET and MR data. Potential workflows are depicted in Fig. 3.4. Synergistic benefits of integrating PET (with its vast variety of specific tracers, its good volume coverage) and MRI (with its high in-plane resolution) are rather compact protocols with a maximum of 30 min scan time. Today, clinical MRI in the heart is realistically a matter of 45–60 min, and all aspects of perfusion, contractile function, and metabolic surrogate parameters are measured sequentially. Thus, integrated PET/MRI could increase patient comfort and throughput and thus cost-effectiveness which potentially offset the significant more expensive costs of the device. Cardiovascular PET/MRI has the advantage that typically only a limited area in the body is investigated which reduces the scan time in difference to complex whole-body protocols in oncological imaging. However, simultaneous PET/MRI imaging is challenging from the operational perspective: it needs to be kept in mind that perfectly matching image data do not come automatically and considerable user interaction is needed. Compared with the highly automated workflows in PET/CT and SPECT/CT, this is a major limitation today. Finally, cross-training of the involved personnel operating the scanner is obligatory which holds also true for professionals planning and interpreting the scan. Consequently, a closer-than-usual collaboration between nuclear medicine physicians, radiologists, cardiologists, and physicists and technologists is mandatory.

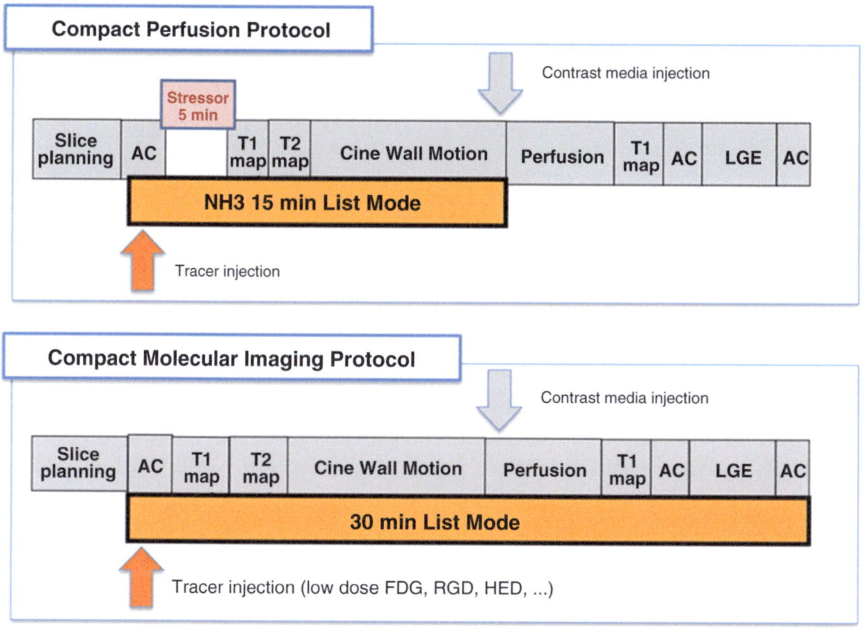

Fig. 3.4 Potential workflows (compact stress/rest perfusion, molecular imaging) for simultaneous PET/MRI

3.3 Cardiac Applications in PET/MRI

3.3.1 Myocardial Perfusion

Awhile being a fundamental advantage of cardiac PET, absolute quantification is one of the major limitations of MRI. MR signal intensities depend on a vast array of parameters such as imaging hardware (transmitters, receivers, amplifiers, gradients, coils, etc.), pulse sequences, as well as many other features which vary between vendors, magnetic field strengths, and scanner models (Fig. 3.4). Although usually irrelevant in morphological imaging, quantification of MR signal is an important step in dynamic MR imaging. Due to its superior time resolution, the true potential in quantitative MRI lies in dynamic data, even if this term is used somewhat differently as compared to nuclear medicine. Basically, it refers to a series of images, where either acquisition parameters varied (such as the inversion time in T1 mapping or the gradients in diffusion imaging) or – more familiar to nuclear cardiology – which are acquired after the injection of MR contrast media.

Perfusion imaging is, as mentioned earlier, a traditional domain of nuclear imaging for the diagnosis of a flow-limiting stenosis in coronary artery disease (CAD), and the investigation of the hemodynamic significance of known CAD is of high clinical relevance. There is increasing evidence that PET MPI offers advantages over the traditional SPECT-based approach due to the absolute quantification of myocardial blood flow (MBF), the validated attenuation correction, and the superior image quality in obese patients [34, 35]. Three PET perfusion tracers have been established: ^{13}N ammonia ($^{13}NH_3$), ^{15}O water, and rubidium (^{82}Rb). $^{13}NH_3$, ^{15}O water, and ^{82}Rb have the advantage of a relatively short half-life, which is about 10 min for $^{13}NH_3$, 122 s for ^{15}O water, and 76 s for ^{82}Rb, which allows for rapid PET MPI scans in rest and under stress. Recently, ^{18}F flurpiridaz was introduced in early trials and has been shown to offer some advantages, e.g. a low positron energy and a half-life with the same logistical advantages as ^{18}F-FDG [36].

But despite the established role of PET MPI, myocardial perfusion imaging using dynamic contrast-enhanced (DCE-) MRI is a research since almost two decades and has shown promising results when compared to PET [5, 37, 38]. MRI perfusion imaging has a much greater availability than cardiac PET, a lower examination cost, and no ionizing radiation. MRI usually offers much greater spatial in-plane resolution than PET, enabling the possibility of voxel-wise quantitative perfusion analysis with a resolution of at least $2\times2\times8\text{mm}^3$ – although still at the price of limited LV coverage [39]. A spatial resolution of three to six slices per cardiac cycle can be achieved with reasonable SNR, surpassing the temporal capabilities of PET imaging. Independent of the competitive ambitions of MRI to take its share in the large market of diagnosing CAD, there is also great potential for integrated systems concerning the creation of synergies. To elucidate that potential, we briefly compare "perfusion" imaging as realized by both modalities.

For PET, the frame rate is usually in the order of 10 s, which is too low to actually observe the tracer's transit through the vascular space. Thus, PET MBF is estimated by observing tracer extraction from the vascular space into those parts of the myocardium where tracer kinetics are slow compared to the minimal frame rate. Retainable tracers as the ones listed above (with the exception of ^{15}O water) are indeed conceptually quite similar to microspheres [40], however adapted for noninvasive application. The main design criterion for those compounds is how efficiently they are extracted from the blood pool and transferred into the myocytes. Depending on the tracer, multi-compartmental modeling is used to map the diffusive extraction from the blood pool and subsequent retention inside the myocytes to simpler rate constants. From the specific model, a first-pass extraction flow constant (often called K_1) is calculated, which can be directly identified with MBF for freely diffusible tracers (^{15}O) or have to be corrected in case of high flow rates ($^{13}NH_3$, ^{82}Rb). In contrast, the underlying principle of myocardial MRI perfusion imaging is the direct observation of indicator convection through the vascular space, enabled by the high temporal resolution of MRI. The mathematical framework for that is the classic indicator-dilution theory as adapted for noninvasive applications by Zierler [41, 42]. This formalism, unlike compartment modeling, does not necessarily impose a priori physiological information about the structure of the tissue. Perfusion flow is described directly as the delivery amplitude of contrast media from the LV lumen (where the AIF is acquired) to the distribution volume of contrast agent in the myocardial tissue. Although rarely applied in myocardial perfusion studies, extraction-based approaches more similar to PET, e.g. the Tofts model [43], are still widely used in cerebral and oncologic studies. It is important to note though that for highly vascularized tissue or high MBFs, the "extraction" of Gd-DTPA from the vascular space is permeability limited and not flow limited [44]. This renders it virtually impossible to extrapolate flow characteristics from Gd-DTPA extraction rates at high flows, which is why an extraction-based approach is usually not suitable for myocardial perfusion imaging at stress.

An additional, highly relevant point concerning MRI perfusion is that gadolinium-based contrast agents distribute in blood plasma, but do not permeate red blood cells (and thus the whole vascular space) as the more diffusible PET tracers do which clearly affects the generated signals (Fig. 3.5). As long as flow patterns of plasma

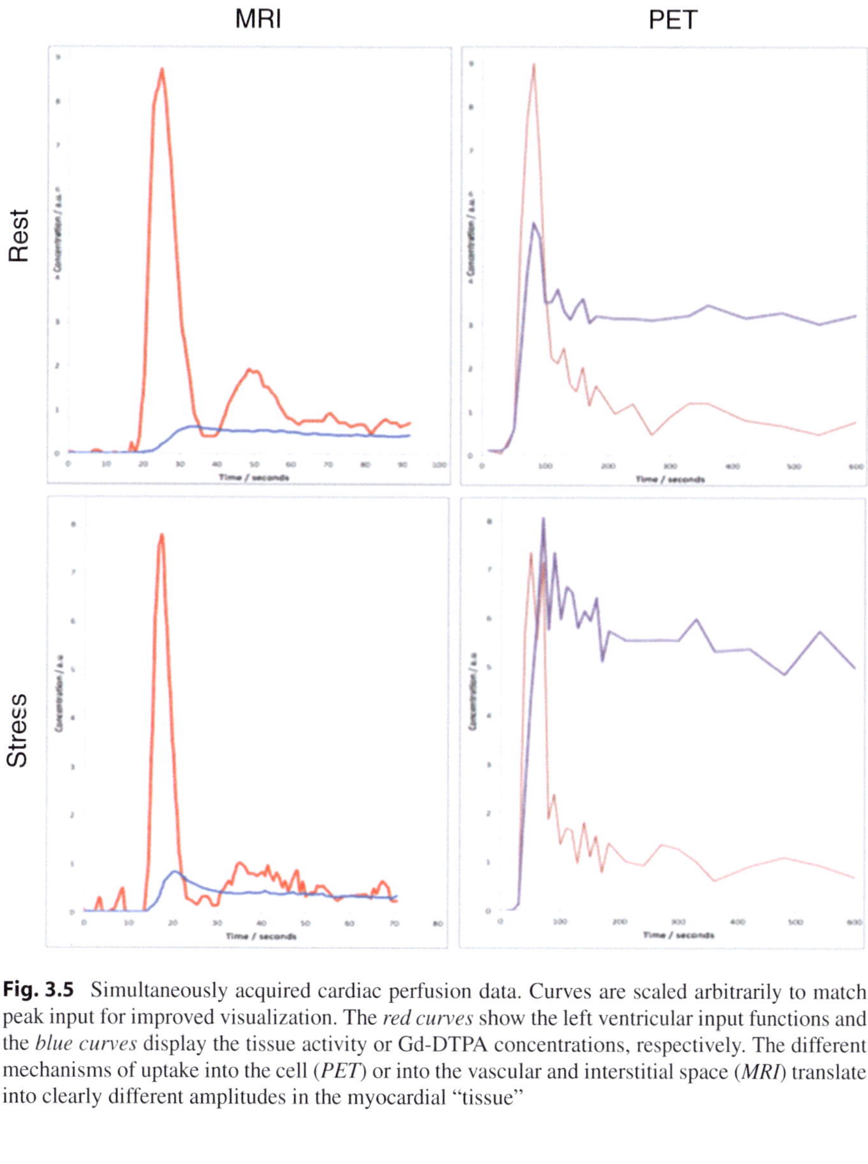

Fig. 3.5 Simultaneously acquired cardiac perfusion data. Curves are scaled arbitrarily to match peak input for improved visualization. The *red curves* show the left ventricular input functions and the *blue curves* display the tissue activity or Gd-DTPA concentrations, respectively. The different mechanisms of uptake into the cell (*PET*) or into the vascular and interstitial space (*MRI*) translate into clearly different amplitudes in the myocardial "tissue"

and blood cells are homogeneous, this has no influence on time-related parameters like mean indicator transit times (MTT). However, there is a need to correct for the effective difference between large-vessel hematocrit and microvascular hematocrit [45] when estimating MBF. This might affect especially stress studies [46, 47].

To which extent this has consequences in a clinical setup is unclear yet but might be one of the reasons for the per-patient variability seen in comparative studies [5]. There are several additional factors stemming from the need to accurately estimate contrast agent concentrations from MRI signal values, making data post processing much more complicated in PET. In a similar fashion as for hematocrit, those factors may affect input functions and tissue curves differently, e.g. water exchange conditions [48], Gd-DTPA relaxivity [49], AIF dispersion [50], and blood flow effects. In conclusion, despite important differences in data structure to PET, new opportunities arise from the spatially and temporally highly resolved assessment of microvascular dynamics from MRI-based flow assessments. Especially for integrated PET/MRI systems, such synergistic approaches hold great promise for future clinical applications in multimodal perfusion imaging.

3.3.2 Cardiac MRI for Tissue Characterization

Targeting the water and its properties is another technique modulating MRI to retrieve "molecular" information. In oncological imaging, using advanced imaging sequences and strong gradients, this avenue was already explored: the apparent diffusion coefficient (ADC) of water [51] is already widely used to characterize tumorous tissue. In general, water is the predominant source of the MR signal and its motility (or diffusion properties) can be used for tissue characterization. Another approach is the delineation of the longitudinal relaxation time T1. This parameter describes the potential of the exited spins to transfer their energy to the surrounding macromolecules. Thus, one of the changes in the microchemical cellular environment was the introduction of MR medical imaging as T1 values differ between healthy and tumorous tissue [52]. The so-called T1 weighting (and its modification, inversion recovery imaging) is still a fundamental imaging sequence in diagnosis imaging as different T1 values will produce different signal intensities, and thus, the contrast between healthy and abnormal tissue is optimized. For inversion recovery imaging, any signal from remote myocardium is nulled and scar tissue is enhanced in late gadolinium enhancement (LGE) [53]. More specifically, it shows areas with a different distribution volume for MR contrast agents. Accordingly, different wash-out kinetics from the interstitial space was shown previously in the acute as in the chronic setting of myocardial infarction [54, 55]. Unfortunately, larger clinical validations are still lacking, but two general modes of T1 mapping in the heart are already used in an increasing number of MRI centers. In the last decade, novel cardiac MR technology allowed the calculation of pixel-wise T1 maps [56]. Native T1 maps were used in imaging regional edema, fibrosis, amyloidosis, Anderson-Fabry disease, intramyocardial hemorrhage, and other structural alterations, where a modified water content and protein environment in the myocardium occurs [6].

In addition, using MR contrast media, pre- and post-contrast T1 maps enable the calculation of the extracellular volume (ECV). It was already shown that the expansion of extracellular matrix has prognostic value [57] and might have an important role in heart failure imaging. Even the term "vulnerable interstitium" was already coined in sudden death patients [58]. Although this is speculative, cardiac PET/MRI might be an excellent platform to validate and improve the characterization of myocardial tissue by integrating this information with tracer signals.

3.3.3 Improving Myocardial Tissue Characterization by 18F-FDG PET/MRI Viability Imaging

Myocardial hibernation is a well-known phenomenon where myocytes shift their metabolism from fatty acids toward glucose after chronic hypoperfusion [59]. Several preclinical and clinical studies have proved the beneficial effects of revascularization which is followed by recovery of the contractile function [60]. Several modalities showed potential to identify hibernating myocardium: dobutamine stress echocardiography, MRI, ^{18}F-FDG PET, and late gadolinium enhancement (LGE) MRI.

Considered as "gold standard" by many imagers, nuclear cardiology offers one of the most commonly applied techniques using ^{18}F-FDG PET as marker of myocardial viability [61]. Typically, ^{18}F-FDG is combined with a flow marker (^{13}N-ammonia, ^{82}Rb, and also ^{99m}Tc-labeled SPECT agents). Based on meta-analyses the sensitivity of ^{18}F-FDG PET to predict functional recovery after revascularization is about 92 %, while the specificity is only 63 % [62]. However, there is evidence that patients with a significant amount of dysfunctional but viable tissue should undergo revascularization as soon as possible as viability is a transient state of the myocytes [63, 64]. Especially from the point of view of spatial resolution, however, MRI offers with delayed gadolinium enhancement (LGE) a readily available approach. MRI spatial resolution is superior to PET (1–3 mm vs. 4–6 mm) which allows the differentiation between transmural and non-transmural infarction [65]. The same advantage helps with a reduced or absent ^{18}F-FDG uptake in thinned myocardium which would potentially be miscategorized as scar by PET. Despite these fundamental differences of the approaches (imaging viable vs. nonviable tissue), a good agreement between both modalities has been demonstrated in a chronic setting [53]. From a practical perspective, LGE is independent of the excretion of insulin and shows advantage in diabetic patients where the clearance of ^{18}F-FDG from the blood is limited and cardiac image quality is poor. However, if a hybrid use of ^{18}F-FDG PET MRI and LGE MRI is beneficial is still subject of research and only limited data is available indicating again good agreement (Fig. 3.6) [20].

In our initial experience in a similar setting, we found a small proportion of myocardial segments in disconcordance between ^{18}F-FDG uptake and transmurality of LGE [66]. However, the clinical relevance for functional recovery in the long-term setting post-acute MI is debatable and warrants further research.

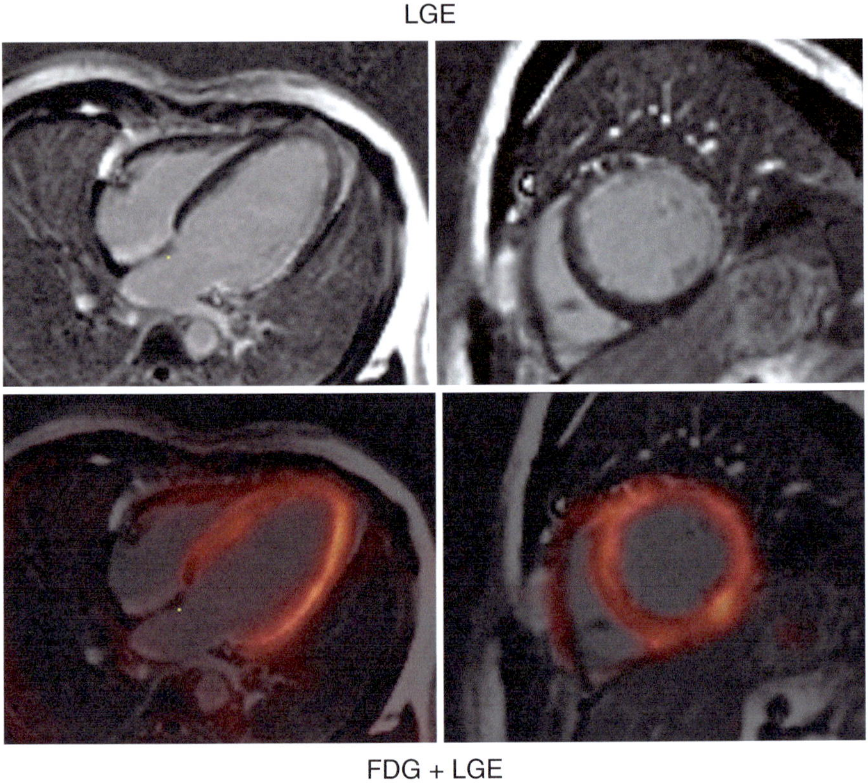

Fig. 3.6 18F-FDG PET/MRI shortly after AMI. Short- and long-axis images of a patient imaged shortly after acute MI with occlusion of the left main using simultaneous ^{18}F-FDG PET/MRI. In the *top row*, the LGE images and, in the *bottom row*, LGE images fused with FDG are shown

3.4 Applications in Cardiovascular Molecular Imaging: Targeting Inflammation

3.4.1 Inflammatory Response After Acute Myocardial Infarction

In the following paragraphs the delineation of (mostly) inflammatory signals is described in our first experience in distinct disease entities. Recent research has focused on the myocardial response to ischemia – with an emphasis on the cardiac inflammatory response after acute MI which is considered a risk factor for deleterious remodeling and finally the development of heart failure. The fact that monocytes migrate rapidly into the myocardium identified them as key components of cardiac inflammation [67–69]. This is a highly complex process and so far is the domain of preclinical research. However, ^{18}F-FDG PET – due to its readily availability – is frequently used in a variety of settings, as activated inflammatory cells show increased expression of glucose transporters which can be visualized

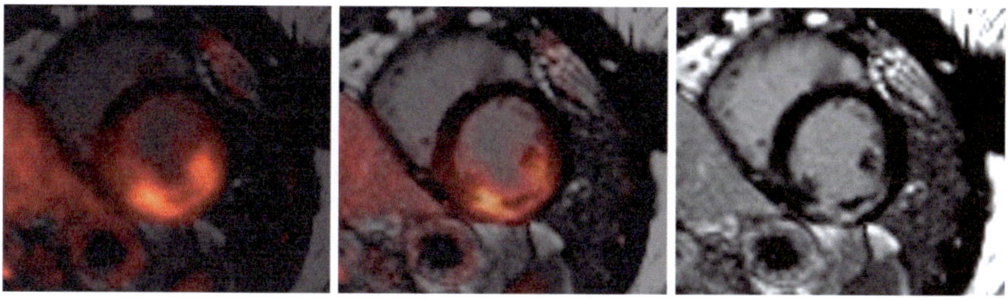

Fig. 3.7 Multimodal characterization of the myocardial tissue after AMI using PET/MRI. Short-axis images of a patient who was imaged shortly after acute MI using simultaneous ^{18}F-FDG PET/MRI. Myocardial scarring can be imaged using LGE MRI. Using fasted/heparin ^{18}F-FDG PET/MRI, the area of postischemic inflammation/ischemic memory can be assessed. Myocardial obstruction is visible at the center of the LGE zone

using ^{18}F-FDG PET. This signal could be supplemented with MRI's capability to image scar formation, microvascular obstruction, edema, hemorrhage, and left ventricular function. A recent preclinical study using a mouse infarct model of myocardial infarction showed that ^{18}F-FDG PET/MRI quantifies the amount of accumulated monocytes in the postischemic heart if the glucose uptake of cardiomyocytes is suppressed [70]. Such a strategy would enable a detailed morphologic characterization of the infarcted heart by PET/MRI and is feasible in humans (Fig. 3.7) [71, 72].

In patients, the glucose metabolism of cardiomyocytes can be suppressed by a high-fat/low-carb diet (the so-called Atkins diet) and/or the administration of unfractionated heparin prior to ^{18}F-FDG injection which is used, e.g., to image sarcoidosis with PET. However, there are limitations as the ^{18}F-FDG uptake is not unique in the heart: as used in conventional viability imaging, ischemically compromised myocardium switches its metabolism from fatty acids toward glucose degradation [73]. In addition, expression of GLUT1 transporters has been demonstrated in postischemic myocardium and can persist over weeks and is responsible for the "ischemic memory" [74, 75]. Thus, ^{18}F-FDG uptake in postischemic myocardium may not solely reflect inflammation but viable cardiomyocytes. However, if this characterization of tissue and its inflammatory state proves to be clinically reliable, it could identify patients at risk for developing heart failure or – even more relevant – it may serve as a tool to guide immunomodulatory therapeutic strategies.

3.4.2 Sarcoidosis

Following the same considerations as above, imaging inflammation in sarcoidosis developed into an attractive approach with PET/CT [76]. Sarcoidosis is a systemic granulomatous disease which is characterized by an intense inflammatory process and inflammatory granulomas, causing post-inflammatory scars. Those may result in conduction abnormalities, arrhythmia, and heart failure. Due to these large risks,

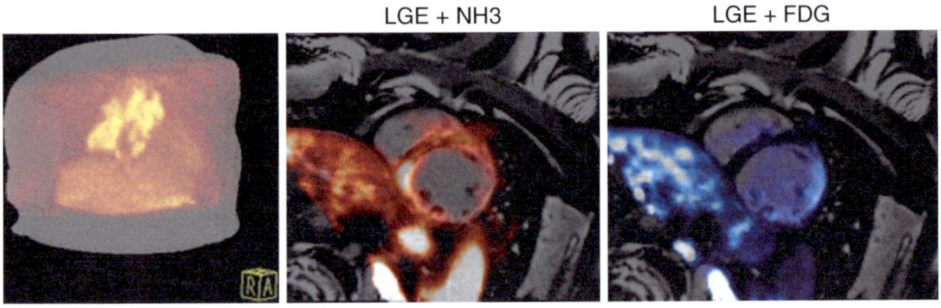

Fig. 3.8 Sarcoidosis. In a patient with acute sarcoidosis, a 3D rendering of the FDG uptake in the thorax (*left*), a fused LGE and NH3 perfusion PET (*middle*), and a fused LGE and FDG PET are depicted

cardiac involvement should be ruled out immediately. The guidelines of the Japanese Ministry of Health and Welfare, which serve as a worldwide standard, do currently not include PET but cardiac MRI or ^{67}Ga scintigraphy. In this particular setting, PET/MRI might be very useful for the initial diagnosis of cardiac sarcoidosis and also could guide therapy. As we showed initially, a combined approach of perfusion (e.g., ^{13}N-ammonia) and inflammation (e.g., ^{18}F-FDG), PET imaging would allow for exact staging of the disease as well as the assessment of the inflammatory status [77]: normal perfusion combined with avid ^{18}F-FDG uptake indicates active inflammation, hypoperfusion and intense glucose metabolism are suggestive for advanced stage, and reduced or absent perfusion and missing ^{18}F-FDG uptake are indicative for end-stage cardiac sarcoidosis. LGE MRI supplements the localization of regional fibrosis and aids the lead placement in the case of ICD implantation (Fig. 3.8).

3.4.3 Plaque Imaging in Atherosclerotic Disease

Finally, leaving the focus on imaging the heart, MRI is competing with CT in angiography if it comes to a characterization of the vessel wall, plaques, and their composition without the use of ionizing radiation [78, 79]. As an example from our group, Gd-contrast enhancement was observed in the vessel wall following myocardial infarction which correlated with the degree of stenosis and resolved in a 3-month follow-up scan possibly representing reduced inflammatory activity [80]. However, imaging the vessel wall requires substantial expertise and tends to be time-consuming. Thus, the combination with PET tracers could be attractive to facilitate imaging atherosclerotic plaques with a large spatial coverage. The dominating tracer is again ^{18}F-FDG, and it is assumed that an increased ^{18}F-FDG uptake is related to an intense macrophage infiltration representing a high vulnerability [81, 82]. Initial clinical work investigating the feasibility of simultaneous ^{18}F-FDG PET/MRI for imaging carotid arteries was demonstrated in six HIV-positive patients representing a population with a known increased risk of atherosclerosis [83]. Unfortunately, ^{18}F-FDG has limitations, and limited clearance from the blood pool and uptake in muscle (including the heart itself) adjacent to the relatively small vessels are among them. Thus, the search for alternatives is ongoing. Recently, 80 patients with myocardial infarction were imaged with ^{18}F-fluoride (^{18}F-NaF) [84]. This tracer shows excellent imaging properties with clear focal uptake. In 93 % of the patients, the highest ^{18}F-NaF uptake was observed in the culprit lesion, while the ^{18}F-FDG uptake was obscured by the unspecific (muscular) myocardial uptake. Furthermore, almost every second patient with stable angina had plaques with focal ^{18}F-NaF uptake which were associated with high-risk features on intravascular ultrasound. Logistically, this agent is available and already in clinical (oncological) use. However, the evidence of usefulness is limited to a single study and future studies have to extend this. Potentially valuable tracers targeting integrins, such as $\alpha_V\beta_3$, have also been investigated in preclinical models and are currently being translated into clinics [85–87], and an initial study showed its feasibility in humans [88]. PET/MRI could also be an attractive platform for this very localized imaging as motion (both respiratory and cardiac) limits the detection. MRI could provide the means of motion detection and correction as already demonstrated in thoracic PET/MRI imaging [89, 90].

3.5 Summary

Today, both PET and MRI are well-recognized methods for the assessment of myocardial perfusion and viability. Integrating these modalities into a system capable of simultaneous acquisitions is a major technological achievement, but it remains to be seen whether this has a real added value in noninvasive cardiac imaging. At present cardiac PET/MRI is an attractive yet expensive research device with two focus areas: cross-validation of new imaging methods under identical experimental conditions and the search for synergistic applications. PET/MRI is currently slowly moving into clinical reality. The main reasons are the high costs, complex workflows, and the mandatory interdisciplinary interaction at a very high level. This results into the conclusion that it remains to be seen whether this new imaging technique is so cost-effective that cardiac imaging will profit from its unique and extraordinary capabilities.

References

1. Shaw LJ, Hendel R, Borges-Neto S, et al. Prognostic value of normal exercise and adenosine (99 m)Tc-tetrofosmin SPECT imaging: results from the multicenter registry of 4,728 patients. J Nucl Med. 2003;44(2):134–9.
2. Slomka PJ, Berman DS, Germano G. New cardiac cameras: single-photon emission CT and PET. Semin Nucl Med. 2014;44(4):232–51.
3. Kolh P, Windecker S. ESC/EACTS myocardial revascularization guidelines 2014. Eur Heart J. 2014;35(46):3235–6.
4. Gaemperli O, Kaufmann PA, Alkadhi H. Cardiac hybrid imaging. Eur J Nucl Med Mol Imaging. 2014;41 Suppl 1:S91–103.

5. Morton G, Chiribiri A, Ishida M, et al. Quantification of absolute myocardial perfusion in patients with coronary artery disease: comparison between cardiovascular magnetic resonance and positron emission tomography. J Am Coll Cardiol. 2012;60(16):1546–55.
6. Moon JC, Messroghli DR, Kellman P, et al. Myocardial T1 mapping and extracellular volume quantification: a Society for Cardiovascular Magnetic Resonance (SCMR) and CMR Working Group of the European Society of Cardiology consensus statement. J Cardiovasc Magn Reson. 2013;15:92.
7. Zaidi H, Ojha N, Morich M, et al. Design and performance evaluation of a whole-body Ingenuity TF PET-MRI system. Phys Med Biol. 2011;56(10):3091–106.
8. Delso G, Furst S, Jakoby B, et al. Performance measurements of the Siemens mMR integrated whole-body PET/MR scanner. J Nucl Med. 2011;52(12):1914–22.
9. Pichler BJ, Judenhofer MS, Catana C, et al. Performance test of an LSO-APD detector in a 7-T MRI scanner for simultaneous PET/MRI. J Nucl Med. 2006;47(4):639–47.
10. Davison H, Ter Voert EE, de Galiza Barbosa F, et al. Incorporation of time-of-flight information reduces metal artifacts in simultaneous positron emission tomography/magnetic resonance imaging: a Simulation Study. Invest Radiol. 2015 Mar 11 [Epub ahead of print]. doi:10.1097/RLI.0000000000000146.
11. Levin C, Deller T, Peterson W, Maramraju SH, Kim C, Prost R. Initial results of simultaneous whole-body ToF PET/MR. J Nucl Med. 2014;55(Supplement 1):660.
12. Martinez-Moller A, Souvatzoglou M, Navab N, Schwaiger M, Nekolla SG. Artifacts from misaligned CT in cardiac perfusion PET/CT studies: frequency, effects, and potential solutions. J Nucl Med. 2007;48(2):188–93.
13. Gould KL, Pan T, Loghin C, Johnson NP, Guha A, Sdringola S. Frequent diagnostic errors in cardiac PET/CT due to misregistration of CT attenuation and emission PET images: a definitive analysis of causes, consequences, and corrections. J Nucl Med. 2007;48(7):1112–21.
14. Souvatzoglou M, Bengel F, Busch R, et al. Attenuation correction in cardiac PET/CT with three different CT protocols: a comparison with conventional PET. Eur J Nucl Med Mol Imaging. 2007;34(12):1991–2000.
15. Koepfli P, Hany TF, Wyss CA, et al. CT attenuation correction for myocardial perfusion quantification using a PET/CT hybrid scanner. J Nucl Med. 2004;45(4):537–42.
16. Martinez-Moller A, Souvatzoglou M, Delso G, et al. Tissue classification as a potential approach for attenuation correction in whole-body PET/MRI: evaluation with PET/CT data. J Nucl Med. 2009;50(4):520–6.
17. Schulz V, Torres-Espallardo I, Renisch S, et al. Automatic, three-segment, MR-based attenuation correction for whole-body PET/MR data. Eur J Nucl Med Mol Imaging. 2011;38(1):138–52.
18. Fürst S, Souvatzoglu M, Rischpler C, Ziegler S, Schwaiger M, Nekolla S. Effects of MR contrast agents on attenuation map generation and cardiac PET quantification in PET/MR. J Nucl Med. 2012;53(Supplement 1):139.
19. Drzezga A, Souvatzoglou M, Eiber M, et al. First clinical experience with integrated whole-body PET/MR: comparison to PET/CT in patients with oncologic diagnoses. J Nucl Med. 2012;53(6):845–55.
20. Nensa F, Poeppel TD, Beiderwellen K, et al. Hybrid PET/MR imaging of the heart: feasibility and initial results. Radiology. 2013;268(2):366–73.
21. Nuyts J, Michel C, Fenchel M, Bal G, Watson C. Completion of a truncated attenuation image from the attenuated PET emission data. IEEE Trans Med Imaging. 2013;32(2):237–46. doi:10.1109/TMI.2012.2220376. Epub 2012 Sep 21.
22. Delso G, Martinez-Moller A, Bundschuh RA, Nekolla SG, Ziegler SI. The effect of limited MR field of view in MR/PET attenuation correction. Med Phys. 2010;37(6):2804–12.
23. Blumhagen JO, Ladebeck R, Fenchel M, Scheffler K. MR-based field-of-view extension in MR/PET: B(0) homogenization using gradient enhancement (HUGE). Magn Reson Med. 2013;70(4):1047–57.
24. Delso G, Martinez-Moller A, Bundschuh RA, et al. Evaluation of the attenuation properties of MR equipment for its use in a whole-body PET/MR scanner. Phys Med Biol. 2010; 55(15):4361–74.

25. Furst S, Souvatzoglou M, Martinez-Moller A, Schwaiger M, Nekolla SG, Ziegler SI. Impact of flexible body surface coil and patient table on PET quantification and image quality in integrated PET/MR. Nuklearmedizin (Nuclear medicine). 2014;53(3):79–87.
26. Paulus DH, Tellmann L, Quick HH. Towards improved hardware component attenuation correction in PET/MR hybrid imaging. Phys Med Biol. 2013;58(22):8021–40.
27. DiFilippo FP, Brunken RC. Do implanted pacemaker leads and ICD leads cause metal-related artifact in cardiac PET/CT? J Nucl Med. 2005;46(3):436–43.
28. Marinskis G, Bongiorni MG, Dagres N, Dobreanu D, Lewalter T, Blomstrom-Lundqvist C. Performing magnetic resonance imaging in patients with implantable pacemakers and defibrillators: results of a European Heart Rhythm Association survey. Europace. 2012;14(12): 1807–9.
29. Cohen JD, Costa HS, Russo RJ. Determining the risks of magnetic resonance imaging at 1.5 tesla for patients with pacemakers and implantable cardioverter defibrillators. Am J Cardiol. 2012;110(11):1631–6.
30. Slomka PJ, Diaz-Zamudio M, Dey D, et al. Automatic registration of misaligned CT attenuation correction maps in Rb-82 PET/CT improves detection of angiographically significant coronary artery disease. J Nucl Cardiol. 2015 Feb 20 [Epub ahead of print]. doi:10.1007/s12350-014-0060-9.
31. Nekolla SG, Martinez-Moller A. Attenuation correction in cardiac PET: to raise awareness for a problem which is as old as PET/CT. J Nucl Cardiol. 2015 Feb 20 [Epub ahead of print]. doi:10.1007/s12350-015-0083-x.
32. Adluru G, Chen L, Kim SE, et al. Three-dimensional late gadolinium enhancement imaging of the left atrium with a hybrid radial acquisition and compressed sensing. J Magn Reson Imaging. 2011;34(6):1465–71.
33. Xue H, Zuehlsdorff S, Kellman P, et al. Unsupervised inline analysis of cardiac perfusion MRI. Med Image Comput Comput Assist Interv. 2009;12(Pt 2):741–9.
34. Flotats A, Bravo PE, Fukushima K, Chaudhry MA, Merrill J, Bengel FM. (82)Rb PET myocardial perfusion imaging is superior to (99 m)Tc-labelled agent SPECT in patients with known or suspected coronary artery disease. Eur J Nucl Med Mol Imaging. 2012;39(8):1233–9.
35. Murthy VL, Di Carli MF. Non-invasive quantification of coronary vascular dysfunction for diagnosis and management of coronary artery disease. J Nucl Cardiol. 2012;19(5):1060–72.
36. Sinusas AJ, Lazewatsky J, Brunetti J, et al. Biodistribution and radiation dosimetry of LMI1195: first-in-human study of a novel 18F-labeled tracer for imaging myocardial innervation. J Nucl Med. 2014;55(9):1445–51.
37. Schwitter J, Nanz D, Kneifel S, et al. Assessment of myocardial perfusion in coronary artery disease by magnetic resonance: a comparison with positron emission tomography and coronary angiography. Circulation. 2001;103(18):2230–5.
38. Ibrahim T, Nekolla SG, Schreiber K, et al. Assessment of coronary flow reserve: comparison between contrast-enhanced magnetic resonance imaging and positron emission tomography. J Am Coll Cardiol. 2002;39(5):864–70.
39. Hsu LY, Groves DW, Aletras AH, Kellman P, Arai AE. A quantitative pixel-wise measurement of myocardial blood flow by contrast-enhanced first-pass CMR perfusion imaging: microsphere validation in dogs and feasibility study in humans. JACC Cardiovasc Imaging. 2012;5(2):154–66.
40. Domenech RJ, Hoffman JI, Noble MI, Saunders KB, Henson JR, Subijanto S. Total and regional coronary blood flow measured by radioactive microspheres in conscious and anesthetized dogs. Circ Res. 1969;25(5):581–96.
41. Zierler KL. Equations for measuring blood flow by external monitoring of radioisotopes. Circ Res. 1965;16:309–21.
42. Zierler K. Indicator dilution methods for measuring blood flow, volume, and other properties of biological systems: a brief history and memoir. Ann Biomed Eng. 2000;28(8):836–48.
43. Tofts PS. Modeling tracer kinetics in dynamic Gd-DTPA MR imaging. J Magn Reson Imaging. 1997;7(1):91–101.

44. Sourbron SP, Buckley DL. On the scope and interpretation of the Tofts models for DCE-MRI. Magn Reson Med. 2011;66(3):735–45.
45. Klitzman B, Duling BR. Microvascular hematocrit and red cell flow in resting and contracting striated muscle. Am J Physiol. 1979;237(4):H481–90.
46. Brands J, van Haare J, Vink H, Vanteeffelen JW. Whole-body recruitment of glycocalyx volume during intravenous adenosine infusion. Physiol Rep. 2013;1(5), e00102.
47. Eliasen P, Amtorp O. Effect of intracoronary adenosine upon regional blood flow, microvascular blood volume and hematocrit in canine myocardium. Int J Microcirc Clin Exp. 1984;3(1):3–12.
48. Donahue KM, Burstein D, Manning WJ, Gray ML. Studies of Gd-DTPA relaxivity and proton exchange rates in tissue. Magn Reson Med. 1994;32(1):66–76.
49. Stanisz GJ, Henkelman RM. Gd-DTPA relaxivity depends on macromolecular content. Magn Reson Med. 2000;44(5):665–7.
50. Calamante F, Gadian DG, Connelly A. Delay and dispersion effects in dynamic susceptibility contrast MRI: simulations using singular value decomposition. Magn Reson Med. 2000;44(3):466–73.
51. Vag T, Heck MM, Beer AJ, et al. Preoperative lymph node staging in patients with primary prostate cancer: comparison and correlation of quantitative imaging parameters in diffusion-weighted imaging and 11C-choline PET/CT. Eur Radiol. 2014;24(8):1821–6.
52. Damadian R, Zaner K, Hor D, DiMaio T, Minkoff L, Goldsmith M. Nuclear magnetic resonance as a new tool in cancer research: human tumors by NMR. Ann N Y Acad Sci. 1973;222:1048–76.
53. Klein C, Nekolla SG, Bengel FM, et al. Assessment of myocardial viability with contrast-enhanced magnetic resonance imaging: comparison with positron emission tomography. Circulation. 2002;105(2):162–7.
54. Klein C, Nekolla SG, Balbach T, et al. The influence of myocardial blood flow and volume of distribution on late Gd-DTPA kinetics in ischemic heart failure. J Magn Reson Imaging. 2004;20(4):588–93.
55. Klein C, Schmal TR, Nekolla SG, Schnackenburg B, Fleck E, Nagel E. Mechanism of late gadolinium enhancement in patients with acute myocardial infarction. J Magn Reson Imaging. 2007;9(4):653–8.
56. Messroghli DR, Radjenovic A, Kozerke S, Higgins DM, Sivananthan MU, Ridgway JP. Modified Look-Locker inversion recovery (MOLLI) for high-resolution T1 mapping of the heart. J Magn Reson Imaging. 2004;52(1):141–6.
57. Wong TC, Piehler KM, Kang IA, et al. Myocardial extracellular volume fraction quantified by cardiovascular magnetic resonance is increased in diabetes and associated with mortality and incident heart failure admission. Eur Heart J. 2014;35(10):657–64.
58. Tamarappoo BK, John BT, Reinier K, et al. Vulnerable myocardial interstitium in patients with isolated left ventricular hypertrophy and sudden cardiac death: a postmortem histological evaluation. J Am Heart Assoc. 2012;1(3), e001511.
59. Ghosh N, Rimoldi OE, Beanlands RS, Camici PG. Assessment of myocardial ischaemia and viability: role of positron emission tomography. Eur Heart J. 2010;31(24):2984–95.
60. Di Carli MF. Predicting improved function after myocardial revascularization. Curr Opin Cardiol. 1998;13(6):415–24.
61. Tillisch J, Brunken R, Marshall R, et al. Reversibility of cardiac wall-motion abnormalities predicted by positron tomography. N Engl J Med. 1986;314(14):884–8.
62. Schinkel AF, Poldermans D, Elhendy A, Bax JJ. Assessment of myocardial viability in patients with heart failure. J Nucl Med. 2007;48(7):1135–46.
63. Bax JJ, Schinkel AF, Boersma E, et al. Early versus delayed revascularization in patients with ischemic cardiomyopathy and substantial viability: impact on outcome. Circulation. 2003;108 Suppl 1:II39–42.
64. Beanlands RS, Ruddy TD, deKemp RA, et al. Positron emission tomography and recovery following revascularization (PARR-1): the importance of scar and the development of a prediction rule for the degree of recovery of left ventricular function. J Am Coll Cardiol. 2002;40(10):1735–43.

65. Kim RJ, Wu E, Rafael A, et al. The use of contrast-enhanced magnetic resonance imaging to identify reversible myocardial dysfunction. N Engl J Med. 2000;343(20):1445–53.
66. Rischpler C, Langwieser N, Souvatzoglou M, et al. PET/MRI early after myocardial infarction: evaluation of viability with late gadolinium enhancement transmurality vs. 18F-FDG uptake. Eur Heart J Cardiovasc Imaging. 2015;16(6):661–9. doi:10.1093/ehjci/jeu317. Epub 2015 Feb 13.
67. Frangogiannis NG, Smith CW, Entman ML. The inflammatory response in myocardial infarction. Cardiovasc Res. 2002;53(1):31–47.
68. Maekawa Y, Anzai T, Yoshikawa T, et al. Prognostic significance of peripheral monocytosis after reperfused acute myocardial infarction: a possible role for left ventricular remodeling. J Am Coll Cardiol. 2002;39(2):241–6.
69. Nahrendorf M, Swirski FK, Aikawa E, et al. The healing myocardium sequentially mobilizes two monocyte subsets with divergent and complementary functions. J Exp Med. 2007;204(12):3037–47.
70. Lee WW, Marinelli B, van der Laan AM, et al. PET/MRI of inflammation in myocardial infarction. J Am Coll Cardiol. 2012;59(2):153–63.
71. Wollenweber T, Roentgen P, Schafer A, et al. Characterizing the inflammatory tissue response to acute myocardial infarction by clinical multimodality noninvasive imaging. Circ Cardiovasc Imaging. 2014;7(5):811–8.
72. Rischpler C, Nekolla SG, Dregely I, Schwaiger M. Hybrid PET/MR imaging of the heart: potential, initial experiences, and future prospects. J Nucl Med. 2013;54(3):402–15.
73. Schwaiger M, Schelbert HR, Ellison D, et al. Sustained regional abnormalities in cardiac metabolism after transient ischemia in the chronic dog model. J Am Coll Cardiol. 1985;6(2):336–47.
74. Egert S, Nguyen N, Schwaiger M. Myocardial glucose transporter GLUT1: translocation induced by insulin and ischemia. J Mol Cell Cardiol. 1999;31(7):1337–44.
75. Taegtmeyer H, Dilsizian V. Imaging myocardial metabolism and ischemic memory. Nat Clin Pract Cardiovasc Med. 2008;5 Suppl 2:S42–8.
76. Blankstein R, Osborne M, Naya M, et al. Cardiac positron emission tomography enhances prognostic assessments of patients with suspected cardiac sarcoidosis. J Am Coll Cardiol. 2014;63(4):329–36.
77. Schneider S, Batrice A, Rischpler C, Eiber M, Ibrahim T, Nekolla SG. Utility of multimodal cardiac imaging with PET/MRI in cardiac sarcoidosis: implications for diagnosis, monitoring and treatment. Eur Heart J. 2014;35(5):312.
78. Fayad ZA, Fuster V, Fallon JT, et al. Noninvasive in vivo human coronary artery lumen and wall imaging using black-blood magnetic resonance imaging. Circulation. 2000;102(5):506–10.
79. Kim WY, Stuber M, Bornert P, Kissinger KV, Manning WJ, Botnar RM. Three-dimensional black-blood cardiac magnetic resonance coronary vessel wall imaging detects positive arterial remodeling in patients with nonsignificant coronary artery disease. Circulation. 2002;106(3):296–9.
80. Ibrahim T, Makowski MR, Jankauskas A, et al. Serial contrast-enhanced cardiac magnetic resonance imaging demonstrates regression of hyperenhancement within the coronary artery wall in patients after acute myocardial infarction. JACC Cardiovasc Imaging. 2009;2(5):580–8.
81. Rudd JH, Warburton EA, Fryer TD, et al. Imaging atherosclerotic plaque inflammation with [18F]-fluorodeoxyglucose positron emission tomography. Circulation. 2002;105(23):2708–11.
82. Davies JR, Rudd JH, Weissberg PL, Narula J. Radionuclide imaging for the detection of inflammation in vulnerable plaques. J Am Coll Cardiol. 2006;47(8 Suppl):C57–68.
83. Ripa RS, Knudsen A, Hag AM, et al. Feasibility of simultaneous PET/MR of the carotid artery: first clinical experience and comparison to PET/CT. Am J Nucl Med Mol Imaging. 2014;4(5):448–58.
84. Joshi NV, Vesey AT, Williams MC, et al. 18F-fluoride positron emission tomography for identification of ruptured and high-risk coronary atherosclerotic plaques: a prospective clinical trial. Lancet. 2014;383(9918):705–13.

85. Saraste A, Laitinen I, Weidl E, et al. Diet intervention reduces uptake of alphavbeta3 integrin-targeted PET tracer 18F-galacto-RGD in mouse atherosclerotic plaques. J Nucl Cardiol. 2012;19(4):775–84.
86. Laitinen I, Notni J, Pohle K, et al. Comparison of cyclic RGD peptides for alphavbeta3 integrin detection in a rat model of myocardial infarction. EJNMMI Res. 2013;3(1):38.
87. Beer AJ, Pelisek J, Heider P, et al. PET/CT imaging of integrin alphavbeta3 expression in human carotid atherosclerosis. JACC Cardiovasc Imaging. 2014;7(2):178–87.
88. Makowski MR, Ebersberger U, Nekolla S, Schwaiger M. In vivo molecular imaging of angiogenesis, targeting alphavbeta3 integrin expression, in a patient after acute myocardial infarction. Eur Heart J. 2008;29(18):2201.
89. Furst S, Grimm R, Hong I, et al. Motion correction strategies for integrated PET/MR. J Nucl Med. 2015;56(2):261–9.
90. Grimm R, Furst S, Souvatzoglou M, et al. Self-gated MRI motion modeling for respiratory motion compensation in integrated PET/MRI. Med Image Anal. 2015;19(1):110–20.

4 Role of PET/CT in Assessing Cardiac Sarcoidosis

Matthieu Pelletier-Galarneau, Brian Mc Ardle, Hiroshi Ohira, Eugene Leung, and Terrence D. Ruddy

4.1 Introduction

Sarcoidosis is a multisystem disease of unknown origin, predominantly affecting young adults, and characterized by compact noncaseating epithelioid cell granulomas. The term *sarkoid* was first introduced in 1899 by Caesar Boeck, a Norwegian dermatologist, to describe benign cutaneous lesions that resembled sarcoma on histopathological examination [1]. With the development and progress of new imaging modalities including positron emission tomography (PET) and magnetic resonance imaging (MRI), there has been a recent increase in interest from clinicians and researchers regarding the diagnosis and treatment of cardiac sarcoidosis.

4.2 Sarcoidosis

4.2.1 Epidemiology and Pathophysiology

The incidence of sarcoidosis is estimated to be 5 per 100,000 person-years in whites, with slight female predominance, and up to 39 per 100,000 person-years in African-Americans [2–4]. However, recent data suggest even higher prevalence, reaching 3–10 and 35–80 per 100,000 person-years in whites and African-Americans, respectively [5]. Underestimation of sarcoidosis incidence is likely due in part to lack of accurate diagnostic tests, leading to under recognition and misdiagnosis of the disease [6]. Even though the exact causes of sarcoidosis are unknown, current evidence

M. Pelletier-Galarneau, MD, MSc (✉) • B. Mc Ardle, MD • H. Ohira, MD • E. Leung, MD, FRCPC • T.D. Ruddy, MD, FRCPC, FACC
Division of Cardiology, University of Ottawa Heart Institute, Canadian Molecular Imaging Center of Excellence (CMICE), Ottawa, ON, Canada
e-mail: mattgalarneau@gmail.com; bmcardle@toh.on.ca; qqyr4ecy9@forest.ocn.ne.jp; euleung@toh.on.ca; TRuddy@ottawaheart.ca

T.H. Schindler et al. (eds.), *Molecular and Multimodality Imaging in Cardiovascular Disease*, DOI 10.1007/978-3-319-19611-4_4

Table 4.1 Different agents that have been linked to increased incidence of sarcoidosis

Infectious agents Virus	Herpes, Epstein-Barr, retrovirus, Coxsackie B virus, cytomegalovirus
Bacteria	*Borrelia burgdorferi*, *Propionibacterium acnes*, *Mycoplasma*
Mycobacteria	*Mycobacterium tuberculosis*
Organic compounds	Clay, pine tree pollen, combustion products
Inorganic compounds	Aluminum, talc, titanium, zirconium

Adapted from [2]

suggests that the disease is the result of inflammation mediated by T lymphocytes and activated macrophages following exposure to specific agents in subjects with genetic predispositions [2, 6–13]. Some agents that have been linked to increased incidence of sarcoidosis are listed in Table 4.1.

4.2.2 Clinical Presentation and Treatment

Presenting symptoms of sarcoidosis typically include dyspnea and cough due to lung involvement as well as systemic symptoms including fatigue, weight loss, and fever. However, sarcoidosis can affect virtually any organ of the human body and can present with a wide variety of symptoms depending on organ involvement (Table 4.2).

Most patients with sarcoidosis present with mild symptoms and will recover spontaneously. Decision to initiate treatment should be based on risk-benefit analysis [14]. The mainstay of sarcoidosis treatment is corticosteroids. Current guidelines recommend the use of 20–40 mg of oral prednisone per day [2], and response to therapy should be assessed within 1–3 months. In case of improvement, prednisone treatment can be tapered down to dosage of 5–15 mg per day for an additional 9–12 months, whereas lack of response suggests irreversible fibrotic disease [14]. Given the nonspecific nature of sarcoidosis symptoms, it can be difficult to accurately monitor response to therapy. The use of cytotoxic medication such as methotrexate and immunomodulatory agents such as tumor necrosis factor alpha has been shown to be a viable therapeutic option in patient not responding to corticosteroids or unable to pursue corticosteroid treatment due to adverse effects [15]. Other therapeutic options include hydroxychloroquine to treat patients with skin involvement and hypercalcemia [14].

4.2.3 Diagnosis of Sarcoidosis

The diagnosis of systemic sarcoidosis is established when there is radiographic evidence of sarcoidosis with compatible clinical features and noncaseating granulomas on biopsy with other causes of granulomas ruled out. Response to corticosteroids is not enough to establish diagnosis of sarcoidosis [14]. There are no specific serum markers for sarcoidosis. C reactive protein (CRP) and erythrocyte sedimentation rate (ESR) are sensitive inflammation markers but are not specific for sarcoidosis. Serum angiotensin-converting enzyme (ACE) levels are elevated in approximately

Table 4.2 Symptoms and signs of sarcoidosis depending on organ involvement

	Clinical presentation
Constitutional	Fever fatigue Weight loss Low-grade fever
Lungs and upper respiratory tract	Dyspnea Cough Dysphagia Chest pain
Lymphatic system	Enlarged lymph nodes
Heart	Palpitation Syncope Dizziness Chest pain
Liver	Abnormal liver function tests Hepatomegaly
Spleen	Splenomegaly
Skin	Papular sarcoidosis Erythema nodosum Lupus pernio
Eyes	Uveitis Retinal vasculitis
Central nervous system	Cranial mononeuropathies Neuroendocrine dysfunction
Musculoskeletal	Acute polyarthritis Chronic arthritis Diffuse myositis
Salivary glands	Painless swelling

60 % of patients with sarcoidosis due to production of ACE by the granulomas [14]. However, serum ACE is neither sensitive nor specific enough to screen patients with suspected sarcoidosis with its positive predictive value of 84 % and negative predictive value of 74 % [16]. Furthermore, serum ACE should not be used to diagnose sarcoidosis or guide therapy [14].

Due to lack of useful serum markers, diagnosis of sarcoidosis relies greatly on imaging. Classical features of sarcoidosis on chest radiographs include mediastinal and hilar lymphadenopathy, parenchymal opacities, and parenchymal fibrosis in more advanced cases [17]. A staging based on chest radiography has been described more than 40 years ago to monitor chest disease in patient with sarcoidosis (Fig. 4.1) [18]. Although this scale shows poor interobserver agreement, especially for advanced disease, it remains widely used due to its prognostic value [19].

Computed tomography (CT) imaging is only indicated when chest radiograph is atypical for sarcoidosis or when patients present with hemoptysis. Lymphadenopathy and parenchymal disease are more readily seen on CT. Classically, parenchymal lesions present as small pulmonary nodules in a peribronchovascular distribution or following the fissures [17]. Lymphadenopathy with coarse calcification or "icing sugar" lymphadenopathies are frequently described in sarcoidosis. In more advanced disease, lung fibrosis is seen.

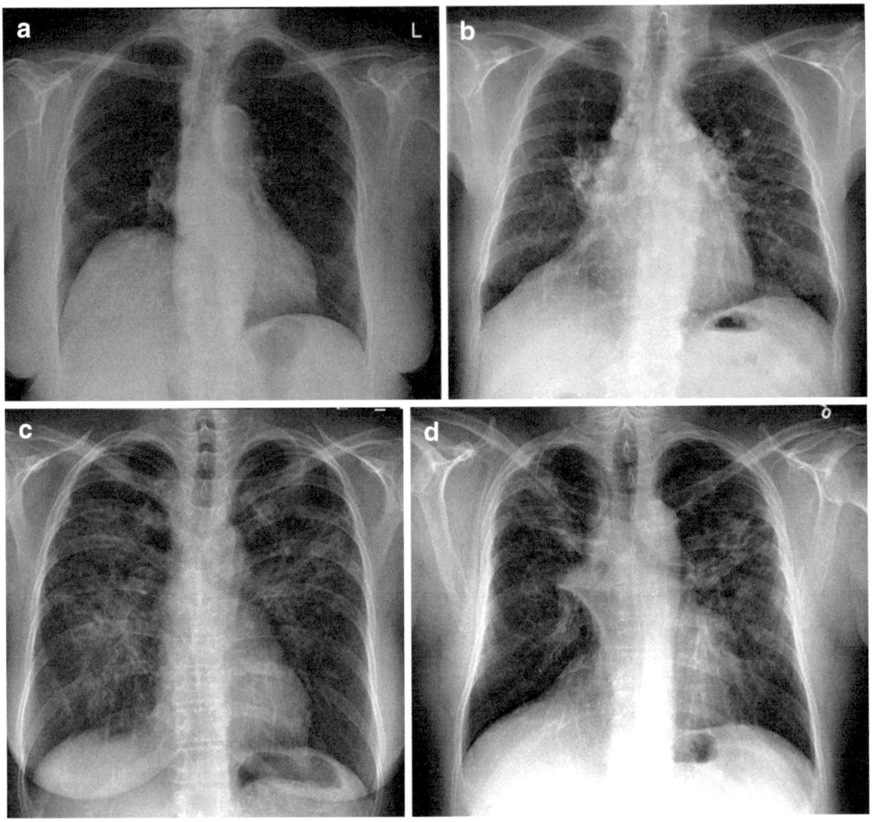

Fig. 4.1 Four stages of sarcoidosis on chest radiographs. (**a**) Stage I: hilar or mediastinal lymphadenopathy. (**b**) Stage II: lymphadenopathy and parenchymal disease. (**c**) Stage III: parenchymal disease alone. (**d**) Stage IV: pulmonary fibrosis

Gallium-67 citrate has been used for the diagnosis, staging, and treatment follow-up of patients with sarcoidosis. Classical findings include the so-called lambda sign, arising from uptake in the mediastinal and hilar lymphadenopathy, and the panda sign, from abnormal parotid and lacrimal gland uptake (Fig. 4.2). However, accuracy of gallium scintigraphy varies greatly from one study to another with reported sensitivity ranging from 60 to 90 % and suboptimal interobserver variability [20–25].

4.2.4 Role of PET/CT in Sarcoidosis

^{18}F-fluorodeoxyglucose (FDG) is a diagnostic PET radiopharmaceutical with half-life of 109.7 min. FDG is a glucose analog that is transported from the blood into the cells by glucose transporters GLUT 1 and GLUT 4. Once intracellular, FDG is then phosphorylated by hexokinase to form FDG-6-phosphate [26]. Unlike glucose, FDG-6-phosphate is not further metabolized, which leads to trapping of the

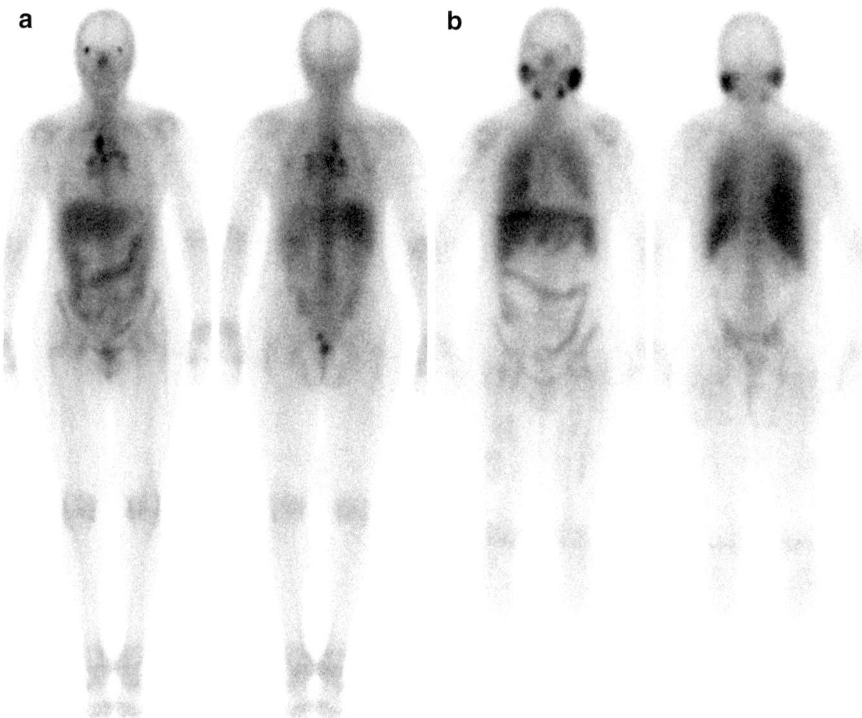

Fig. 4.2 Gallium-67 scintigraphy of two different patients with sarcoidosis. (**a**) Increased activity in the mediastinal and hilar lymph nodes gives the characteristic lambda sign. (**b**) Uptake in the parotid and submandibular salivary glands as well as diffuse lung uptake due to sarcoidosis

radiopharmaceutical into the cells (Fig. 4.3). Uptake of FDG is proportional to glucose metabolism, and therefore, increased FDG uptake is seen in several conditions including infection, inflammation, and malignancies.

FDG-PET has several practical and technical advantages over ^{67}Ga, including favorable tracer kinetics, lower radiation exposure, and better quality images [27]. FDG-PET is more accurate and allows better evaluation of extrapulmonary involvement compared to ^{67}Ga [25, 28].

4.2.4.1 Evaluation of Disease Extent

FDG-PET imaging permits whole-body assessment in a single-step examination. A large proportion of patients with suspected pulmonary sarcoidosis have extrapulmonary involvement visualized on FDG-PET [29]. Frequent extrapulmonary sites include the bone, spleen, liver, and abdominal lymph nodes [30]. Accurate determination of the spread of active disease with FDG-PET provides an explanation for persistent disabling symptoms and has been shown to influence patient management [29, 31]. Moreover, identification of sites of extrapulmonary sarcoidosis can identify potential biopsy sites (Fig. 4.4) [29].

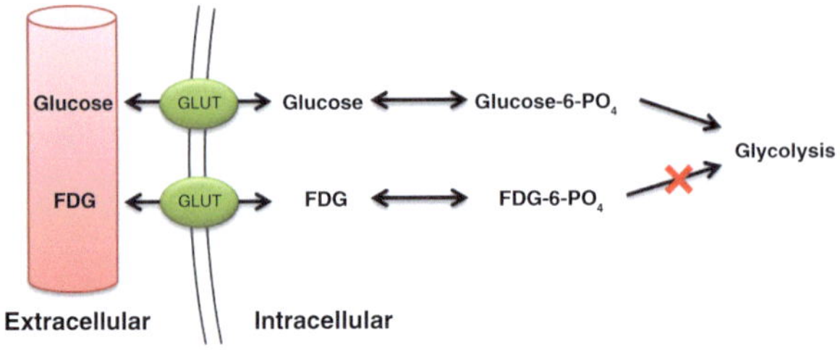

Fig. 4.3 Mechanism of uptake and trapping of FDG

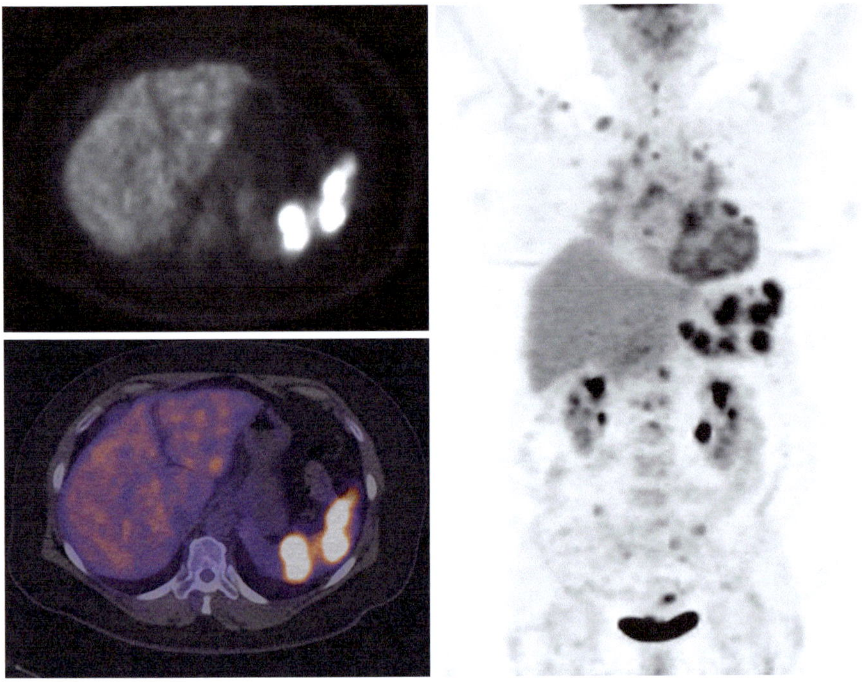

Fig. 4.4 Whole-body FDG-PET scan with selected axial slice in a patient with known thoracic sarcoidosis demonstrating abnormal uptake corresponding to sarcoidosis involvement of the spleen, thoracolumbar spine, and heart as well as in pelvic lymph nodes

4.2.4.2 FDG-PET as a Marker of Disease Activity and in Assessment of Therapy Response

The goal of treatment in sarcoidosis is to treat reversible granulomatous inflammation. Still, there is currently no gold standard method for monitoring inflammatory activity in patients with sarcoidosis. Because of the serious side effects associated with sarcoidosis therapy, it is important to differentiate active and treatable inflammation from quiescent fibrosis. Sarcoidosis often presents with nonspecific systemic symptoms such as fatigue. Monitoring of these nonspecific symptoms does not allow to assess disease progression or response to therapy [32]. Besides, some patients are completely asymptomatic. Serum ACE is also used to monitor response to treatment but does not accurately reflect inflammatory activity [33]. Changes on conventional anatomical imaging, including x-ray and high-resolution CT, are not reliable markers of active inflammation, as they can remain positive even without active disease [34]. On the contrary, PET was shown to provide additional value to assess inflammatory activity in patients with pulmonary fibrosis [35]. Bronchoalveolar lavage (BAL) is an important tool in diagnosis of pulmonary sarcoidosis, but is not recommended for assessment of treatment response [36]. The prognostic value of BAL depends on the number of T lymphocytes, neutrophils, and mast cells [37–39]. Although gallium-67 has been used to detect active granulomas, it lacks correlation with BAL lymphocyte counts [23, 40]. Because FDG accumulates in inflammatory cells and allows imaging of active inflammation, FDG-PET could be used to monitor response to therapy (Figs. 4.4 and 4.5) [41]. FDG-PET has been shown to be a useful adjunct to other diagnostic methods for detecting active inflammation, especially in patients with persistent symptoms and normal ACE levels [31]. FDG-PET is also used to monitor response to therapy. So far, only few studies, most retrospective and with a small sample size, have looked at FDG-PET before and after corticosteroid therapy [20, 42–45] and TNF-α inhibitor therapy [46, 47]. FDG-PET post therapy was shown to correlate with symptoms [44, 46] as well as corticosteroid dosage [42]. It also correlates with endoscopic findings in patients with sinonasal sarcoidosis [45]. On the other hand, FDG-PET does not correlate with serum ACE, serum IL-2R, or pulmonary function tests (PFT) [20, 44, 46, 47]. These findings suggest that FDG-PET could provide useful information to assess response to treatment and adjust steroid dosage.

4.3 Cardiac Sarcoidosis

4.3.1 Epidemiology

In the United States, myocardial involvement is recognized in approximately 25 % of patients with sarcoidosis [48]. In the Japanese population, the prevalence of cardiac involvement in patients with sarcoidosis is significantly greater, reaching 58 % [49–51]. Cardiac sarcoidosis is characterized by noncaseating granulomas in the myocardium surrounded by lymphocytes [52]. The left ventricular free wall and septum are the most frequently affected myocardial regions [49, 52].

4.3.2 Clinical Presentation and Treatment

Patients with cardiac sarcoidosis may have different presentations depending on the extension and location of the disease [14]. They can present with conduction abnormalities due to direct infiltration of inflammatory cell and/or scar formation. These can also manifest as atrioventricular block or bundle branch block [49]. Atrioventricular block affects approximately 25 % of patients with cardiac sarcoidosis and is caused by

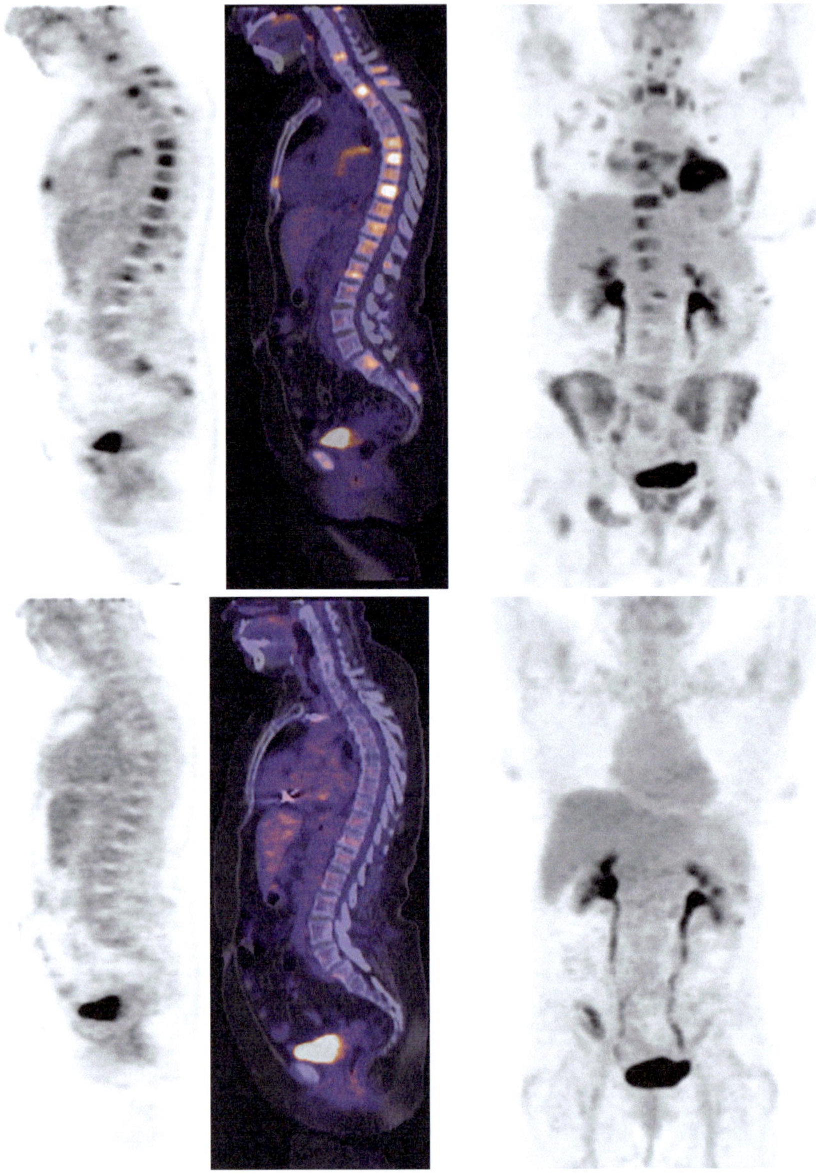

Fig. 4.5 Whole-body FDG-PET scan with selected sagittal slice and maximum intensity projection (MIP) of a patient with extensive sarcoidosis in the heart and bone. Follow-up scan after corticosteroid therapy demonstrates normal biodistribution of FDG, consistent with response to treatment

inflammation or scar in the basal septum [53, 54]. Diagnosis of cardiac sarcoidosis should be considered in young patients with atrioventricular heart block of unknown etiology [54, 55]. Patients with cardiac sarcoidosis can also present with congestive heart failure due to extensive infiltration of the myocardium by granulomas [49, 56].

As with pulmonary sarcoidosis, cardiac inflammation from sarcoidosis is typically treated with corticosteroids. Several uncontrolled series and small sample retrospective studies suggest that steroids may be valuable to treat cardiac sarcoidosis [53, 54, 57–59]. Thus far, there are no randomized controlled trials available to confirm these results and treatment of cardiac sarcoidosis with corticosteroids remains controversial [60]. Initiation of corticosteroid therapy, even with antiarrhythmic drugs, does not prevent arrhythmic event [61]. Pacemakers and ICD are often required when there is extensive involvement of the conduction system or when there is significant heart failure [60]. A systematic review of corticosteroid therapy in cardiac sarcoidosis revealed a wide range of steroid regimens, with prednisone dosage of 20–60 mg daily or 50–60 mg on alternate day [62]. In small single-center retrospective studies, corticosteroid therapy was associated with maintenance of LV function in patients with normal function at diagnosis and improvement of ejection fraction in patients with mild to moderate LV dysfunction [58, 59, 63]. However, no improvement was observed in patients with severe LV dysfunction. As regards to ventricular arrhythmias, some studies showed benefits of immunosuppression therapy [59, 64, 65], whereas others showed no benefit or worsening [61, 66]. As for LV dysfunction, immunosuppressive therapy appears more beneficial in early phase of disease [58, 59]. There is, however, currently not enough data to establish mortality benefit from steroid therapy [62].

4.3.3 PET Imaging

4.3.3.1 Patient Preparation

The myocardium can metabolize different substrates, including free fatty acids, glucose, pyruvate, and ketone bodies. Under physiological conditions, the heart metabolizes mainly free fatty acids and glucose, with free fatty acids accounting for 60–90 % of the energy substrates [67–69]. The source of energy used by the myocardium depends mainly on free fatty acids and glucose plasma concentration and insulin levels [70]. In order to obtain diagnostic FDG-PET images for assessing active cardiac sarcoidosis, pretest preparation is required to suppress physiological uptake in the normal myocardium. Adequate suppression of physiological myocardial FDG uptake is crucial to maximize diagnostic accuracy (Fig. 4.6).

Fasting

When fasting, the myocardial metabolism is shifted and 90 % of its energy comes from metabolism of free fatty acids [71]. For this reason, prolonged fasting is routinely used to suppress physiological myocardial glucose uptake. Several protocols have been described using different fasting time to suppress physiological myocardial FDG uptake, typically between 5 and 18 h [72–75]. To maximize specificity of myocardial FDG uptake, current guidelines recommend fasting for at least 12 h [76].

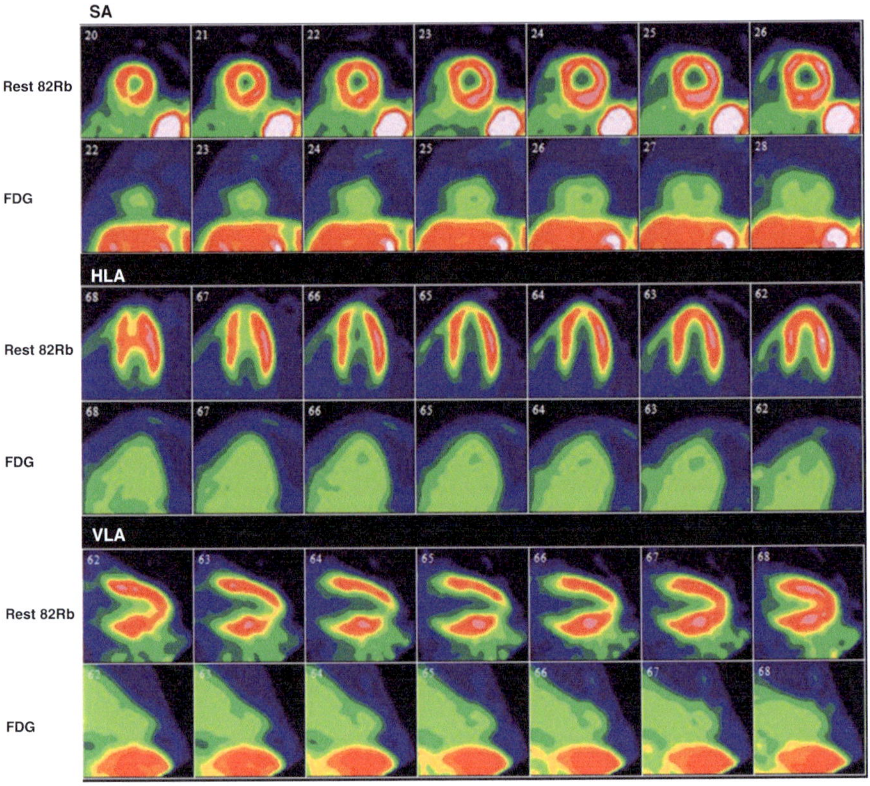

Fig. 4.6 Rest rubidium-82 and FDG-PET scan of a patient with suspected cardiac sarcoidosis. After adequate suppression of physiological myocardial uptake, there is no significant FDG uptake in the myocardium with only blood pool activity, representing a negative study for cardiac sarcoidosis

Diet

Twelve-hour fasting alone can lead to variable myocardial FDG uptake and additional measures are important to consider to minimize physiological uptake [76]. Changing diet prior to imaging has been shown to be at least as effective as fasting to suppress physiological myocardial uptake [72]. Indeed, the fatty acid-glucose cycle, known as the Randle cycle, indicates that glucose loading suppresses fatty acid utilization and that fatty acid loading suppresses glucose utilization by the myocardium [77]. Different low-carbohydrate diets and low-carbohydrate high-fat (LCHF) diets have been used to minimize myocardial FDG uptake (Table 4.3). In a small randomized study, Cheng et al. showed that a simple low-carbohydrate diet in combination with prolonged fasting of 6 h provided adequate myocardial suppression of FDG uptake, while addition of fatty acid loading did not, suggesting that low carbohydrate might be preferable [78]. Others suggested that high-fat meal 3–6 h or 1 h prior to imaging provided adequate myocardial suppression [79]. Harisankar et al. demonstrated that LCHF diet is superior to prolonged fasting of 12 h to

Table 4.3 Review of different patient preparation to minimize physiological myocardial uptake of FDG

Authors	Year	*N*	Patients	Fasting	Diet	Fat	Carbohydrates
Lum et al. [82]	2002	69	Cancer staging	Overnight	Low carbohydrate	N/A	N/A
Williams and Kolodny [79]	2008	161	Cancer staging	3–6 h	Very high fat, low carbohydrate, protein permitted	N/A	N/A
Cheng et al. [78]	2010	63	Cancer staging	6 h	Low carbohydrate	N/A	<5 g
Wykrzykowska et al. [83]	2009	32	Cancer staging with suspected CAD	Overnight	Very high fat, low carbohydrate, protein permitted	N/A	<5 g
Harisankar et al. [80]	2011	120	Coronary artery disease	12 h	Low carbohydrate, high fat, protein permitted	20.8 g	1.2 g
Coulden et al. [84]	2012	120	Cancer staging	Overnight	Low carbohydrate	N/A	<3 g
Kobayashi et al. [85]	2013	14	Healthy volunteers	6 h	24 h low-carbohydrate diet with high-fat meal	9 g	1 g
Soussan et al. [81]	2013	58	Cardiac sarcoidosis	4 h	Low-carbohydrate high-fat meal 4 h	N/A	N/A

Table 4.4 Example of the LCHF recommendations provided to the patients prior to FDG imaging at the University of Ottawa Heart Institute

Do eat	Do not eat
Beverages: Mineral water, seltzer, water, clear liquids without milk or sugar, coffee, tea, and herbal tea (without milk or sugar) *Eggs*: Fried, scrambled prepared without milk, omelet prepared without milk or vegetables *Condiments* and *seasonings*: Anything that does not contain sugar *Fats/oils*: Animal fats that are part of the meat you eat, butter, margarine *Sweeteners*: Aspartame, NutraSweet, Sweet'N Low, Equal *Fish*: any fish Fatty unsweetened fish (fried or broiled but not grilled) *Meats*: Fatty unsweetened (fried or broiled but not grilled) red meat, bacon, meat only sausages, bacon, ham *Poultry*: Fatty unsweetened chicken and turkey (fried or broiled but not grilled) *Shellfish*: Any non-processed shellfish *Low-carbohydrate vegetables*: Cucumber, broccoli, lettuce, celery, mushroom, radish, asparagus, green pepper, cabbage, spinach *Sweeteners*: Aspartame, NutraSweet, Sweet'N Low, Equal	*No sugar*: Sugar in any form is strictly forbidden (including natural sugars in fruit) *No starches*: Pasta, breads, bagels, cereals, crackers, cookies, muffins, rice, potatoes *No candy*: Candy, chewing gum, mints, cough drops *No processed products*: Processed foods such as deli meats. These products often contain hidden sugars *No Splenda substitutes* *No milk or milk products* *No cheese or cheese products* *No peanut butter or nuts* *No alcohol* *No fruit* *No vegetables with higher carbohydrate content*

suppress myocardial FDG uptake [80]. More recently, Soussan et al. demonstrated that a LCHF diet for the dinner and breakfast preceding imaging followed by 4 h fasting provided sufficient myocardial suppression of uptake for the diagnosis of cardiac sarcoidosis [81]. There is currently no evidence that clearly established usefulness of LCHF diet over low carbohydrate alone. Furthermore, there is no data on improvement of diagnosis of cardiac sarcoidosis using such diets. Nevertheless, because diet modification is an easily applicable measure, it is routine to follow a diet with less than 5 g of carbohydrate, with or without high-fat meal prior to imaging. Table 4.4 shows an example of the LCHF recommendations provided to the patients prior to FDG imaging.

Heparin

Nuutila et al. showed that increased free fatty acid serum levels induced by heparin infusion were associated with decreased myocardial FDG uptake in healthy volunteers [86]. The protocol used in their study consisted of two 200 IU boluses

Table 4.5 Oral diabetic medication that should be continued or held on the day of PET scan based on the University of Ottawa Heart Institute protocol

Oral medication that should be continued on the day of the PET scan	Oral medication that should be held on the day of the PET scan
Exenatide (Byetta)	Acarbose (Glucobay)
Linagliptin (Trajenta)	Gliclazide (Diamicron)
Liraglutide (Victoza)	Gliclazide MR (Diamicron MR)
Metformin (Glucophage or Glumetza)	Glimepiride (Amaryl)
Pioglitazone (Actos)	Glyburide (Diabeta)
Rosiglitazone (Avandia)	Repaglinide (Gluconorm)
Saxagliptin (Onglyza)	
Sitagliptin (Januvia)	

of unfractionated heparin, injected intravenously, 90 min before FDG injection and at time of injection, with continuous infusion of 15 IU/min starting 90 min prior to FDG injection. The increased in FFA levels is mediated via activation of the lipoprotein and hepatic lipase [87]. Heparin injection is now routinely done to suppress myocardial FDG uptake, and typical dosage is 50 IU/kg divided in one or two intravenous bolus injections [25, 74, 88, 89], without reports of increased bleeding risk [25, 89]. However, using heparin infusion alone to suppress myocardial uptake is not sufficient since approximately half of the patients still present diffuse myocardial FDG uptake following heparin injection and 6 h fasting [89, 90]. Administration of unfractionated heparin prior to injection of FDG has not been shown to improve detection of cardiac sarcoidosis yet. Nevertheless, many centers have implemented heparin injection in their imaging protocol to maximize diagnostic accuracy.

Diabetic Patients

While many studies on patient preparation prior for FDG imaging exclude patients with diabetes [80, 82, 83, 85], others include only very small number of patients with diabetes [78]. In the small number of studies that do include patients with diabetes, there are discrepancies between the protocols with some suggesting to continue diabetic medication [79], while others are prescribing to hold diabetic medication on the day of the scan [81]. Currently, there are no data addressing specifically the optimal pretest preparation of patients with diabetes prior to FDG-PET in the context of cardiac sarcoidosis.

Different centers have different protocols to image diabetic patients. At the University of Ottawa Heart Institute, diabetic patients are scheduled as the first case of the day, following 12 h fasting and low-carbohydrate high-fat diet, to minimize patient discomfort and glycemic issues. It is recommended that diabetic patients monitor their blood sugar levels following their usual routine with one measurement obtained the morning of the PET scan. If the glycemia falls to less than 4 mmol/L, patients are instructed to drink juice or take glucose to raise their sugar level to higher than 4 mmol/L. Some oral medications should be held on the morning of the scan, while others should be continued (Table 4.5).

In many cases, usual doses of long-acting and intermediate-acting insulin can be continued the night before the PET scan. Short-acting insulin dosage and premixed insulin may need to be reduced the evening before the scan given the low-carbohydrate diet. Since the patients will be fasting on the day of the test, the usual breakfast dose of short-acting insulin should not be taken. Finally, for patients with type 1 diabetes using an insulin pump, basal insulin should be continued on the day of the test.

4.3.4 Imaging Protocol

Imaging protocol includes three components: (1) cardiac rest perfusion scan, (2) whole-body FDG scan, and (3) dedicated cardiac FDG scan. The imaging protocol used at the University of Ottawa Heart Institute (UOHI) is illustrated in Fig. 4.7.

Cardiac rest perfusion scan is typically performed using PET perfusion tracers such as rubidium-82 or ammonia-N13 and follows regular procedure guidelines for rest myocardial perfusion [91]. With Rb-82, dosages of 10–20 MBq/kg up to 2,200 MBq are used and ECG-gated images are acquired over 4–8 min after injection. Ammonia-N13 rest images are acquired over 15–30 min approximately 5 min after intravenous injection of 5–10 MBq/kg (up to 750 MBq). Images are reconstructed using CT-based attenuation correction and displayed in the usual short and long axes.

Approximately 1 h after intravenous injection of 5 MBq/kg (up to 550 MBq) of ^{18}F-FDG, whole-body PET scan is acquired. The patient is positioned supine with his or her arms up above his head. A low-dose CT for attenuation correction and localization is first acquired. Then, whole-body FDG-PET images are acquired from the base of the skull to mid thighs, 3 min per bed position. Following

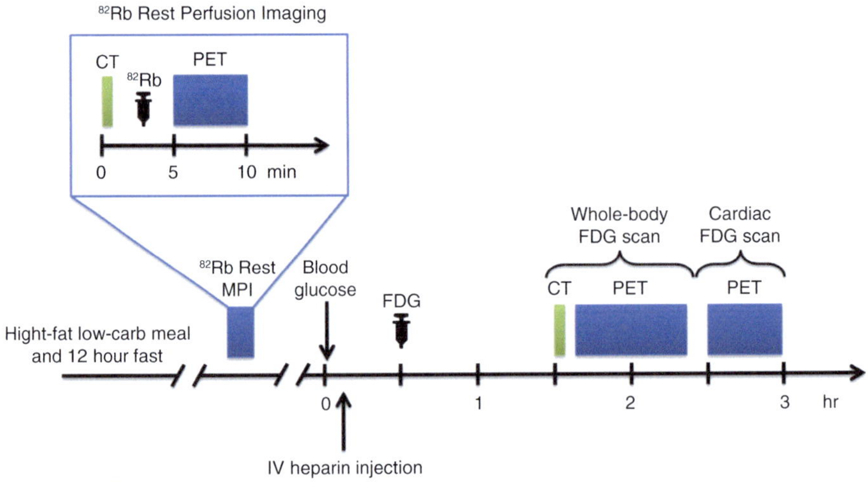

Fig. 4.7 Typical imaging protocol combining rest Rb-82 perfusion imaging and whole-body and dedicated cardiac FDG-PET scan

whole-body imaging, dedicated cardiac PET scan is performed. This acquisition includes a static and, if available, ECG-gated acquisitions. Images are reconstructed by OSEM with attenuation correction and displayed along the perfusion images in the usual short and long axes (Fig. 4.6).

4.3.5 Image Interpretation

Cardiac FDG interpretation must ensure adequate patient preparation. Indeed, poor patient preparation can result in equivocal study due to physiological myocardial FDG uptake. For interpretation, cardiac FDG-PET images are displayed along with rest perfusion images with conventional cardiac display software in the usual short and long axes. Ishimaru et al. described four patterns of FDG uptake: none, focal, focal on diffuse, and diffuse (Fig. 4.8) [89]. This classification has been adopted by other studies and is now frequently used [88, 92]. Focal and focal on diffuse uptake patterns are considered suspicious for cardiac sarcoidosis, whereas diffuse or absence of uptake are considered negative. In order to increase specificity of the diagnostic test, correlation with clinical history is crucial in the interpretation of FDG-PET scan. The interventricular septum is known to be frequently affected in patients with CS and is associated with second- and third-degree atrioventricular block [53, 54]. Therefore, uptake in that region in a patient presenting with atrioventricular block is highly suspicious for sarcoidosis (Fig. 4.9) [93].

Similarly, if the onset site of VT demonstrates focal FDG uptake on FDG-PET, the likelihood that the uptake represents active cardiac sarcoidosis is increased [76]. Although not routinely used, quantification of heterogeneity of uptake can be used to increased specificity. Quantification of heterogeneity of uptake using SUV

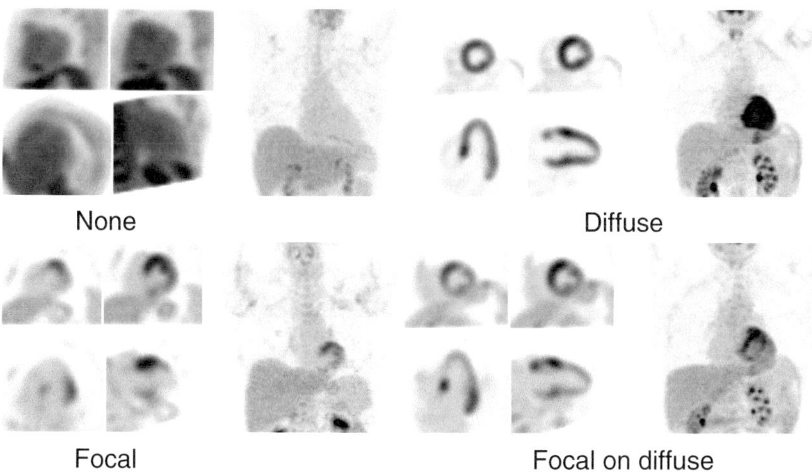

Fig. 4.8 Four different patterns of myocardial FDG uptake: none, diffuse, focal, and focal on diffuse

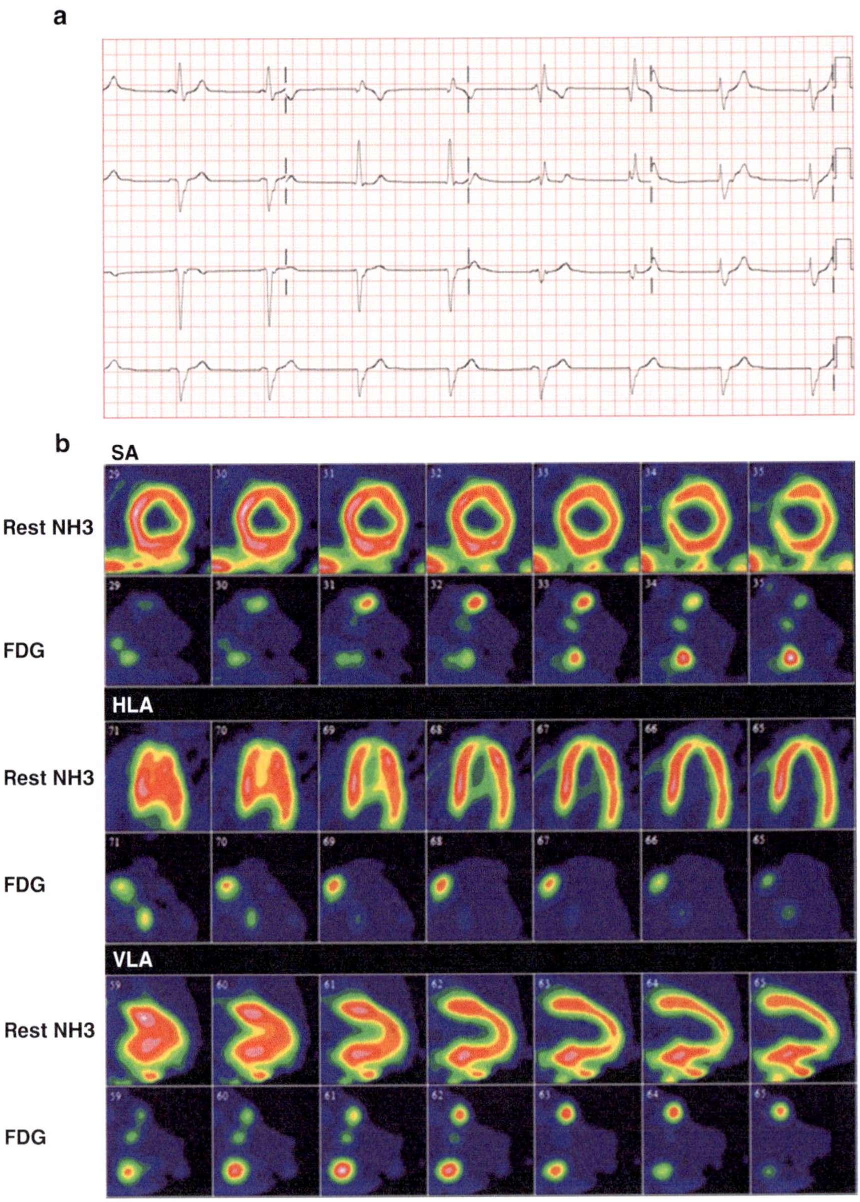

Fig. 4.9 (**a**) ECG of a patient without known history of sarcoidosis presenting with complete atrioventricular block and junctional escape beat with right bundle branch block. (**b**) Subsequent FDG-PET/CT with ammonia-N13 rest imaging shows focal increased uptake in the basal septal wall, right ventricular insertion, as well as right ventricular free wall

coefficient of variation has been shown to be significantly higher in patients with CS compared to normal healthy subjects and in patients with DCM [92].

Image interpretation should include comparison with perfusion images. This allows detection of myocardial scar and assessment of active sarcoidosis in these

Table 4.6 Interpretation criteria combining rest perfusion imaging and FDG findings

Rest perfusion	FDG	Interpretation
Normal	No uptake	Negative for CS
Normal	Diffuse	Diffuse FDG most likely due to suboptimal patient preparation
Normal	Focal	Could represent early disease
Defect	No uptake	Perfusion defect represents scar from sarcoidosis or other etiology
Defect	Focal in area of perfusion defect	Active inflammation with scar in the same location
Defect	Focal on diffuse with focal in area of perfusion defect	Active inflammation with scar in the same location with either diffuse inflammation or suboptimal preparation
Defect	Focal in area of normal perfusion	Presence of both scar and inflammation in different segments of the myocardium

Adapted from Blankstein et al. [95]

areas [94]. Interpretation criteria including perfusion images are summarized in Table 4.6 [95]. Finally, whole-body FDG-PET scan should be reviewed to assess for extracardiac sarcoidosis and other incidental findings. Detection of extrathoracic sarcoidosis can facilitate and accelerate the diagnosis of sarcoidosis by identifying potential biopsy sites [29]. It must be noted that imaging represents one of the criteria used for the diagnosis of cardiac sarcoidosis and diagnosis cannot be established solely on the base of a positive FDG-PET scan.

4.3.6 Role of FDG-PET in Cardiac Sarcoidosis

4.3.6.1 Diagnosis of Cardiac Sarcoidosis

Revision of the original Japanese Ministry of Health and Welfare (JMHW) guidelines for the diagnosis of cardiac sarcoidosis was presented by the joint committee of the Japan Society of Sarcoidosis and Other Granulomatous Disorders and the Japanese College of Cardiology in 2006 (Table 4.7) [96]. These new guidelines, simply referred as the JMHW guidelines, are currently used in many studies as a gold standard for cardiac sarcoidosis. Although FDG-PET is not explicitly included in these criteria, gallium-67 scintigraphy is often substituted by FDG-PET. According to these criteria, diagnosis of CS requires histopathological or clinical diagnosis of extracardiac sarcoidosis. Endomyocardial biopsy has limited sensitivity due to sampling method and heterogeneous myocardial involvement [97]. Unlike amyloidosis, cardiac involvement with sarcoidosis is typically patchy; therefore, even in the cases of negative endomyocardial biopsy, the diagnostic of cardiac sarcoidosis can still be established in the appropriate clinical setting [76]. Because of poor correlation between imaging findings and JMHW diagnosis of CS, some authors have suggested that JMHW has limited sensitivity for detection of CS [88, 95, 98].

More recently, the Heart Rhythm Society (HRS), in collaboration with many organisms including the World Association for Sarcoidosis and Other Granulomatous Disorders (WASOG), published an expert consensus recommendation on criteria

Table 4.7 2006 revised JMHW guidelines for the diagnosis of cardiac sarcoidosis presented by the joint committee of the Japan Society of Sarcoidosis and Other Granulomatous Disorders and the Japanese College of Cardiology [96]

1. Histological diagnosis Cardiac sarcoidosis is confirmed when cardiac biopsy specimens demonstrate noncaseating epithelioid cell granuloma with histological or clinical diagnosis of extracardiac sarcoidosis
2. Clinical diagnosis group Cardiac sarcoidosis is diagnosed without endomyocardial biopsy or in the absence of typical granulomas on cardiac biopsy when histological or clinical diagnosis of extracardiac sarcoidosis is established and a combination of major or minor diagnostic criteria has been satisfied as follows: (a) ≥2 of the 4 following major criteria are satisfied Advanced atrioventricular block Basal thinning of the ventricular septum Positive cardiac gallium uptake* Left ventricular ejection fraction <50 % *or* (b) 1 of the 4 major criteria and ≥2 of the following minor criteria are satisfied: Abnormal electrocardiogram findings including ventricular tachycardia, multifocal frequent premature ventricular contractions, complete right bundle branch block, abnormal Q waves, or abnormal axis deviation Abnormal echocardiogram demonstrating regional wall motion abnormalities, ventricular aneurysm, or unexplained increase in wall thickness Perfusion defects detected by myocardial scintigraphy Delayed gadolinium enhancement of the myocardium on cardiac MRI scanning Interstitial fibrosis or monocyte infiltration greater than moderate grade by endomyocardial biopsy

Table 4.8 Expert consensus recommendation from the Heart Rhythm Society on criteria for the diagnosis of cardiac sarcoidosis [99]

1. Histological diagnosis from myocardial tissue CS is diagnosed in the presence of noncaseating granuloma on histological examination of myocardial tissue with no alternative cause identified (including negative organismal stains if applicable)
2. Clinical diagnosis from invasive and noninvasive studies: It is probable that there is CS if: (a) There is a histological diagnosis of extracardiac sarcoidosis *and* (b) One or more of the following is present: Steroid +/− immunosuppressant responsive cardiomyopathy or atrioventricular block Unexplained reduced LVEF (o40 %) Unexplained sustained (spontaneous or induced) VT Mobitz type II second-degree heart block or third-degree heart block Patchy uptake on dedicated cardiac PET (in a pattern consistent with CS) Late gadolinium enhancement on cardiac MRI (in a pattern consistent with CS) Positive gallium uptake (in a pattern consistent with CS) *and* (c) Other causes for the cardiac manifestation(s) have been reasonably excluded

for the diagnosis of cardiac sarcoidosis (Table 4.8) [99]. Imaging modalities recommended in these guidelines include FDG-PET, Ga-67 scintigraphy, and cardiac MRI. Furthermore, these criteria are more stringent, requiring histological diagnosis of cardiac or extracardiac sarcoidosis.

4.3.6.2 Diagnostic Accuracy

Establishing diagnostic accuracy for cardiac sarcoidosis (CS) of any imaging modality is challenging because of lack of a proper gold standard. Ideally, diagnostic accuracy studies would use myocardial biopsy on all subjects. However, this gold standard is invasive and has a poor sensitivity below 25 % due to the heterogeneity of myocardial involvement [100, 101]. Because of this, studies tend to have small sample size and/or rely on JMWH criteria as their gold standard. A meta-analysis reviewing seven studies with a total of 164 patients reported sensitivity of FDG-PET scan for cardiac sarcoidosis ranging from 79 to 100 % with pooled sensitivity of 89 % [74]. They reported a wide range of specificity values from 38 to 100 % with pooled specificity of 78 %. It was hypothesized that this wide range of specificity is due to physiological myocardial uptake leading to false-positive studies and low sensitivity of the use of JMHW criteria as gold standard [74].

FDG-PET vs Gallium 67

As for other sites of extrapulmonary sarcoidosis, sensitivity of Ga-67 to detect cardiac sarcoidosis is very low, ranging from 15 to 40 % [25, 75, 102]. In a retrospective study including 76 patients with suspected cardiac sarcoidosis using the 1993 JMHW criteria as their gold standard, fasting FDG-PET sensitivity and specificity were 85 % and 90 %, respectively, compared to 15 % and 80 % for Ga-67 scintigraphy [75]. These results reinforce the importance of revising JMHW diagnostic criteria to incorporate FDG-PET instead of Ga-67.

Pitfalls

The wide range of reported specificity of FDG-PET to detect cardiac sarcoidosis has been attributed in part to a suboptimal gold standard [74]. Additionally, other conditions can render false-positive results. One of the major causes of false-positive study is related to poor patient preparation. Without preparation, uptake in the myocardium is usually diffuse but can be focal or focal on diffuse [103]. Respect of protocol can be optimized by good communication with patients and an interview to ensure adequate preparation prior to imaging. Nevertheless, even after proper fasting, normal myocardium can demonstrate uptake with regional disparities, with the lateral and inferior wall containing more activity compared to the septum and anterior wall [104]. Indeed, lateral wall uptake in a normal heart following adequate preparation was reported and is thought to represent a normal variation [74, 88, 89], possibly related to regional substrate availability (Fig. 4.10) [92].

Dilated cardiomyopathy (DCM) can also present as focal on diffuse FDG uptake, possibly due to myocardial cell loss or regional fibrosis. Consequently, in the appropriate clinical context, DCM should be included in the differential diagnosis of a positive FDG-PET study [92]. Other causes of myocarditis, cardiac amyloidosis, infection, and myocardial metastases can also demonstrate abnormal myocardial uptake. Finally, patients with pulmonary hypertension can demonstrate increased right ventricular FDG [105, 106], mimicking RV involvement.

FDG-PET is a sensitive examination to detect CS, and therefore, there are few circumstances under which FDG-PET will be falsely negative [74]. Patient receiving

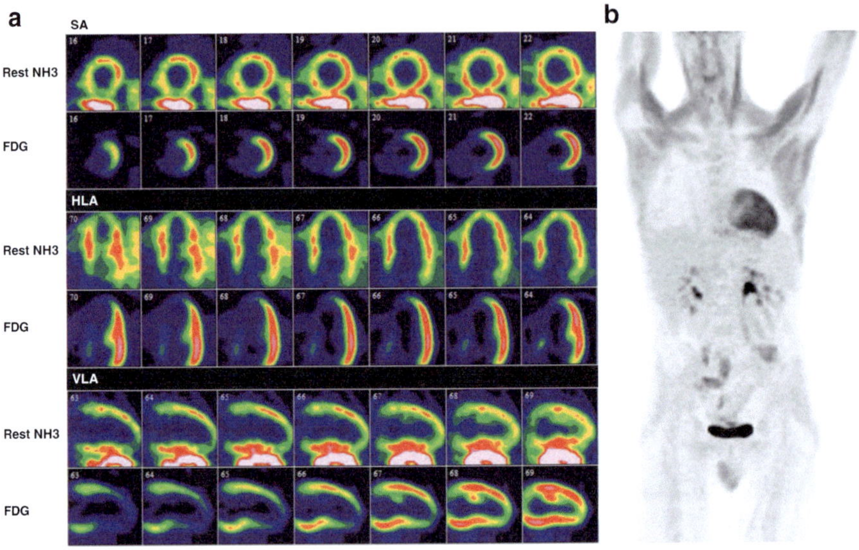

Fig. 4.10 (**a**) Rest ammonia-N13 and FDG-PET scan of a patient with suspected cardiac sarcoidosis. After following fasting and HCLF diet to suppress physiological myocardial uptake, there is FDG uptake in the lateral wall of the left ventricle, representing a normal variant. (**b**) Anterior projection of maximal intensity projection showing no evidence of extracardiac sarcoidosis. Note the diffuse uptake in muscle of the upper extremities, in keeping with recent strenuous activity

corticosteroids or with "burned-out" sarcoidosis can have a negative FDG-PET scan [107]. In the case of burned-out sarcoidosis, rest perfusion scan will demonstrate a perfusion defect in the area of granulomatous scar [95]. Finally, another potential cause of false negative is related to the size of the area of inflammation. Although spatial resolution of FDG-PET is significantly greater than [67] Ga scintigraphy, it remains lower than MRI and very small foci of inflammation could be missed.

4.3.6.3 Prognostic Value of PET/CT

Cardiac involvement in sarcoidosis can lead to congestive heart failure due to progressive infiltration of the myocardium by granulomas [49, 56]. In a survey conducted in the United Kingdom, the 5-year survival rate of patients with sarcoidosis and suspected cardiac involvement was 40 %, with most of these patients receiving steroid treatments [108]. In a more recent study by Yazaki et al., the 5-year survival rate of patients treated for cardiac sarcoidosis and systolic impairment was 75 %, while the 5-year survival rate reached 90 % in patients treated for cardiac sarcoidosis with normal systolic function [56]. These results suggest that identification and treatment of patients with active cardiac sarcoidosis before the occurrence of systolic dysfunction is fundamental in the prevention of adverse outcomes. Unfortunately, approximately half of the patients with cardiac sarcoidosis are asymptomatic [109]. Furthermore, the severity of pulmonary involvement assessed either by imaging or PFTs does not correlate with the presence of CS [109, 110]. Therefore, identification of patients with CS before occurrence of systolic dysfunction can be challenging. For this reason, it is

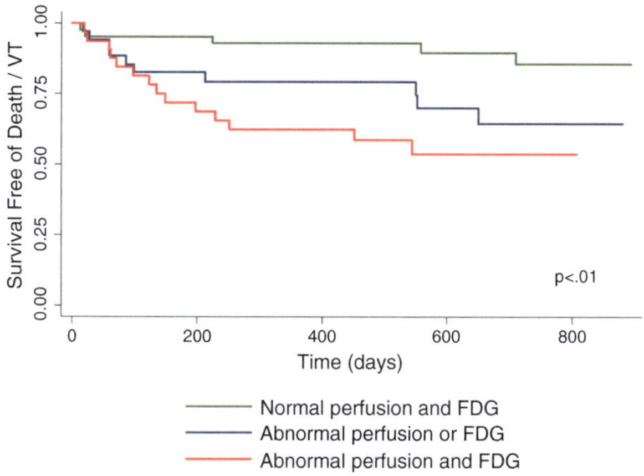

Fig. 4.11 Survival free of death or ventricular tachycardia stratified by perfusion and FDG-PET results, demonstrating that combination of perfusion abnormality and abnormal FDG-PET uptake is associated with increased risk of death and ventricular tachycardia (Reprinted from Blankstein et al. [95] with permission from the author and Elsevier)

thought that imaging could play a central role in the identification of patients with CS and could lead to prevention of adverse outcome.

Other complications of patients with cardiac sarcoidosis are ventricular arrhythmias and sudden death [49]. Patients with cardiac sarcoidosis diagnosed based on the JMHW presenting with unsustained VT display significantly higher FDG uptake when compared with those with AV blocks and asymptomatic controls [111]. Conversely, patients demonstrating both perfusion abnormality and inflammation on FDG-PET have threefold increased rate of event rate (VT or sudden death) [95]. Blankstein et al. demonstrated, using a multivariable model including left ventricular ejection fraction (LVEF), JMHW criteria, and pattern of abnormality on PET scan, that the presence of both abnormal FDG uptake and perfusion abnormalities had the strongest link to death or VT (Fig. 4.11) [95]. Furthermore, they showed that risk was greater when there was RV involved [95]. There is likely a relationship between arrhythmias and FDG findings, but there is currently only sparse data on prognostic value of FDG-PET in CS, and therefore, current guidelines on ICD implantation in patients with CS do not rely specifically on FDG-PET [99].

FDG-PEt allows detection of CS before functional and structural changes are detectable, allowing early diagnosis and appropriate management. Furthermore, close monitoring of patients with myocardial inflammation demonstrated on FDG-PET is warranted and may prevent progressive cardiac disease [109].

4.3.6.4 Assessment of Response to Therapy

Another potential role of FDG-PET in CS is the assessment of response to therapy. Because FDG accumulates in active inflammation and not fibrosis [41], it could be used to evaluate response to therapy on serial studies. Several studies showed that following steroid therapy, there is a decrease in FDG uptake in both extracardiac

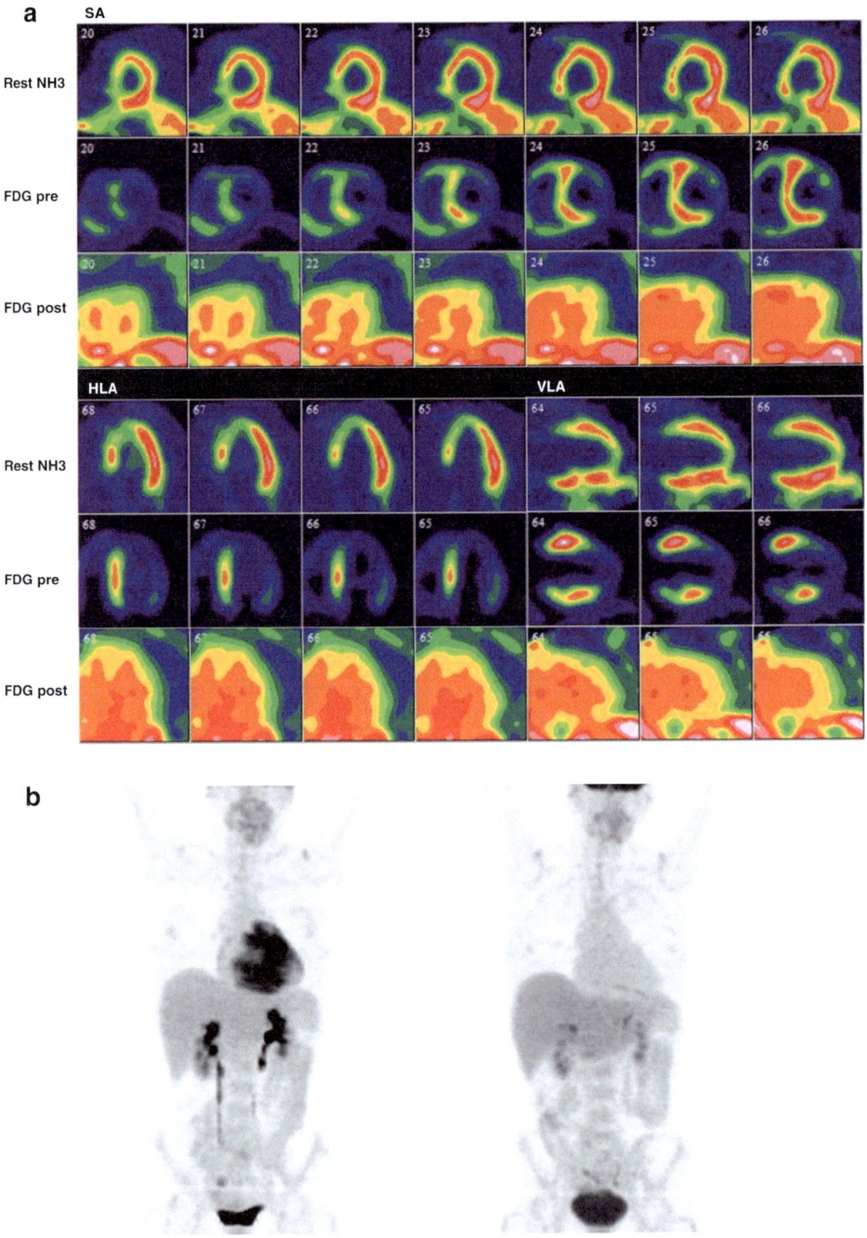

Fig. 4.12 (**a**) Baseline rest ammonia-N13 perfusion images with (**b**) corresponding FDG-PET images of a patient with diagnosis of cardiac sarcoidosis. Following a treatment of 9 months of corticosteroid, a FDG-PET study was repeated 13 months following baseline evaluation, showing no evidence of active inflammation in the myocardium. The LVEF, as measured by radionuclide ventriculography prior to each FDG-PET scan, remained unchanged, from 53 to 51 %

lesions [20, 42–45] and cardiac lesions (Fig. 4.12) [73]. Resolution of FDG uptake in the basal septum has been associated with resolution of third-degree atrioventricular block and progression of FDG uptake after steroid tapering was associated with VT in case reports [112, 113].

In a retrospective study of 23 patients with cardiac sarcoidosis treated with immunosuppressive therapies guided by serial PET scans, reduction in the intensity and extent of inflammation, as quantified by FDG uptake, was associated with an increase in LVEF [107]. These results reinforce the potential role of FDG-PET in guiding the duration and intensity of immunosuppressive treatment. Nonetheless, further validation of the role of FDG-PET in assessment of response to therapy by prospective trials is necessary.

4.3.7 When to Consider PET/CT in Patients with Sarcoid Disease

Metha et al. studied prevalence of cardiac symptoms, ECG findings, Holter monitoring, and transthoracic echocardiography findings of 62 patients with known sarcoidosis [109]. Description of abnormalities studied is presented in Table 4.9. They showed that patients with cardiac sarcoidosis had more cardiac symptoms and more findings on Holter monitoring and on transthoracic echocardiography compared to patients without cardiac sarcoidosis. All patients with cardiac sarcoidosis had symptoms or at least one abnormal test result [109]. Based on these results, the HRS expert consensus recommends screening of patients with established extracardiac sarcoidosis with clinical symptoms, ECG and echocardiography; [99] if one or more of these screening tests is abnormal, the patient is then referred for further cardiac imaging with FDG-PET or cardiac MRI.

Table 4.9 Screening tests with accompanying abnormalities associated with cardiac sarcoidosis

Screening test	Description of abnormalities
Cardiac symptoms	Significant palpitation Presyncope Syncope
Abnormal ECG	RBBB LBBB Second- or third-degree AV block Q waves in two consecutive leads Ventricular tachycardia
Abnormal Holter monitoring	Supraventricular tachycardia Excessive PVCs AV block Ventricular tachycardia
Echocardiography findings	LV systolic dysfunction Segmental wall motion abnormalities LV diastolic dysfunction RV systolic dysfunction

4.3.8 When to Consider PET/CT in Patients Without Evidence of Sarcoid Disease

Multiple studies have reported cardiac manifestations as the initial presentation of patients with sarcoidosis [54, 114]. These patients were younger than 55 years old and initially presented with new onset of unexplained atrioventricular block and VT [115]. Nery et al. prospectively evaluated patients younger than 60 years old who presented with unexplained second- or third-degree atrioventricular block, with no previous history of sarcoidosis [55]. Of the 32 patients studied, CS was diagnosed in 11 (34 %) subjects and 11/11 were subsequently diagnosed with extracardiac sarcoidosis. Similar results were obtained in patients presenting with sustained VT of unknown etiology [116]. Nery et al. prospectively evaluated patients presenting with monomorphic VT of unknown etiology, excluding patients with idiopathic VT, ischemic VT, or known sarcoidosis. In their sample, 6 out of 14 (28 %) patients had CS as the underlying etiology. Based on these results, it is recommended to perform advanced cardiac imaging with FDG-PET or cardiac MRI in patients younger than 60 years old presenting with unexplained second- or third-degree atrioventricular block, and it could be useful in patients with VT of unknown etiology [99].

4.4 Future Directions

The rationale behind detection of patient with cardiac sarcoidosis is prevention of life-threatening arrhythmias and to preserve left ventricular function. Over the past decade, FDG-PET has been playing a central role in detecting cardiac sarcoidosis. Nevertheless, the current criteria used in the diagnosis of CS require further refinement. For example, an optimal pretest preparation protocol should be determined and image interpretation should be standardized. Additionally, understanding physiological uptake after preparation is central to improve accuracy. Some authors reported the possibility of FDG uptake in areas without inflammation due to regional substrate availability [92]. Furthermore, very little data is available on accuracy of FDG-PET in patients with insulin resistance. Given the high prevalence of diabetes and that corticosteroids can induce insulin resistance, many patients referred for FDG-PET imaging may present with insulin resistance. For this reason, understanding the effects of insulin resistance on FDG-PET accuracy and optimization of pretest preparation in these patients is necessary.

Although promising results have emerged so far, further prospective studies to establish the role of FDG uptake in therapy monitoring are needed. Using FDG-PET to differentiate between quiescent granulomas and active inflammation could be used to adjust therapy dosage, and decision to discontinue treatment could be based on assessment of inflammation rather than fixed time periods.

New hybrid imaging systems combining PET and MRI are now available, allowing combination of tissue characterization capabilities of MRI with PET. Two reports have highlighted the complementary role of PET and MRI in cardiac sarcoidosis with PET-MRI hybrid imaging [117, 118].

Although FDG-PET is an effective tool in the diagnosis of CS, FDG remains a nonspecific marker and interpretation of results should always be conducted in light of clinical information. Some authors have described combination of FDG with other PET tracers including 11C-methionine [119, 120], fluorine-18-alpha-methyltyrosine (FMT) [121], and 18F-fluorothymidine (FLT) [122] to improve specificity of FDG imaging in extracardiac sarcoidosis. Clinical trials are under way to assess the potential role of 68Ga-DOTANOC, a neuroendocrine tumor marker, in cardiac sarcoidosis. To this day, only anecdotal reports are available on imaging sarcoidosis with other tracers than FDG. In order to replace FDG in clinical practice, a new PET tracer would need to be more specific and less dependent on patient preparation and not require on-site cyclotron. Until then, FDG-PET remains an accurate and efficient way of imaging patients for sarcoidosis.

References

1. Boeck C. Multiple benign sarkoid of the skin. J Cutan Genitourinary Dis. 1899;17:543–50.
2. Statement on sarcoidosis. Joint Statement of the American Thoracic Society (ATS), the European Respiratory Society (ERS) and the World Association of Sarcoidosis and Other Granulomatous Disorders (WASOG) adopted by the ATS Board of Directors and by the ERS Executive Committee, February 1999. Am J Respir Crit Care Med. 1999;160:736–55.
3. Henke CE, Henke G, Elveback LR, et al. The epidemiology of sarcoidosis in Rochester, Minnesota: a population-based study of incidence and survival. Am J Epidemiol. 1986;123:840–5.
4. Bresnitz EA, Strom BL. Epidemiology of sarcoidosis. Epidemiol Rev. 1983;5:124–56.
5. Erdal BS, Clymer BD, Yildiz VO, et al. Unexpectedly high prevalence of sarcoidosis in a representative U.S. Metropolitan population. Respir Med. 2012;106:893–9.
6. Hennessy TW, Ballard DJ, DeRemee RA, et al. The influence of diagnostic access bias on the epidemiology of sarcoidosis: a population-based study in Rochester, Minnesota, 1935–1984. J Clin Epidemiol. 1988;41:565–70.
7. Buck AA, Sartwell PE. Epidemiologic investigations of sarcoidosis. II. Skin sensitivity and environmental factors. Am J Hyg. 1961;74:152–73.
8. Buck AA, McKusick VA. Epidemiologic investigations of sarcoidosis. III. Serum proteins; syphilis; association with tuberculosis: familial aggregation. Am J Hyg. 1961;74:174–88.
9. Buck AA. Epidemiologic investigations of sarcoidosis. IV. Discussion and summary. Am J Hyg. 1961;74:189–202.
10. Hills SE, Parkes SA, Baker SB. Epidemiology of sarcoidosis in the Isle of Man–2: Evidence for space-time clustering. Thorax. 1987;42:427–30.
11. Prezant DJ, Dhala A, Goldstein A, et al. The incidence, prevalence, and severity of sarcoidosis in New York City firefighters. Chest. 1999;116:1183–93.
12. Kajdasz DK, Lackland DT, Mohr LC, Judson MA. A current assessment of rurally linked exposures as potential risk factors for sarcoidosis. Ann Epidemiol. 2001;11:111–7.
13. Kucera GP, Rybicki BA, Kirkey KL, et al. Occupational risk factors for sarcoidosis in African-American siblings. Chest. 2003;123:1527–35.
14. Iannuzzi MC, Rybicki BA, Teirstein AS. Sarcoidosis. N Engl J Med. 2007;357:2153–65.
15. Baughman RP, Lower EE. Novel therapies for sarcoidosis. Semin Respir Crit Care Med. 2007;28:128–33.
16. Studdy PR, Bird R. Serum angiotensin converting enzyme in sarcoidosis–its value in present clinical practice. Ann Clin Biochem. 1989;26(Pt 1):13–8.
17. Prabhakar HB, Rabinowitz CB, Gibbons FK, et al. Imaging features of sarcoidosis on MDCT, FDG PET, and PET/CT. AJR Am J Roentgenol. 2008;190:S1–6.

18. Scadding JG. Prognosis of intrathoracic sarcoidosis in England. A review of 136 cases after five years' observation. Br Med J. 1961;2:1165–72.
19. Baughman RP, Shipley R, Desai S, et al. Changes in chest roentgenogram of sarcoidosis patients during a clinical trial of infliximab therapy: comparison of different methods of evaluation. Chest. 2009;136:526–35.
20. Braun JJ, Kessler R, Constantinesco A, Imperiale A. 18 F-FDG PET/CT in sarcoidosis management: review and report of 20 cases. Eur J Nucl Med Mol Imaging. 2008;35:1537–43.
21. Abrar ML, Agrawal K, Bhattacharya A, Mittal BR. Diffuse lung uptake in stress myocardial perfusion scintigraphy with Thallium-201 in a patient with sarcoidosis. Indian J Nucl Med. 2013;28:57.
22. Lebtahi R, Crestani B, Belmatoug N, et al. Somatostatin receptor scintigraphy and gallium scintigraphy in patients with sarcoidosis. J Nucl Med. 2001;42:21–6.
23. Beaumont D, Herry JY, Sapene M, et al. Gallium-67 in the evaluation of sarcoidosis: correlations with serum angiotensin-converting enzyme and bronchoalveolar lavage. Thorax. 1982;37:11–8.
24. Klech H, Kohn H, Kummer F, Mostbeck A. Assessment of activity in sarcoidosis. Sensitivity and specificity of 67Gallium scintigraphy, serum ACE levels, chest roentgenography, and blood lymphocyte subpopulations. Chest. 1982;82:732–8.
25. Nishiyama Y, Yamamoto Y, Fukunaga K, et al. Comparative evaluation of 18 F-FDG PET and 67Ga scintigraphy in patients with sarcoidosis. J Nucl Med. 2006;47:1571–6.
26. Phelps ME, Hoffman EJ, Selin C, et al. Investigation of [18 F]2-fluoro-2-deoxyglucose for the measure of myocardial glucose metabolism. J Nucl Med. 1978;19:1311–9.
27. Basu S, Zhuang H, Torigian DA, et al. Functional imaging of inflammatory diseases using nuclear medicine techniques. Semin Nucl Med. 2009;39:124–45.
28. Mañá J. Nuclear imaging. 67Gallium, 201thallium, 18 F-labeled fluoro-2-deoxy-D-glucose positron emission tomography. Clin Chest Med. 1997;18:799–811.
29. Cremers JP, Van Kroonenburgh MJ, Mostard RL, et al. Extent of disease activity assessed by 18 F-FDG PET/CT in a Dutch sarcoidosis population. Sarcoidosis Vasc Diffuse Lung Dis. 2014;31:37–45.
30. Ambrosini V, Zompatori M, Fasano L, et al. 18 F-FDG PET/CT for the assessment of disease extension and activity in patients with sarcoidosis: results of a preliminary prospective study. Clin Nucl Med. 2013;38:e171–7.
31. Sobic-Saranovic D, Grozdic I, Videnovic-Ivanov J, et al. The utility of 18 F-FDG PET/CT for diagnosis and adjustment of therapy in patients with active chronic sarcoidosis. J Nucl Med. 2012;53:1543–9.
32. De Vries J, Rothkrantz-Kos S, van Dieijen-Visser MP, Drent M. The relationship between fatigue and clinical parameters in pulmonary sarcoidosis. Sarcoidosis Vasc Diffuse Lung Dis. 2004;21:127–36.
33. Schoenberger CI, Line BR, Keogh BA, et al. Lung inflammation in sarcoidosis: comparison of serum angiotensin-converting enzyme levels with bronchoalveolar lavage and gallium-67 scanning assessment of the T lymphocyte alveolitis. Thorax. 1982;37:19–25.
34. Nunes H, Brillet P-Y, Valeyre D, et al. Imaging in sarcoidosis. Semin Respir Crit Care Med. 2007;28:102–20.
35. Mostard RLM, Vöö S, van Kroonenburgh MJPG, et al. Inflammatory activity assessment by F18 FDG-PET/CT in persistent symptomatic sarcoidosis. Respir Med. 2011;105:1917–24.
36. Drent M, Mansour K, Linssen C. Bronchoalveolar lavage in sarcoidosis. Semin Respir Crit Care Med. 2007;28:486–95.
37. Bjermer L, Rosenhall L, Angström T, Hällgren R. Predictive value of bronchoalveolar lavage cell analysis in sarcoidosis. Thorax. 1988;43:284–8.
38. Keogh BA, Hunninghake GW, Line BR, Crystal RG. The alveolitis of pulmonary sarcoidosis. Evaluation of natural history and alveolitis-dependent changes in lung function. Am Rev Respir Dis. 1983;128:256–65.
39. Lin YH, Haslam PL, Turner-Warwick M. Chronic pulmonary sarcoidosis: relationship between lung lavage cell counts, chest radiograph, and results of standard lung function tests. Thorax. 1985;40:501–7.

40. Turner-Warwick M, McAllister W, Lawrence R, et al. Corticosteroid treatment in pulmonary sarcoidosis: do serial lavage lymphocyte counts, serum angiotensin converting enzyme measurements, and gallium-67 scans help management? Thorax. 1986;41:903–13.
41. Treglia G, Taralli S, Giordano A. Emerging role of whole-body 18 F-fluorodeoxyglucose positron emission tomography as a marker of disease activity in patients with sarcoidosis: a systematic review. Sarcoidosis Vasc Diffuse Lung Dis. 2011;28:87–94.
42. Brudin LH, Valind SO, Rhodes CG, et al. Fluorine-18 deoxyglucose uptake in sarcoidosis measured with positron emission tomography. Eur J Nucl Med. 1994;21:297–305.
43. Teirstein AS, Machac J, Almeida O, et al. Results of 188 whole-body fluorodeoxyglucose positron emission tomography scans in 137 patients with sarcoidosis. Chest. 2007;132:1949–53.
44. Sobic-Saranovic DP, Grozdic IT, Videnovic-Ivanov J, et al. Responsiveness of FDG PET/CT to treatment of patients with active chronic sarcoidosis. Clin Nucl Med. 2013;38:516–21.
45. Imperiale A, Riehm S, Braun JJ. Interest of [18 F]FDG PET/CT for treatment efficacy assessment in aggressive phenotype of sarcoidosis with special emphasis on sinonasal involvement. Q J Nucl Med Mol Imaging. 2013;57:177–86.
46. Keijsers RGM, Verzijlbergen JF, van Diepen DM, et al. 18 F-FDG PET in sarcoidosis: an observational study in 12 patients treated with infliximab. Sarcoidosis Vasc Diffuse Lung Dis. 2008;25:143–9.
47. Milman N, Graudal N, Loft A, et al. Effect of the TNF-α inhibitor adalimumab in patients with recalcitrant sarcoidosis: a prospective observational study using FDG-PET. Clin Respir J. 2012;6:238–47.
48. Silverman KJ, Hutchins GM, Bulkley BH. Cardiac sarcoid: a clinicopathologic study of 84 unselected patients with systemic sarcoidosis. Circulation. 1978;58:1204–11.
49. Matsui Y, Iwai K, Tachibana T, et al. Clinicopathological study of fatal myocardial sarcoidosis. Ann N Y Acad Sci. 1976;278:455–69.
50. Tadamura E, Yamamuro M, Kubo S, et al. Effectiveness of delayed enhanced MRI for identification of cardiac sarcoidosis: comparison with radionuclide imaging. AJR Am J Roentgenol. 2005;185:110–5.
51. Sekhri V, Sanal S, Delorenzo LJ, et al. Cardiac sarcoidosis: a comprehensive review. Arch Med Sci. 2011;7:546–54.
52. Roberts WC, McAllister HA, Ferrans VJ. Sarcoidosis of the heart. A clinicopathologic study of 35 necropsy patients (group 1) and review of 78 previously described necropsy patients (group 11). Am J Med. 1977;63:86–108.
53. Banba K, Kusano KF, Nakamura K, et al. Relationship between arrhythmogenesis and disease activity in cardiac sarcoidosis. Heart Rhythm. 2007;4:1292–9.
54. Kandolin R, Lehtonen J, Kupari M. Cardiac sarcoidosis and giant cell myocarditis as causes of atrioventricular block in young and middle-aged adults. Circ Arrhythm Electrophysiol. 2011;4:303–9.
55. Nery PB, Beanlands RS, Nair GM, et al. Atrioventricular block as the initial manifestation of cardiac sarcoidosis in middle-aged adults. J Cardiovasc Electrophysiol. 2014;25:875–81.
56. Yazaki Y, Isobe M, Hiroe M, et al. Prognostic determinants of long-term survival in Japanese patients with cardiac sarcoidosis treated with prednisone. Am J Cardiol. 2001;88: 1006–10.
57. Chapelon-Abric C, de Zuttere D, Duhaut P, et al. Cardiac sarcoidosis: a retrospective study of 41 cases. Medicine (Baltimore). 2004;83:315–34.
58. Kato Y, Morimoto S, Uemura A, et al. Efficacy of corticosteroids in sarcoidosis presenting with atrioventricular block. Sarcoidosis Vasc Diffuse Lung Dis. 2003;20:133–7.
59. Yodogawa K, Seino Y, Ohara T, et al. Effect of corticosteroid therapy on ventricular arrhythmias in patients with cardiac sarcoidosis. Ann Noninvasive Electrocardiol. 2011;16:140–7.
60. Doughan AR, Williams BR. Cardiac sarcoidosis. Heart. 2006;92:282–8.
61. Winters SL, Cohen M, Greenberg S, et al. Sustained ventricular tachycardia associated with sarcoidosis: assessment of the underlying cardiac anatomy and the prospective utility of programmed ventricular stimulation, drug therapy and an implantable antitachycardia device. J Am Coll Cardiol. 1991;18:937–43.

62. Sadek MM, Yung D, Birnie DH, et al. Corticosteroid therapy for cardiac sarcoidosis: a systematic review. Can J Cardiol. 2013;29:1034–41.
63. Chiu C-Z, Nakatani S, Zhang G, et al. Prevention of left ventricular remodeling by long-term corticosteroid therapy in patients with cardiac sarcoidosis. Am J Cardiol. 2005;95:143–6.
64. Jefic D, Joel B, Good E, et al. Role of radiofrequency catheter ablation of ventricular tachycardia in cardiac sarcoidosis: report from a multicenter registry. Heart Rhythm. 2009;6:189–95.
65. Futamatsu H, Suzuki J, Adachi S, et al. Utility of gallium-67 scintigraphy for evaluation of cardiac sarcoidosis with ventricular tachycardia. Int J Cardiovasc Imaging. 2006;22:443–8.
66. Hiramitsu S, Morimoto S, Uemura A, et al. National survey on status of steroid therapy for cardiac sarcoidosis in Japan. Sarcoidosis Vasc Diffuse Lung Dis. 2005;22:210–3.
67. Liedtke AJ. Alterations of carbohydrate and lipid metabolism in the acutely ischemic heart. Prog Cardiovasc Dis. 1981;23:321–36.
68. Camici P, Ferrannini E, Opie LH. Myocardial metabolism in ischemic heart disease: basic principles and application to imaging by positron emission tomography. Prog Cardiovasc Dis. 1989;32:217–38.
69. Stanley WC, Lopaschuk GD, Hall JL, McCormack JG. Regulation of myocardial carbohydrate metabolism under normal and ischaemic conditions. Potential for pharmacological interventions. Cardiovasc Res. 1997;33:243–57.
70. Stanley WC, Recchia FA, Lopaschuk GD. Myocardial substrate metabolism in the normal and failing heart. Physiol Rev. 2005;85:1093–129.
71. Wisneski JA, Gertz EW, Neese RA, Mayr M. Myocardial metabolism of free fatty acids. Studies with 14C-labeled substrates in humans. J Clin Invest. 1987;79:359–66.
72. Ohira H, Tsujino I, Yoshinaga K. ^{18}F-Fluoro-2-deoxyglucose positron emission tomography in cardiac sarcoidosis. Eur J Nucl Med Mol Imaging. 2011;38:1773–83.
73. Yamagishi H, Shirai N, Takagi M, et al. Identification of cardiac sarcoidosis with (13) N-NH(3)/(18)F-FDG PET. J Nucl Med. 2003;44:1030–6.
74. Youssef G, Leung E, Mylonas I, et al. The use of 18 F-FDG PET in the diagnosis of cardiac sarcoidosis: a systematic review and metaanalysis including the Ontario experience. J Nucl Med. 2012;53:241–8.
75. Langah R, Spicer K, Gebregziabher M, Gordon L. Effectiveness of prolonged fasting 18f-FDG PET-CT in the detection of cardiac sarcoidosis. J Nucl Cardiol. 2009;16:801–10.
76. Ishida Y, Yoshinaga K, Miyagawa M, et al. Recommendations for (18)F-fluorodeoxyglucose positron emission tomography imaging for cardiac sarcoidosis: Japanese Society of Nuclear Cardiology recommendations. Ann Nucl Med. 2014;28:393–403.
77. Frayn KN. The glucose-fatty acid cycle: a physiological perspective. Biochem Soc Trans. 2003;31:1115–9.
78. Cheng VY, Slomka PJ, Ahlen M, et al. Impact of carbohydrate restriction with and without fatty acid loading on myocardial 18 F-FDG uptake during PET: a randomized controlled trial. J Nucl Cardiol. 2010;17:286–91.
79. Williams G, Kolodny GM. Suppression of myocardial 18 F-FDG uptake by preparing patients with a high-fat, low-carbohydrate diet. AJR Am J Roentgenol. 2008;190:W151–6.
80. Harisankar CNB, Mittal BR, Agrawal KL, et al. Utility of high fat and low carbohydrate diet in suppressing myocardial FDG uptake. J Nucl Cardiol. 2011;18:926–36.
81. Soussan M, Brillet P-Y, Nunes H, et al. Clinical value of a high-fat and low-carbohydrate diet before FDG-PET/CT for evaluation of patients with suspected cardiac sarcoidosis. J Nucl Cardiol. 2013;20:120–7.
82. Lum DP, Wandell S, Ko J, Coel MN. Reduction of myocardial 2-deoxy-2-[18 F]fluoro-D-glucose uptake artifacts in positron emission tomography using dietary carbohydrate restriction. Mol Imaging Biol. 2002;4:232–7.
83. Wykrzykowska J, Lehman S, Williams G, et al. Imaging of inflamed and vulnerable plaque in coronary arteries with 18 F-FDG PET/CT in patients with suppression of myocardial uptake using a low-carbohydrate, high-fat preparation. J Nucl Med. 2009;50:563–8.

84. Coulden R, Chung P, Sonnex E, et al. Suppression of myocardial 18 F-FDG uptake with a preparatory "Atkins-style" low-carbohydrate diet. Eur Radiol. 2012;22:2221–8.
85. Kobayashi Y, Kumita S, Fukushima Y, et al. Significant suppression of myocardial 18 F-fluorodeoxyglucose uptake using 24-h carbohydrate restriction and a low-carbohydrate, high-fat diet. J Cardiol. 2013;62:314–9.
86. Nuutila P, Koivisto VA, Knuuti J, et al. Glucose-free fatty acid cycle operates in human heart and skeletal muscle in vivo. J Clin Invest. 1992;89:1767–74.
87. Persson E. Lipoprotein lipase, hepatic lipase and plasma lipolytic activity. Effects of heparin and a low molecular weight heparin fragment (Fragmin). Acta Med Scand. 1988;724(Suppl):1–56.
88. Ohira H, Tsujino I, Ishimaru S, et al. Myocardial imaging with 18 F-fluoro-2-deoxyglucose positron emission tomography and magnetic resonance imaging in sarcoidosis. Eur J Nucl Med Mol Imaging. 2008;35:933–41.
89. Ishimaru S, Tsujino I, Takei T, et al. Focal uptake on 18 F-fluoro-2-deoxyglucose positron emission tomography images indicates cardiac involvement of sarcoidosis. Eur Heart J. 2005;26:1538–43.
90. Morooka M, Moroi M, Uno K, et al. Long fasting is effective in inhibiting physiological myocardial 18 F-FDG uptake and for evaluating active lesions of cardiac sarcoidosis. EJNMMI Res. 2014;4:1.
91. Strauss HW, Miller DD, Wittry MD, et al. Procedure guideline for myocardial perfusion imaging 3.3. J Nucl Med Technol. 2008;36:155–61.
92. Tahara N, Tahara A, Nitta Y, et al. Heterogeneous myocardial FDG uptake and the disease activity in cardiac sarcoidosis. JACC Cardiovasc Imaging. 2010;3:1219–28.
93. Manabe O, Ohira H, Yoshinaga K, et al. Elevated (18)F-fluorodeoxyglucose uptake in the interventricular septum is associated with atrioventricular block in patients with suspected cardiac involvement sarcoidosis. Eur J Nucl Med Mol Imaging. 2013;40:1558–66.
94. Skali H, Schulman AR, Dorbala S. 18 F-FDG PET/CT for the assessment of myocardial sarcoidosis. Curr Cardiol Rep. 2013;15:1–11.
95. Blankstein R, Osborne M, Naya M, et al. Cardiac positron emission tomography enhances prognostic assessments of patients with suspected cardiac sarcoidosis. J Am Coll Cardiol. 2014;63:329–36.
96. Diagnostic standard and guidelines for sarcoidosis. Jpn J Sarcoidosis Granulomatous Disorders [in Japanese]. 2007;27:89–102.
97. Deng JC, Baughman RP, Lynch JP. Cardiac involvement in sarcoidosis. Semin Respir Crit Care Med. 2002;23:513–27.
98. Patel MR, Cawley PJ, Heitner JF, et al. Detection of myocardial damage in patients with sarcoidosis. Circulation. 2009;120:1969–77.
99. Birnie DH, Sauer WH, Bogun F, et al. HRS expert consensus statement on the diagnosis and management of arrhythmias associated with cardiac sarcoidosis. Heart Rhythm. 2014;11:1305–23.
100. Cooper LT, Baughman KL, Feldman AM, et al. The role of endomyocardial biopsy in the management of cardiovascular disease: a scientific statement from the American Heart Association, the American College of Cardiology, and the European Society of Cardiology. Circulation. 2007;116:2216–33.
101. Ardehali H, Howard DL, Hariri A, et al. A positive endomyocardial biopsy result for sarcoid is associated with poor prognosis in patients with initially unexplained cardiomyopathy. Am Heart J. 2005;150:459–63.
102. Okumura W, Iwasaki T, Toyama T, et al. Usefulness of fasting 18 F-FDG PET in identification of cardiac sarcoidosis. J Nucl Med. 2004;45:1989–98.
103. Khandani AH, Isasi CR, Donald Blaufox M. Intra-individual variability of cardiac uptake on serial whole-body 18 F-FDG PET. Nucl Med Commun. 2005;26:787–91.
104. Gropler RJ, Siegel BA, Lee KJ, et al. Nonuniformity in myocardial accumulation of fluorine-18-fluorodeoxyglucose in normal fasted humans. J Nucl Med. 1990;31:1749–56.
105. De Keizer B, Scholtens AM, van Kimmenade RRJ, de Jong PA. High FDG uptake in the right ventricular myocardium of a pulmonary hypertension patient. J Am Coll Cardiol. 2013;62:1724.

106. Can MM, Kaymaz C, Tanboga IH, et al. Increased right ventricular glucose metabolism in patients with pulmonary arterial hypertension. Clin Nucl Med. 2011;36:743–8.
107. Osborne MT, Hulten EA, Singh A, et al. Reduction in 18 F-fluorodeoxyglucose uptake on serial cardiac positron emission tomography is associated with improved left ventricular ejection fraction in patients with cardiac sarcoidosis. J Nucl Cardiol. 2014;21:166–74.
108. Fleming HA, Bailey SM. The prognosis of sarcoid heart disease in the United Kingdom. Ann N Y Acad Sci. 1986;465:543–50.
109. Mehta D, Lubitz SA, Frankel Z, et al. Cardiac involvement in patients with sarcoidosis: diagnostic and prognostic value of outpatient testing. Chest. 2008;133:1426–35.
110. Judson MA, Baughman RP, Teirstein AS, et al. Defining organ involvement in sarcoidosis: the ACCESS proposed instrument. ACCESS Research Group. A Case Control Etiologic Study of Sarcoidosis. Sarcoidosis Vasc Diffuse Lung Dis. 1999;16:75–86.
111. Mc Ardle BA, Birnie DH, Klein R, et al. Is there an association between clinical presentation and the location and extent of myocardial involvement of cardiac sarcoidosis as assessed by ^{18}F- fluorodoexyglucose positron emission tomography? Circ Cardiovasc Imaging. 2013;6:617–26.
112. Takeda N, Yokoyama I, Hiroi Y, et al. Positron emission tomography predicted recovery of complete A-V nodal dysfunction in a patient with cardiac sarcoidosis. Circulation. 2002;105:1144–5.
113. Pandya C, Brunken RC, Tchou P, et al. Detecting cardiac involvement in sarcoidosis: a call for prospective studies of newer imaging techniques. Eur Respir J. 2007;29:418–22.
114. Uusimaa P, Ylitalo K, Anttonen O, et al. Ventricular tachyarrhythmia as a primary presentation of sarcoidosis. Eurospace. 2008;10:760–6.
115. Nery PB, Leung E, Birnie DH. Arrhythmias in cardiac sarcoidosis: diagnosis and treatment. Curr Opin Cardiol. 2012;27:181–9.
116. Nery PB, Mc Ardle BA, Redpath CJ, et al. Prevalence of cardiac sarcoidosis in patients presenting with monomorphic ventricular tachycardia. Pacing Clin Electrophysiol. 2014;37:364–74.
117. White JA, Rajchl M, Butler J, et al. Active cardiac sarcoidosis: first clinical experience of simultaneous positron emission tomography–magnetic resonance imaging for the diagnosis of cardiac disease. Circulation. 2013;127:e639–41.
118. Schneider S, Batrice A, Rischpler C, et al. Utility of multimodal cardiac imaging with PET/MRI in cardiac sarcoidosis: implications for diagnosis, monitoring and treatment. Eur Heart J. 2014;35:312.
119. Yamada Y, Uchida Y, Tatsumi K, et al. Fluorine-18-fluorodeoxyglucose and carbon-11-methionine evaluation of lymphadenopathy in sarcoidosis. J Nucl Med. 1998;39:1160–6.
120. Hain SF, Beggs AD. C-11 methionine uptake in granulomatous disease. Clin Nucl Med. 2004;29:585–6.
121. Kaira K, Oriuchi N, Otani Y, et al. Diagnostic usefulness of fluorine-18-alpha-methyltyrosine positron emission tomography in combination with 18 F-fluorodeoxyglucose in sarcoidosis patients. Chest. 2007;131:1019–27.
122. Kim S-K, Im HJ, Kim W, et al. F-18 fluorodeoxyglucose and F-18 fluorothymidine positron emission tomography/computed tomography imaging in a case of neurosarcoidosis. Clin Nucl Med. 2010;35:67–70.

Multimodality Imaging of Cardiac Amyloidosis

5

Sharmila Dorbala

5.1 Background

Systemic amyloidoses are a group of protein misfolding disorders that are typified by the extracellular deposition of insoluble, non-branching, amyloid fibrils with a common beta-pleated sheet structure [1, 2]. Misfolding of over 25 unique precursor proteins can cause amyloidosis. Amyloid fibrils from the precursor proteins—immunoglobulin light chains (primary or AL) and the transthyretin protein (TTR)—usually involve the heart. AL amyloidosis is a plasma cell dyscrasia with an overproduction of abnormal kappa or lambda immunoglobulin light chains that aggregate into AL fibrils. ATTR amyloidosis, however, results from aggregation of either native (senile systemic amyloidosis) or variant TTR protein (familial amyloidosis) produced by the liver of individuals with mutations of the TTR gene (>100 single nucleotide polymorphisms and 80 confirmed mutations described) [3]. Senile systemic amyloidosis affects older individuals (>70 years) and almost always affects the heart. Variant TTR protein can cause familial amyloid cardiomyopathy, familial amyloid neuropathy, or mixed disease (cardiomyopathy and neuropathy) and younger individuals (fourth decade of life or later) may manifest clinical symptoms [4].

Most individuals with cardiac amyloidosis present with heart failure, from diastolic or systolic dysfunction, as their first symptom. But, due to the multitude of symptoms from systemic disease—involvement of the gastrointestinal tract,

S. Dorbala, MD, MPH, FACC
Noninvasive Cardiovascular Imaging Program, Departments of Radiology and Medicine (Cardiology), Brigham and Women's Hospital, Harvard University, Boston, MA, USA

Cardiac Amyloidosis Program, Department of Medicine, Brigham and Women's Hospital, Harvard Medical School Boston, MA, USA

Brigham and Women's Hospital, Harvard Medical School, Boston, MA, USA
e-mail: SDORBALA@PARTNERS.ORG

T.H. Schindler et al. (eds.), *Molecular and Multimodality Imaging in Cardiovascular Disease*, DOI 10.1007/978-3-319-19611-4_5

peripheral and autonomic nervous system, heart, or kidneys—recognition of amyloidosis (and cardiac involvement) is typically delayed. Also, the clinical features of AL and ATTR cardiac amyloidosis are so similar that the two entities cannot be distinguished from one another on clinical grounds alone. Their prognosis and management, however, are vastly different [5, 6]. Individuals with AL cardiac amyloidosis, if untreated, have a median survival of 18–24 months; [1] highly effective AL chemotherapy directed against the clonal plasma cells, with or without stem cell transplantation, is poorly tolerated by individuals with cardiac involvement [7]. On the other hand, until recently, no specific therapies were available for ATTR amyloidosis. Currently, several novel agents (tafamidis or diflunisal) are under development to stabilize the tetrameric form of TTR and prevent it from becoming a monomer which is more prone to aggregate [3]. Other treatment approaches include antisense oligonucleotides to silence the TTR gene (Alnylam compound or Isis pharmaceuticals compound), small interfering RNA molecules to reduce the production of the mutant TTR from the liver, or agents to dissolve the amyloid fibrils from the various organs (doxycycline/TUDCA) [3]. Liver transplantation removes the source of the variant TTR and replaces it with normal TTR and is a major treatment option in individuals with familial amyloid cardiomyopathy [3]. ATTR amyloidosis, however, can recur following liver transplantation [8]. Due to the distinct clinical course and treatment options for AL and ATTR amyloidosis, early diagnosis of cardiac amyloidosis as well as typing of AL or ATTR disease are critical [9].

5.2 Diagnosis of Cardiac Amyloidosis

Cardiac amyloidosis is usually suspected clinically and evaluated by a variety of diagnostic tests. A 12-lead ECG and 2D transthoracic echocardiography are common first tests; they are followed by advanced imaging with cardiac magnetic resonance imaging or radionuclide imaging when clinical suspicion for cardiac amyloidosis is high. Each of these tests provides insights into specific pathophysiological processes in the heart of individuals with amyloidosis (Table 5.1).

The most definitive diagnosis, however, is by endomyocardial biopsy. After the amyloid deposits are identified on histology (Congo red or sulfated Alcian blue staining), the precursor protein for the fibrils is identified by immunohistochemistry staining for kappa and lambda light chains or transthyretin. Transthyretin protein is further analyzed to distinguish variant TTR from wild-type TTR. But, none of these tests is diagnostic on its own, including endomyocardial biopsy which may rarely be false negative due to sampling error [9]. The information obtained from each of these tests is integrated with clinical data to diagnose amyloidosis, to plan management, and to screen family members of individuals with genetic forms of amyloidosis.

Table 5.1 Typical imaging features in cardiac amyloidosis

ECG	Low voltage: <5 mm in limb leads and <10 mm in the chest leads
Echocardiogram	Thick LV and RV myocardium
	Sparkling/granular appearance
	Increased LV mass
	Small LV cavity size
	LV wall thickness-to-ECG voltage ratio
	Biatrial enlargement
	Pericardial effusions
	Restrictive filling pattern Mitral E/A TDI Pulmonary venous inflow (S> > D) RVTDI
	LV longitudinal systolic strain with apical sparing—apical-to-basal strain ratio >2.1
CMR	Above structural features Late gadolinium enhancement—diffuse, patchy, subendocardial LGE in the left ventricle, atria, and the right ventricle Expanded ECV Nulling of myocardial signal prior to blood pool signal on T1 scout
Radionuclide imaging	Tc-99m DPD uptake—ATTR amyloidosis Tc-99m PYP uptake—ATTR amyloidosis C-11 PiB uptake—AL and ATTR amyloidosis F-18 florbetapir uptake—AL and ATTR amyloidosis

LV left ventricle, *RV* right ventricle, *ECG* electrocardiogram, *TDI* tissue Doppler imaging, *LGE* late gadolinium enhancement, *ECV* extracellular volume, *ATTR* transthyretin amyloidosis, *AL* light chain amyloidosis, *DPD* = 3,3-diphosphono-1,2-propanodicarboxylic acid, *PYP* = pyrophosphate; *PiB* = Pittsburgh B compound.

5.2.1 ECG

A classic finding of cardiac amyloidosis is the paradox of a low-voltage ECG (<0.1 mV in all the chest leads or <0.05 mV in all the standard limb leads) in individuals with increased LV wall thickening (Fig. 5.1). Unfortunately, this predicts amyloidosis in only 56 % of individuals with cardiac amyloidosis [10]. These low-voltage ECG patterns are most common in individuals with AL rather than ATTR amyloidosis [6, 11]. Adding to this enigma, individuals with amyloidosis may manifest normal ECG voltage or even high ECG voltage meeting criteria for LVH (especially with senile systemic amyloidosis and coexistent hypertension) [12]. The precise reasons for the low-voltage ECG are not known, but, myocyte atrophy and/or local myotoxicity from circulating AL and amyloid fibril component interactions are possible causal factors [6]. Other significant ECG findings in cardiac amyloidosis patients include pseudoinfarction patterns (66–69 %), atrial fibrillation (5–27 %),

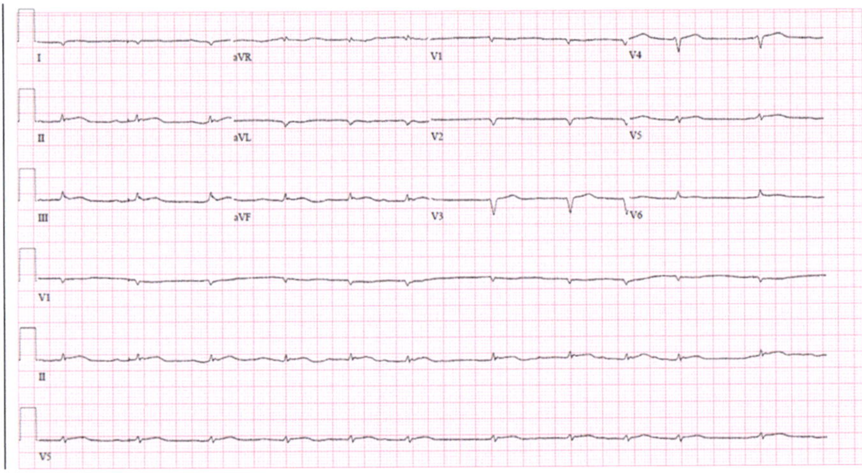

Fig. 5.1 Typical ECG in cardiac amyloidosis. A 60-year-old man with AL cardiac amyloidosis has atrial fibrillation, low-voltage ECG in precordial and limb leads, and pseudo Q-waves

first-degree AV block, RBBB, or LBBB (4–33 %) [10, 13, 14]. A 12-lead ECG, though an appropriate first step, is not sufficiently diagnostic on its own. Further evaluation with advanced imaging is often necessary.

5.2.2 Echocardiography

Echocardiography, in cardiac amyloidosis, is fundamental to establish the diagnosis, to define the magnitude of myocardial dysfunction, to guide management, and to define prognosis [15–24]. A comprehensive advanced transthoracic 2D echocardiogram study for cardiac amyloidosis includes assessment of (1) cardiac structure by 2D imaging (Fig. 5.2), (2) valve function by color and spectral Doppler imaging, (3) myocardial relaxation by tissue Doppler imaging of the right and left ventricle, and (4) myocardial deformation by 2D tissue Doppler or speckle tracking longitudinal and radial strain imaging of the left and the right ventricles. Transesophageal echocardiography may be frequently performed, prior to cardioversion, in individuals with atrial fibrillation which is common in cardiac amyloidosis.

The classic 2D echocardiographic features of sparkling myocardium and increased left ventricular (LV) wall thickness (Fig. 5.2a, b) typically indicate advanced myocardial infiltration with amyloid. Unlike left ventricular myocardial hypertrophy from increased afterload (hypertensive heart disease or aortic stenosis), the increased wall thickness in amyloidosis represents amyloid deposits, usually parallels disease burden, and is associated with low-voltage ECG [10]. The sparkling myocardial appearance, present in about 25 % of individuals [10], is not specific for amyloidosis and may be seen with other forms of hypertrophic diseases. Increased LV wall thickness (>12 mm), decreased LV end-diastolic and end-systolic

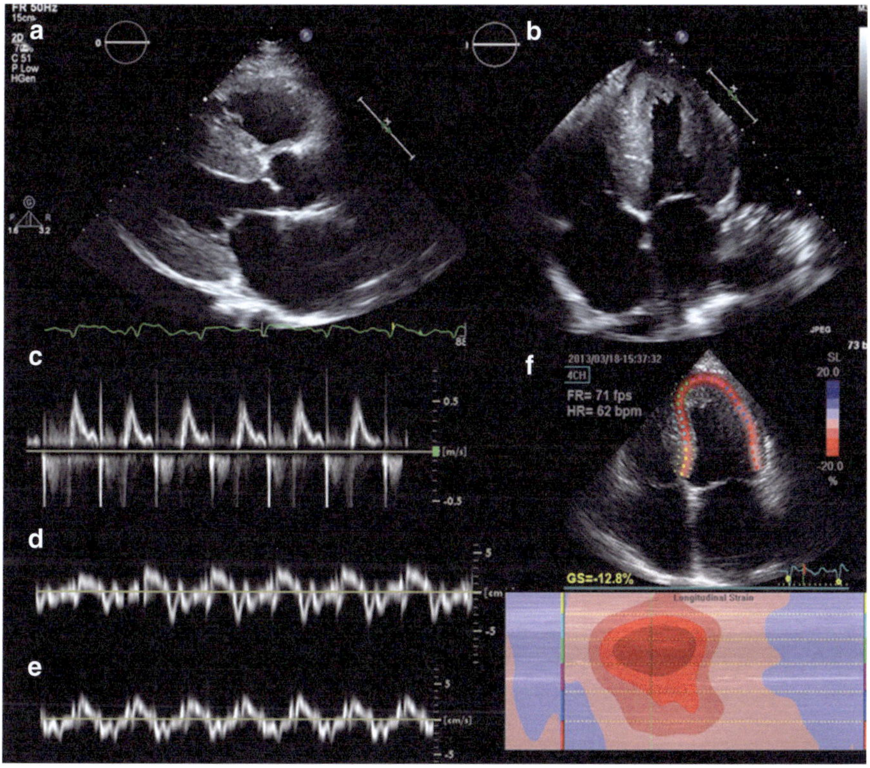

Fig. 5.2 Typical echocardiographic features of cardiac amyloidosis. Increased left ventricular wall thickness with sparkling myocardium on parasternal long-axis (**a**), apical four-chamber views (**b**) and restrictive filling pattern on the mitral inflow (**c**), and mitral annular tissue Doppler imaging (*TDI*, (**d**) septal, (**e**) lateral). Panel (**f**) shows typical longitudinal systolic strain pattern with apical sparing (*red in the center* of the bulls eye plot represents preserved apical strain)

volumes, biatrial enlargement, right ventricular (RV) hypertrophy, pericardial effusions, thickening of the interatrial septum (a specific feature) [24], and increased atrioventricular valve thickening characterize cardiac amyloidosis [6, 10, 25].

Imaging of myocardial relaxation by spectral and tissue Doppler imaging demonstrates classic features of restrictive heart disease (Fig. 5.2c–e): E/A reversal, short deceleration time, high E-wave velocity, and reduced pulmonary venous systolic velocity [26]. Tissue Doppler imaging as well as pulmonary inflow parameters are more sensitive than the mitral inflow parameters to identify earlier stages of restriction [15]. While the mitral early diastolic tissue Doppler velocities (e') are reduced early, before onset of overt congestive heart failure (CHF), peak S-wave velocity on pulmonary venous flow and mitral inflow E-wave deceleration time are later manifestations and are seen in individuals with overt CHF [20]. Objective evidence of abnormalities in diastolic filling portends worse outcomes [27], incremental to LV wall thickening and fractional shortening [17].

Left ventricular myocardial deformation, global longitudinal strain, using 2D tissue Doppler or speckle tracking, is a sensitive and early marker of myocardial systolic dysfunction. Abnormalities in longitudinal strain, with a classic pattern of apical sparing on 2D (Fig. 5.2f) [20] or 3D strain imaging [28], may precede an overt decline of LV ejection fraction. Although the ratio of longitudinal strain at the apex to base (>2.1) may distinguish amyloid heart disease from other forms of LV hypertrophy, there is significant overlap [28, 29].

The right ventricle is almost universally thickened in cardiac amyloidosis. Reductions in RV longitudinal strain as well as tricuspid annular plane systolic excursion (TAPSE) are early markers of cardiac amyloidosis [27, 30] and independent predictors of cardiac death [27].

Although echocardiography is almost invariably the initial test in most individuals with symptoms suggestive of cardiac amyloidosis, it remains insensitive to detect early disease. Also, echocardiography cannot definitively diagnose cardiac amyloidosis from other hypertrophic heart diseases and cannot distinguish AL from ATTR amyloidosis. When the echocardiogram shows classic features, in individuals with biopsy-proven systemic AL amyloidosis, cardiac amyloidosis is diagnosed, and an endomyocardial biopsy is spared. On the other hand, if echocardiogram is classic and systemic, AL amyloidosis is excluded by serum-free light chain assay and serum/urine immunofixation studies, ATTR amyloidosis is possible. Prior to endomyocardial biopsy to confirm ATTR amyloidosis, advanced imaging with cardiac MRI or radionuclide imaging may be performed [9].

5.2.3 Cardiac Magnetic Resonance Imaging

Cardiac magnetic resonance imaging (CMR) is a powerful method to image cardiac structure, function, and amyloid deposition. Clinically, CMR is typically considered in individuals with echocardiograms that are suspicious but not typical for amyloidosis or in individuals with high clinical suspicion, irrespective of echocardiogram results (gene-positive individuals with symptoms or at the age when disease onset is expected). Standard CMR sequences for cardiac amyloidosis include (1) cine images in the standard long-axis and short-axis views to study cardiac structure, systolic function, calculate LV wall thickness and mass; (2) late gadolinium enhancement imaging (about 5 min after injection of gadolinium) in axial, short-, and long-axis views; (3) optimal myocardial inversion time is assessed about 4 min after injection of gadolinium (0.05 mmol/kg of gadolinium at 3 cc/s) to identify specific patterns of myocardial nulling in amyloid as opposed to left ventricular myocardial hypertrophy; and (4) T1 mapping native (precontrast) and post-gadolinium contrast T1 mapping to calculate extracellular volume (ECV).

CMR, with excellent spatial resolution, can characterize the classic phenotypic changes of cardiac amyloidosis, including increased LV and RV wall thickness, myocardial mass, biatrial enlargement, pericardial effusions, and pleural effusions (Fig. 5.3a, b) [31–34].

Cardiac amyloid deposits can substantially alter myocardial tissue characteristics. Intravenous gadolinium administration markedly reduces the myocardial longitudinal relaxation times (T-1) [32], corresponding to histological distribution of amyloid deposits, with significantly lower T-1 times in the subendocardium compared to the subepicardium [32]. Also, the myocardial T-1 times correlated with myocardial amyloid mass as assessed by left ventricular mass and parameters of diastolic dysfunction [32].

Late gadolinium enhancement (LGE), especially in the subendocardial region, is common (80–90 %) in biopsy-proven advanced cardiac amyloidosis [32–35]. Several patterns of late gadolinium enhancement (diffuse or focal subendocardial, focal or diffuse myocardial patterns) are described, but LGE of the papillary muscle [34] and atria is a distinctive feature of cardiac amyloidosis (Fig. 5.3c, d) [33, 35]. Of note, in cardiac amyloidosis, identifying an appropriate nulling of the normal

a

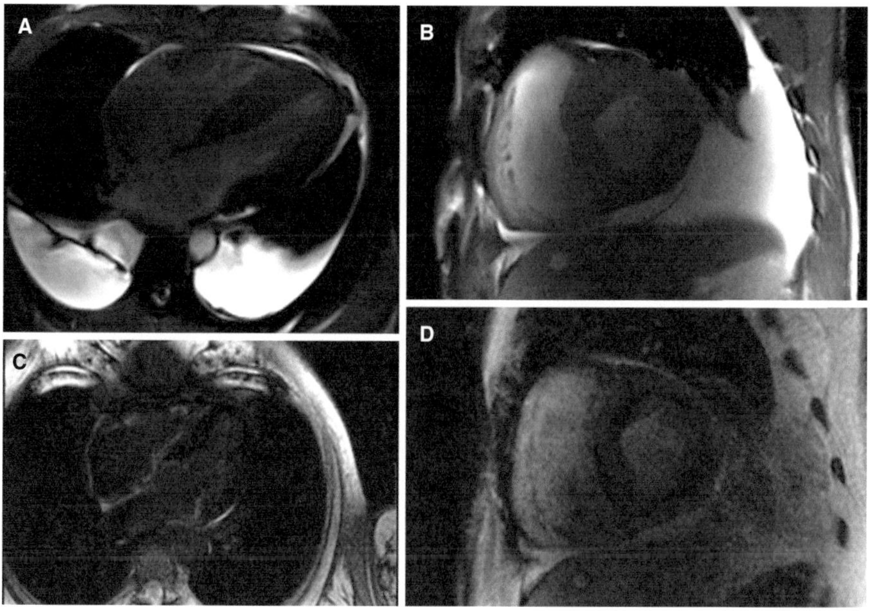

Fig. 5.3 (**a**) Cardiac magnetic resonance imaging features of cardiac amyloidosis. Typical features of cardiac amyloidosis on CMR are shown. Left ventricular wall thickness is increased concentrically with and small ventricular cavity and bilateral pleural effusions [*A* (apical four-chamber view) and *B* (mid-ventricular short-axis view)]. The late gadolinium enhancement (*LGE*) images in *C* (apical four-chamber view) show subendocardial LGE in the right ventricle and the right atrium (different patient than in *A*); *D* demonstrates diffuse LGE of the left ventricle (same patient as in *A*). Typical TI (inversion time) scout images in cardiac amyloidosis are shown in panel *B* (reproduced with permission from Ref. [35]). (**b**) The images demonstrate that, in contrast to individuals with hypertensive left ventricular hypertrophy in whom the blood pool signal nulls prior to the myocardial signal (*top panel*), in individuals with cardiac amyloidosis (*bottom panel*), the myocardial signal nulls prior to the blood pool signal consistent with diffuse late gadolinium enhancement

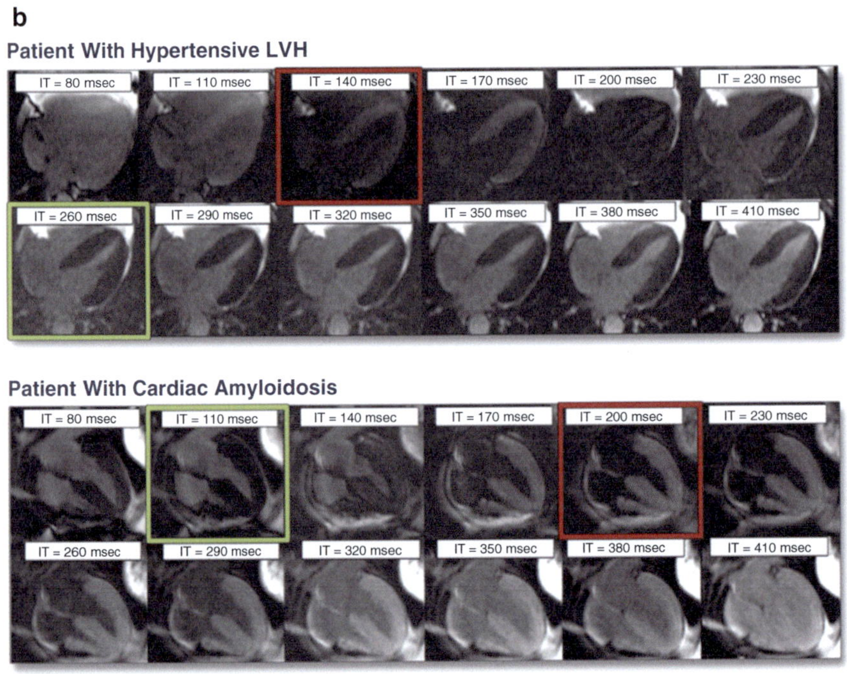

Fig. 5.3 (continued)

myocardium can be a challenge and may provide a false-negative result if an incorrect inversion time (TI inversion time) is used. However, when imaged appropriately, global transmural and subendocardial LGE patterns correlate with left ventricular mass index and cardiac amyloid burden on histology [33]. Furthermore, in one study of 47 patients with suspected cardiac amyloidosis, presence of LGE was predictive of worse survival [35].

Furthermore, in cardiac amyloidosis, on post-gadolinium contrast images, the myocardium nulls prior to blood pool on the TI-scout images; this unique feature distinguishes cardiac amyloidosis from hypertensive left ventricular hypertrophy (Fig. 5.4) [36].

For the TI scout, a sequence of images are obtained in the mid-ventricular short-axis view and a four-chamber view, using a breath-hold, inversion-recovery cine steady-state free precession (SSFP) pulse sequences, with sequential images of the phases of the cardiac cycle acquired at increasing time from the inversion pulse in 40 ms increments starting at 80 ms [34, 36]. The TI time where 50 % of the normal myocardium nulls prior to the blood pool has been used as the optimal TI time for obtaining the late gadolinium enhancement images [34]. A rapid visual assessment of TI time was helpful to identify cardiac amyloidosis individuals at high risk of mortality [36]. Also, 20–30 % of individuals with AL cardiac amyloidosis have renal dysfunction; a CMR technique that does not require gadolinium contrast, native T-1, is of great interest.

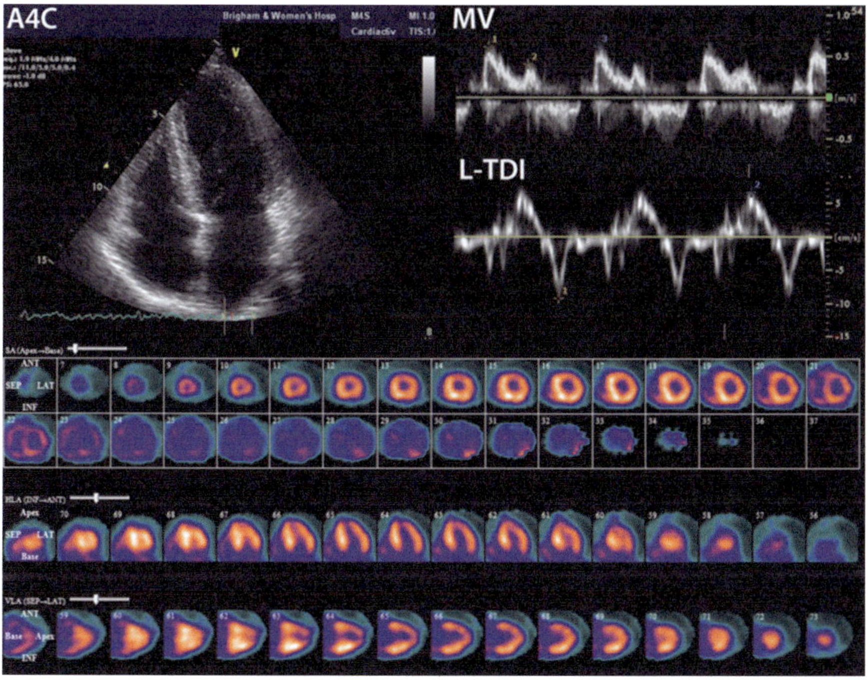

Fig. 5.4 Technetium-99m pyrophosphate imaging in familial transthyretin cardiac amyloidosis. Echocardiogram and technetium-99m pyrophosphate (PYP) images of a 55-year-old woman positive for Ala60 TTR variant and a family history of TTR amyloid cardiomyopathy and neuropathy. The echocardiogram shows relatively normal wall thickness, normal E/A ratio, but significantly impaired lateral mitral annular systolic and diastolic motion by tissue Doppler imaging (*TDI*). In the bottom panel, the Tc-99m PYP images in short axis (*top*), vertical long axis (*middle*), and horizontal long axis (*bottom*) demonstrate moderate, diffusely increased radiotracer uptake in the left and right ventricles suggesting early cardiac involvement

Native (precontrast) T-1 relaxation times were significantly increased in patients with cardiac amyloidosis compared to healthy volunteers [(AL 1140±61 ms vs. healthy 958±20 ms) [37] (ATTR 1097±43 ms vs. healthy 967±34 ms) [38]]. Individuals with AL and ATTR cardiac amyloidosis also have significantly higher T-1 compared to individuals with left ventricular hypertrophy from aortic stenosis [37] or hypertrophic cardiomyopathy [38]. In a study of patients with AL cardiac amyloidosis, increased T-1 time was observed in all patients with LGE [37]. Increased T-1 time correlated with disease burden and was linearly related to myocardial mass ($r=0.58$, $p<0.001$) and inversely related to left ventricular ejection fraction ($r=-0.57$, $p<0.001$) and diastolic function (E/E' ratio; $r=0.44$, $p=0.001$). A higher native T-1 (1,044 ms) also predicted a higher hazard of mortality (HR 5.09, 95 % CI 1.09–23.7, $p=0.04$) in patients with AL amyloidosis [39]. Despite the advantages of not using gadolinium contrast, native T-1 mapping has certain challenges: (1) it measures signal from the myocardium and the interstitial space, (2) it cannot differentiate edema from amyloid, and (3) normal reference values are not standardized and may vary by the type of scanner used [40].

Using advanced techniques, myocardial T-1 times measured by post-gadolinium contrast can quantify expanded myocardial ECV from various cardiovascular pathologies including amyloid deposits [41, 42]. Indeed, ECV is significantly expanded in cardiac amyloidosis (mean ECV 0.44 ± 0.12) compared to healthy controls (mean ECV 0.25 ± 0.02, $p < 0.001$) [39]. Expanded ECV [41, 42] and prolonged T1 relaxation times [37] are directly related to myocardial amyloid burden; they correlate directly with LV mass [37], restrictive features (TDI "S" wave) [41, 42], elevated cardiac biomarker levels (BNP and troponin levels) [41], myocardial uptake of Tc-99m DPD (a specific radiotracer that images ATTR amyloid in the heart) [37], and inversely with left ventricular ejection fraction [37, 41]. Moreover, ECV predicted mortality after accounting for echocardiographic features of diastolic dysfunction, EF, and NT pro BNP levels (HR 4.4.1; 95 % CI 1.35–14.4, $p < 0.0001$) [39]. Although there are no data, being quantitative metrics, T1 mapping and ECV may serve as valuable tools to longitudinally assess the fate of cardiac amyloid burden in response to therapy.

CMR, however, may be limited in individuals with atrial fibrillation or claustrophobia; gadolinium-based contrast agents are contraindicated in individuals with renal dysfunction, and CMR is contraindicated in individuals with certain cardiac devices (pacemakers, ICD). When feasible, CMR plays a major role in the evaluation of individuals with suspected cardiac amyloidosis. In individuals with biopsy-proven systemic AL amyloidosis, classic CMR findings are virtually diagnostic of cardiac amyloidosis. CMR features, however, cannot definitively distinguish AL amyloidosis from ATTR amyloidosis. Therefore, when cardiac amyloidosis is suspected for the first time based on CMR findings, serum-free light chain assay and serum and urine immunofixation are recommended to exclude systemic AL amyloidosis [9]. If those evaluations are negative, to identify ATTR cardiac amyloidosis, either an endomyocardial biopsy or a radionuclide study using technetium-99m pyrophosphate (Tc-99m PYP) is the next step.

5.2.4 Radionuclide Imaging of Cardiac Amyloidosis

Targeted radionuclide imaging of amyloidosis is a robust method to image cardiac amyloid deposition. Radionuclide imaging is typically considered for the diagnosis of amyloidosis in individuals with a high clinical suspicion for ATTR cardiac amyloidosis. More recently, it is also being used for identifying ATTR amyloidosis when echocardiography or CMR are highly suggestive of amyloidosis, but endomyocardial biopsy is not planned, as in elderly individuals with senile systemic amyloidosis. Radionuclide imaging of cardiac amyloidosis is possible with (1) bone imaging SPECT agents (technetium-99m (Tc-99m) pyrophosphate/Tc-99m 3,3-diphosphono-1,2-propanodicarboxylic acid (DPD)), (2) neuronal imaging agents (I-123 meta iodo benzyl guanidine, mIBG), (3) amyloid-binding SPECT agents (I-123 serum amyloid protein-SAP, Tc-99m aprotinin), and (4) amyloid-binding PET agents (C-11 Pittsburgh B compound, PiB, F-18 florbetapir).

5.2.5 Bone Imaging Agents

Radionuclide imaging with Tc-99m PYP or Tc-99m DPD has been used since the 1980s [43], but has recently reemerged as a dominant method for cardiac ATTR amyloid imaging. Extensive literature supports the utility of Tc-99m DPD and PYP imaging to diagnose cardiac amyloidosis [44–46] and to stratify risk of major adverse cardiac events (MACE). The precise mechanism of myocardial uptake of bone imaging agents is not known, but a calcium-mediated mechanism of uptake has been proposed [46]. Tc-99m PYP or DPD (15–20 mCi) is administered intravenously followed by planar or SPECT imaging (preferred) 2.5 h later (Table 5.2). The myocardial radiotracer uptake is semiquantitatively interpreted in relation to sternal uptake into four grades: 0 = no uptake, 1 = less than sternal uptake, 2 = equal to sternal uptake, and 3 = greater than sternal uptake (attenuation of bone uptake) [44]. When available, quantitation on SPECT/CT images may be preferable to avoid overlap from bone radiotracer uptake [47].

Tc-99m PYP and DPD are highly sensitive (>90 %) to diagnose cardiac ATTR amyloidosis [47]. Further, two studies demonstrated that Tc-99m DPD [44] and Tc-99m PYP [46] were able to noninvasively differentiate between AL and TTR amyloidosis, with all TTR patients showing DPD/PYP uptake and none of the AL patients showing DPD/PYP uptake. A heart-to-contralateral lung Tc-99m PYP ratio of 1.5 distinguished AL from ATTR cardiac amyloidosis with 97 % sensitivity and 100 % specificity [46]. In another study, however, low-level Tc-99m DPD uptake was detected in about a third of individuals with AL amyloidosis, but none with significant uptake [45]. Hutt et al. [47] demonstrated significant uptake of Tc-99m DPD in the heart and in the muscles of individuals with wild-type and V122I ATTR patients. These authors suggest that if Tc-99m DPD uptake is ≥ grade 2 with typical soft tissue, the scan is diagnostic for ATTR cardiac amyloidosis, and a confirmatory endomyocardial biopsy may be avoided [47]. Finally, Tc-99m DPD imaging may identify early cardiac amyloidosis in gene-positive individuals without apparent structural cardiac changes by echocardiography (Fig. 5.5).

Table 5.2 Tc-99m PYP study protocol for suspected cardiac transthyretin amyloidosis

Tc-99m PYP is injected intravenously (20–25 mCi) and 20 min imaging is performed after 2.5 h
Planar or chest SPECT (preferred) imaging may be performed
Normal individuals have no myocardial uptake and no blood pool activity at 2.5 h
Individuals with TTR amyloidosis demonstrate significant, biventricular, diffuse myocardial uptake
Myocardial radiotracer uptake is graded on a 0–3 scale 0 = no myocardial uptake 1 < bone uptake 2 = bone uptake and 3 > bone uptake
Heart-to-contralateral lung ratio can be computed

SPECT single-photon emission computed tomography

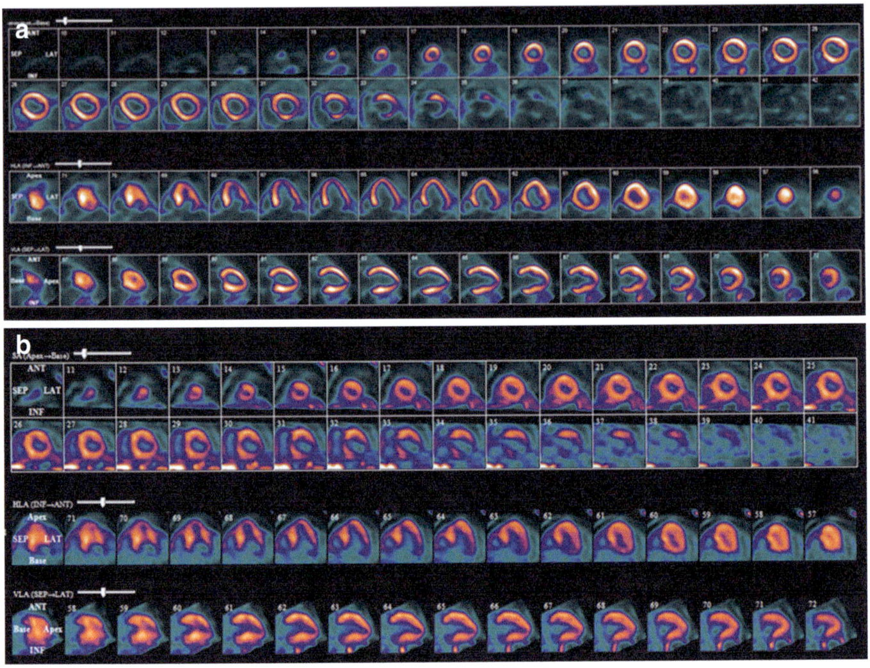

Fig. 5.5 Imaging cardiac amyloidosis with PET radiotracers. F-18 florbetapir PET in a 65-year-old man with light chain cardiac amyloidosis (**a**) and in a 72-year-old man with transthyretin cardiac amyloidosis (**b**). The short-axis (*top*), vertical long-axis (*middle*), and horizontal long-axis (*bottom*) images demonstrate intense and diffusely increased radiotracer uptake in the left and right ventricles

Increased myocardial Tc-99m DPD uptake is directly related to myocardial amyloid burden; it correlates linearly with LV mass on echocardiography [45] and to prolongation of myocardial T-1 relaxation times (CMR), markers of amyloid burden [38]. Furthermore, in 63 patients with hereditary ATTR cardiac amyloidosis, increased heart-to-whole body ratio in conjunction with increased wall thickness was associated with a higher risk of major adverse cardiovascular events [48]. Notably, unlike echocardiography and CMR, Tc-99m PYP or DPD cannot be used as screening test for cardiac amyloidosis—a negative PYP study does not rule out AL cardiac amyloidosis [9]. To address that, a number of amyloid-binding SPECT radiotracers as well as neuronal imaging agents have been tested.

5.3 Imaging Cardiac Sympathetic Denervation with I-123 MIBG

Certain forms of familial ATTR amyloidoses predominantly affect the nervous system with or without concomitant cardiac involvement [3]. A SPECT radiotracer I-123mIBG is a norepinephrine analog that has been successfully used to directly image cardiac adrenergic innervation [49]. Myocardial denervation identified by

I-123 mIBG imaging is an early marker of cardiac amyloidosis in individuals with familial amyloid polyneuropathy (ATTRm) [50] [51] as well as in AL amyloidosis [52]. Delahaye et al. [50] studied 17 patients with biopsy-proven familial amyloid polyneuropathy and found that cardiac I-123 mIBG uptake was significantly decreased in familial amyloid polyneuropathy patients, with no difference in washout rates despite preserved left ventricular systolic function and cardiac perfusion. Imaging myocardial denervation, however, remains an indirect method to image early familial cardiac amyloidosis. Therefore, more recently, the focus has shifted to the use of SPECT bone imaging agents to amyloid-binding SPECT and PET agents to identify early cardiac amyloidosis.

5.4 Amyloid-Binding SPECT Radiotracers

I-123-labeled serum amyloid P component, SAP [53], and Tc-99m-labeled aprotinin [54, 55], are amyloid-binding SPECT tracers. I-123 SAP binds to amyloid fibrils irrespective of precursor protein and can quantify whole-body amyloid load in individuals with systemic AL amyloidosis [53]. But, it has limited availability and a limited signal-to-noise ratio which precludes its use for cardiac imaging [53]. Clinical experience with Tc-99m-labeled aprotinin is more limited, likely due to its limited binding affinity to myocardial amyloid [54, 56, 57]. Furthermore, due to the imaging characteristics, quantitation of radiotracer uptake is challenging with SPECT amyloid radiotracers. This challenge is addressed by the novel amyloid-binding PET radiotracers—C-11 Pittsburgh B compound (PiB), F-18 florbetapir, F-18 florbetaben, and F-18 flutemetamol. Though these radiotracers were originally developed for imaging beta amyloid in the brain, recent pilot studies demonstrate an exciting role for C-11 PiB [58, 59] and F-18 florbetapir [60] for cardiac amyloidosis imaging.

5.5 Amyloid-Binding PET Radiotracers

C-11 Pittsburgh B compound [58, 59] and F-18 florbetapir [60], amyloid-binding PET tracers, appear to nonselectively image AL and ATTR cardiac amyloidosis (Fig. 5.6a, b). In a pilot study of 15 patients (amyloidosis = 10 and healthy controls = 5), Antoni et al. [46] demonstrated that all patients with cardiac amyloid and none of the healthy control subjects demonstrated myocardial C-11 PiB uptake. The myocardial retention of C-11 PiB was significantly higher in amyloid compared to healthy hearts (0.054/min vs. 0.025/min, $p = 0.0007$) [46]. Similar results were demonstrated with F-18 florbetapir, with a significantly higher myocardial retention of F-18 florbetapir by patients with cardiac amyloidosis compared to healthy controls (Fig. 5.6).

F-18 florbetapir myocardial retention index trended higher in patients with AL compared to ATTR cardiac amyloidosis [60]. The median target-to-background (blood pool) ratio of mean SUV (standardized uptake value) was also significantly higher in the amyloid when compared with the control subjects [1.84 (1.64–2.50) vs.

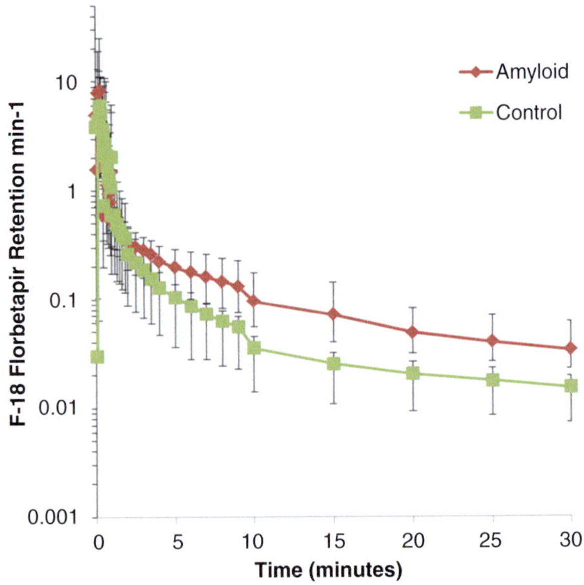

Fig. 5.6 Myocardial retention of F-18 florbetapir in control and amyloid subjects. The mean F-18 florbetapir myocardial retention index was significantly greater in subjects with cardiac amyloidosis (*red line*) compared to control subjects without cardiac amyloidosis (*green line*). The error bars represent the range of values

1.26 (0.91–1.36), $P=0.001$]. Furthermore, in one subject with cardiac AL amyloidosis and the systemic AL amyloidosis in remission, myocardial florbetapir uptake was significantly lower than in individuals with active systemic AL amyloidosis [60]. These findings were confirmed with C-11 PiB imaging in another study of 22 patients with 5 patients who were treated for AL amyloidosis [59]. The maximal myocardial to blood pool target-to-background ratio was significantly higher in amyloidosis patients compared to controls [median 3.86 (range 1.68–19.92) vs. 0.97 (range 0.76–1.23), $p<0.001$]. Notably, five individuals who received chemotherapy for systemic AL amyloidosis demonstrated a significantly lower target-to-background ratio [median 10.39 (range 1.69–19.92) vs. 2.29 (range 1.68–3.81), $p<0.014$]. The results of the three pilot studies together suggest that amyloid imaging with C-11 PiB and F-18 florbetapir may have a potential role for quantitative targeted amyloid imaging. Further studies are warranted to understand if these agents may be helpful to assess myocardial response to antiamyloid therapy.

Conclusions

Significant developments have expanded our understanding of the pathogenesis, evaluation, and management of patients with cardiac amyloidosis. Several novel therapies are dramatically reducing circulating light chains or transthyretin levels and offer the potential to improve outcomes of individuals with cardiac amyloidosis. However, a clinical diagnosis of cardiac amyloidosis can be challenging. Symptoms are confusing due to systemic illness. Typical low-voltage ECG is neither sensitive nor specific. Echocardiography is typically the initial test in symptomatic individuals. If echocardiography is typical, a histological diagnosis by endomyocardial biopsy (for ATTR) or tissue biopsy (AL) is the next step. Advanced CMR and radionuclide imaging make possible, for the first time, accurate and quantitative imaging of whole heart amyloid burden. Indeed, but, CMR cannot distinguish AL from ATTR amyloidosis. Cardiac SPECT with bone imaging agents offer a significant advantage in that regard. They specifically identify cardiac ATTR amyloidosis and may mitigate the need for an endomyocardial biopsy in certain individuals. Cardiac SPECT bone imaging agents are sensitive and specific for ATTR cardiac amyloidosis and may mitigate the need for an endomyocardial biopsy in some of these individuals. Future imaging-guided clinical trials will determine whether advances in imaging can aid in the development of novel antiamyloid therapies that can improve the lives of individuals with this devastating disease.

References

1. Falk RH. Diagnosis and management of the cardiac amyloidoses. Circulation. 2005;112: 2047–60.
2. Merlini G, Bellotti V. Molecular mechanisms of amyloidosis. N Engl J Med. 2003;349:583–96.
3. Ruberg FL, Berk JL. Transthyretin (ttr) cardiac amyloidosis. Circulation. 2012;126:1286–300.
4. Quarta CC, Buxbaum JN, Shah AM, Falk RH, Claggett B, Kitzman DW, Mosley TH, Butler KR, Boerwinkle E, Solomon SD. The amyloidogenic v122i transthyretin variant in elderly black americans. N Engl J Med. 2015;372:21–9.
5. Dubrey SW, Cha K, Skinner M, LaValley M, Falk RH. Familial and primary (al) cardiac amyloidosis: echocardiographically similar diseases with distinctly different clinical outcomes. Heart. 1997;78:74–82.
6. Rapezzi C, Merlini G, Quarta CC, et al. Systemic cardiac amyloidoses: disease profiles and clinical courses of the 3 main types. Circulation. 2009;120:1203–12.
7. Merlini G, Wechalekar AD, Palladini G. Systemic light chain amyloidosis: an update for treating physicians. Blood. 2013;121:5124–30.
8. Dubrey SW, Davidoff R, Skinner M, Bergethon P, Lewis D, Falk RH. Progression of ventricular wall thickening after liver transplantation for familial amyloidosis. Transplantation. 1997;64:74–80.
9. Falk RH, Quarta CC, Dorbala S. How to image cardiac amyloidosis. Circ Cardiovasc Imaging. 2014;7:552–62.
10. Rahman JE, Helou EF, Gelzer-Bell R, et al. Noninvasive diagnosis of biopsy-proven cardiac amyloidosis. J Am Coll Cardiol. 2004;43:410–5.
11. Murtagh B, Hammill SC, Gertz MA, Kyle RA, Tajik AJ, Grogan M. Electrocardiographic findings in primary systemic amyloidosis and biopsy-proven cardiac involvement. Am J Cardiol. 2005;95:535–7.
12. Seward JB, Casaclang-Verzosa G. Infiltrative cardiovascular diseases: cardiomyopathies that look alike. J Am Coll Cardiol. 2010;55:1769–79.
13. Rapezzi C, Quarta CC, Obici L, et al. Disease profile and differential diagnosis of hereditary transthyretin-related amyloidosis with exclusively cardiac phenotype: an Italian perspective. Eur Heart J. 2013;34:520–8.
14. Rapezzi C, Quarta CC, Guidalotti PL, et al. Role of (99m)tc-dpd scintigraphy in diagnosis and prognosis of hereditary transthyretin-related cardiac amyloidosis. JACC Cardiovasc Imaging. 2011;4:659–70.
15. Klein AL, Hatle LK, Burstow DJ, et al. Doppler characterization of left ventricular diastolic function in cardiac amyloidosis. J Am Coll Cardiol. 1989;13:1017–26.
16. Klein AL, Hatle LK, Burstow DJ, et al. Comprehensive doppler assessment of right ventricular diastolic function in cardiac amyloidosis. J Am Coll Cardiol. 1990;15:99–108.

17. Klein AL, Hatle LK, Taliercio CP, et al. Prognostic significance of doppler measures of diastolic function in cardiac amyloidosis. A doppler echocardiography study. Circulation. 1991;83:808–16.
18. Klein AL, Hatle LK, Taliercio CP, et al. Serial doppler echocardiographic follow-up of left ventricular diastolic function in cardiac amyloidosis. J Am Coll Cardiol. 1990;16:1135–41.
19. Buss SJ, Emami M, Mereles D, et al. Longitudinal left ventricular function for prediction of survival in systemic light-chain amyloidosis: incremental value compared with clinical and biochemical markers. J Am Coll Cardiol. 2012;60:1067–76.
20. Koyama J, Ray-Sequin PA, Davidoff R, Falk RH. Usefulness of pulsed tissue doppler imaging for evaluating systolic and diastolic left ventricular function in patients with al (primary) amyloidosis. Am J Cardiol. 2002;89:1067–71.
21. Koyama J, Ray-Sequin PA, Falk RH. Prognostic significance of ultrasound myocardial tissue characterization in patients with cardiac amyloidosis. Circulation. 2002;106:556–61.
22. Koyama J, Ray-Sequin PA, Falk RH. Longitudinal myocardial function assessed by tissue velocity, strain, and strain rate tissue doppler echocardiography in patients with al (primary) cardiac amyloidosis. Circulation. 2003;107:2446–52.
23. Ogiwara F, Koyama J, Ikeda S, Kinoshita O, Falk RH. Comparison of the strain doppler echocardiographic features of familial amyloid polyneuropathy (fap) and light-chain amyloidosis. Am J Cardiol. 2005;95:538–40.
24. Siqueira-Filho AG, Cunha CL, Tajik AJ, Seward JB, Schattenberg TT, Giuliani ER. M-mode and two-dimensional echocardiographic features in cardiac amyloidosis. Circulation. 1981;63:188–96.
25. Carroll JD, Gaasch WH, McAdam KP. Amyloid cardiomyopathy: characterization by a distinctive voltage/mass relation. Am J Cardiol. 1982;49:9–13.
26. Nagueh SF, Appleton CP, Gillebert TC, et al. Recommendations for the evaluation of left ventricular diastolic function by echocardiography. J Am Soc Echocardiogr. 2009;22:107–33.
27. Cappelli F, Porciani MC, Bergesio F, et al. Right ventricular function in al amyloidosis: characteristics and prognostic implication. Eur Heart J Cardiovasc Imaging. 2012;13:416–22.
28. Baccouche H, Maunz M, Beck T, et al. Differentiating cardiac amyloidosis and hypertrophic cardiomyopathy by use of three-dimensional speckle tracking echocardiography. Echocardiography. 2012;29:668–77.
29. Phelan D, Collier P, Thavendiranathan P, et al. Relative apical sparing of longitudinal strain using two-dimensional speckle-tracking echocardiography is both sensitive and specific for the diagnosis of cardiac amyloidosis. Heart. 2012;98:1442–8.
30. Bellavia D, Pellikka PA, Dispenzieri A, et al. Comparison of right ventricular longitudinal strain imaging, tricuspid annular plane systolic excursion, and cardiac biomarkers for early diagnosis of cardiac involvement and risk stratification in primary systematic (al) amyloidosis: a 5-year cohort study. Eur Heart J Cardiovasc Imaging. 2012;13:680–9.
31. Fattori R, Rocchi G, Celletti F, Bertaccini P, Rapezzi C, Gavelli G. Contribution of magnetic resonance imaging in the differential diagnosis of cardiac amyloidosis and symmetric hypertrophic cardiomyopathy. Am Heart J. 1998;136:824–30.
32. Maceira AM, Joshi J, Prasad SK, et al. Cardiovascular magnetic resonance in cardiac amyloidosis. Circulation. 2005;111:186–93.
33. Syed IS, Glockner JF, Feng D, et al. Role of cardiac magnetic resonance imaging in the detection of cardiac amyloidosis. JACC Cardiovasc Imaging. 2010;3:155–64.
34. Vogelsberg H, Mahrholdt H, Deluigi CC, et al. Cardiovascular magnetic resonance in clinically suspected cardiac amyloidosis: noninvasive imaging compared to endomyocardial biopsy. J Am Coll Cardiol. 2008;51:1022–30.
35. Austin BA, Tang WH, Rodriguez ER, et al. Delayed hyper-enhancement magnetic resonance imaging provides incremental diagnostic and prognostic utility in suspected cardiac amyloidosis. JACC Cardiovasc Imaging. 2009;2:1369–77.
36. White JA, Kim HW, Shah D, et al. CMR imaging with rapid visual t1 assessment predicts mortality in patients suspected of cardiac amyloidosis. JACC Cardiovasc Imaging. 2014;7:143–56.
37. Karamitsos TD, Piechnik SK, Banypersad SM, et al. Noncontrast t1 mapping for the diagnosis of cardiac amyloidosis. JACC Cardiovasc Imaging. 2013;6:488–97.

38. Fontana M, Banypersad SM, Treibel TA, et al. Native T1 mapping in transthyretin amyloidosis. JACC Cardiovasc Imaging. 2014;7:157–65.
39. Banypersad SM, Fontana M, Maestrini V, et al. T1 mapping and survival in systemic light-chain amyloidosis. Eur Heart J. 2014;36(4):244–51.
40. Fontana M, Chung R, Hawkins PN, Moon JC. Cardiovascular magnetic resonance for amyloidosis. Heart Fail Rev. 2015;20(2):133–44.
41. Banypersad SM, Sado DM, Flett AS, et al. Quantification of myocardial extracellular volume fraction in systemic al amyloidosis: an equilibrium contrast cardiovascular magnetic resonance study. Circ Cardiovasc Imaging. 2013;6:34–9.
42. Mongeon FP, Jerosch-Herold M, Coelho-Filho OR, Blankstein R, Falk RH, Kwong RY. Quantification of extracellular matrix expansion by cmr in infiltrative heart disease. JACC Cardiovasc Imaging. 2012;5:897–907.
43. Falk RH, Lee VW, Rubinow A, Hood Jr WB, Cohen AS. Sensitivity of technetium-99m-pyrophosphate scintigraphy in diagnosing cardiac amyloidosis. Am J Cardiol. 1983;51:826–30.
44. Perugini E, Guidalotti PL, Salvi F, et al. Noninvasive etiologic diagnosis of cardiac amyloidosis using 99mtc-3,3-diphosphono-1,2-propanodicarboxylic acid scintigraphy. J Am Coll Cardiol. 2005;46:1076–84.
45. Rapezzi C, Quarta CC, Guidalotti PL, et al. Usefulness and limitations of 99mtc-3, 3-diphosphono-1,2-propanodicarboxylic acid scintigraphy in the aetiological diagnosis of amyloidotic cardiomyopathy. Eur J Nucl Med Mol Imaging. 2011;38:470–8.
46. Bokhari S, Castano A, Pozniakoff T, Deslisle S, Latif F, Maurer MS. (99m)tc-pyrophosphate scintigraphy for differentiating light-chain cardiac amyloidosis from the transthyretin-related familial and senile cardiac amyloidoses. Circ Cardiovasc Imaging. 2013;6:195–201.
47. Hutt DF, Quigley AM, Page J, et al. Utility and limitations of 3,3-diphosphono-1, 2-propanodicarboxylic acid scintigraphy in systemic amyloidosis. Eur Heart J Cardiovasc Imaging. 2014;15:1289–98.
48. Rapezzi C, Guidalotti P, Salvi F, Riva L, Perugini E. Usefulness of 99mtc-dpd scintigraphy in cardiac amyloidosis. J Am Coll Cardiol. 2008;51:1509–10.
49. Travin MI. Cardiac autonomic imaging with SPECT tracers. J Nucl Cardiol. 2013;20:128–43.
50. Delahaye N, Dinanian S, Slama MS, et al. Cardiac sympathetic denervation in familial amyloid polyneuropathy assessed by iodine-123 metaiodobenzylguanidine scintigraphy and heart rate variability. Eur J Nucl Med. 1999;26:416–24.
51. Noordzij W, Glaudemans AW, van Rheenen RW, et al. (123)i-labelled metaiodobenzylguanidine for the evaluation of cardiac sympathetic denervation in early stage amyloidosis. Eur J Nucl Med Mol Imaging. 2012;39:1609–17.
52. Hongo M, Urushibata K, Kai R, et al. Iodine-123 metaiodobenzylguanidine scintigraphic analysis of myocardial sympathetic innervation in patients with al (primary) amyloidosis. Am Heart J. 2002;144:122–9.
53. Hawkins PN, Lavender JP, Pepys MB. Evaluation of systemic amyloidosis by scintigraphy with 123i-labeled serum amyloid p component. N Engl J Med. 1990;323:508–13.
54. Aprile C, Marinone G, Saponaro R, Bonino C, Merlini G. Cardiac and pleuropulmonary al amyloid imaging with technetium-99m labelled aprotinin. Eur J Nucl Med. 1995;22:1393–401.
55. Han S, Chong V, Murray T, et al. Preliminary experience of 99mtc-aprotinin scintigraphy in amyloidosis. Eur J Haematol. 2007;79:494–500.
56. Cardoso I, Pereira PJ, Damas AM, Saraiva MJ. Aprotinin binding to amyloid fibrils. Eur J Biochem. 2000;267:2307–11.
57. Minamimoto R, Kubota K, Ishii K, et al. Re-evaluating the potentials and limitations of (99m) tc-aprotinin scintigraphy for amyloid imaging. Am J Nucl Med Mol Imaging. 2013;3:261–71.
58. Antoni G, Lubberink M, Estrada S, et al. In vivo visualization of amyloid deposits in the heart with 11c-pib and pet. J Nucl Med. 2013;54:213–20.
59. Lee SP, Lee ES, Choi H, et al. (11)C-pittsburgh b PET imaging in cardiac amyloidosis. JACC Cardiovasc Imaging. 2015;8:50–9.
60. Dorbala S, Vangala D, Semer J, et al. Imaging cardiac amyloidosis: a pilot study using (18) f-florbetapir positron emission tomography. Eur J Nucl Med Mol Imaging. 2014;41:1652–62.

6 Concepts of PET, SPECT, and MRI in the Assessment of Myocardial Viability Leading to PET/MRI Application

Ines Valenta, Xiaoli Zhang, and Thomas Hellmut Schindler

6.1 Hibernating-Stunning Myocardium: Pathophysiology, Diagnosis, and Clinical Considerations

The prevalence of heart failure is continuously rising in view of the increasingly elderly population and improved survival of acute coronary syndrome (ACS) patients [1]. Although heart failure can be related to various causes such as idiopathic cardiomyopathy (CMP), valvular disease, hypertensive, and diabetic heart disease, ischemic heart disease is the predominant cause of the majority of patients with heart failure symptoms [2]. In the United States, more than four million people suffer from heart failure [3] that poses a considerable public health concern. While there is an ongoing progress in the treatment of heart failure with beta-blockers, angiotensin-converting enzyme (ACE) inhibitors, angiotensin II type 1 receptor (AT-1) blockers, and aldosterone to beneficially influence morbidity and mortality, 5-year mortality rate for heart failure still remains as high as 50 %. Although the left-ventricular remodeling process is related to an activation of the myocardial renin-angiotensin system (RAS), development of interstitial myocardial fibrosis, toxic catecholamine actions, stimulation of matrix metalloproteinase's [4], and

I. Valenta, MD
Department of Radiology SOM, Nuclear Medicine, Johns Hopkins University, Baltimore, MA, USA
e-mail: ines_valenta@hotmail.com

T.H. Schindler, MD (✉)
Johns Hopkins University, Radiology School of Medicine, Cardiovascular Nuclear Medicine, Baltimore, MD, USA
e-mail: tschind3@jhmi.edu

X. Zhang, MD, PhD
Department of Nuclear Medicine, State Key Laboratory of Cardiovascular Disease, Fuwai Hospital, National Center for Cardiovascular Diseases, Chinese Academy of Medical Sciences and Peking Union Medical College, Beijing, People's Republic of China
e-mail: xlzhanig69@yahoo.com

T.H. Schindler et al. (eds.), *Molecular and Multimodality Imaging in Cardiovascular Disease*, DOI 10.1007/978-3-319-19611-4_6

maladaptive cellular and molecular alterations [5], which commonly leads to progressive worsening of left-ventricular function, ischemic heart disease may be the underlying cause to initiate and accelerate this deleterious process. Repetitive ischemia during times of increased metabolic demand or exercise induces cummulative myocardial stunning that over time may manifest clinically as left-ventricular dysfunction with heart failure symptoms (Fig. 6.1) [6]. Thus, repetitive episodes of a dysbalance between oxygen supply and myocardial oxygen demand may lead to cumulative stunning that represents a predecessor of chronic postischemic left-ventricular dysfunction [7, 8].

When this myocardial "stunning" proceeds to myocardial ischemia at rest, then it is commonly referred to as myocardial "hibernation" in *akinetic* or even *dyskinetic* segments (Fig. 6.1) [6, 9–11]. This accord with observations in an animal experimental model of hibernating myocardium that signify reductions in resting flow or perfusion in viable myocardium may be appreciated as a consequence rather than a cause of adaptive myocardial remodeling [12–14]. The decrease of resting myocardial perfusion or flow in the hibernating-stunning myocardium has been suggested to reflect the development of metabolic alterations, including a downregulation of mitochondrial oxygen consumption, or an adaption to the dysbalance between oxygen demand and supply to avoid structural disintegration and/or cellular death of the myocytes and tissue fibrosis. In a clinical investigation with PET perfusion and viability assessment, Zhang et al. [15] could unravel that reduced myocardial perfusion at rest was accompanied by a commensurate decrease in absolute myocardial blood flow (MBF) and on average less severe in viable than nonviable myocardium. Yet, there was a considerable variety in perfusion and MBF values between individuals and myocardial regions, so that the severity in reduced resting flow could not fully differentiate between viable and nonviable myocardium (Fig. 6.2).

Of particular interest, the relative FDG uptake in the viable regions was linearly related to the resting MBF, while this was not observed in the nonviable regions (Fig. 6.3). Such observations put forth that the higher the amount of viable myocardium, the higher is the resting MBF to adequately meet increases in oxygen demand. In addition, the extraction of FDG and, thus, of glucose in the viable myocardium

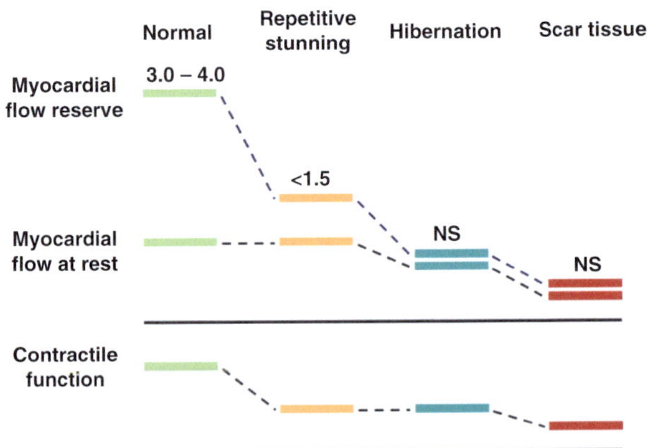

Fig. 6.1 Myocardial flow reserve, resting flow, and spectrum of contractile dysfunction. Progressive worsening of contractile function with reductions in myocardial flow reserve and resting flow

correlated inversely with the myocardial flow reserve (MFR) (Fig. 6.4). The more severe the reduction of MFR, the highest was the FDG extraction and, therefore, the myocardial glucose utilization. This strongly outlines that a severe impairment of the MFR rather than a stenosis-related, downstream reduction in resting coronary flow as a major determinant of myocardial viability. This consideration also agrees with an experimental animal model of myocardial hibernation, where FDG uptake was highest in myocardial territories with MFRs of less than 1.5 [16]. Severe reductions of MFR, therefore, are an important determinant for the stimulation of an adaptive myocardial process consistent with myocardial hibernation [16]. Such an initial adaptive process, however, may ultimately advance to myocardial cell death and tissue fibrosis, if coronary flow is not restored in a timely fashion [17–19].

Stunned and/or hibernating myocardium may completely or partially recover its function again in a substantial number of patients, in whom coronary flow is restored by interventional or surgical revascularization as evidenced by numerous clinical investigations [9, 10, 20, 21]. Imaging of this so-called "hibernating-stunning" or ischemically compromised but viable and dysfunctional myocardium has evolved as a critical step of the clinical assessment of ischemic heart failure patients

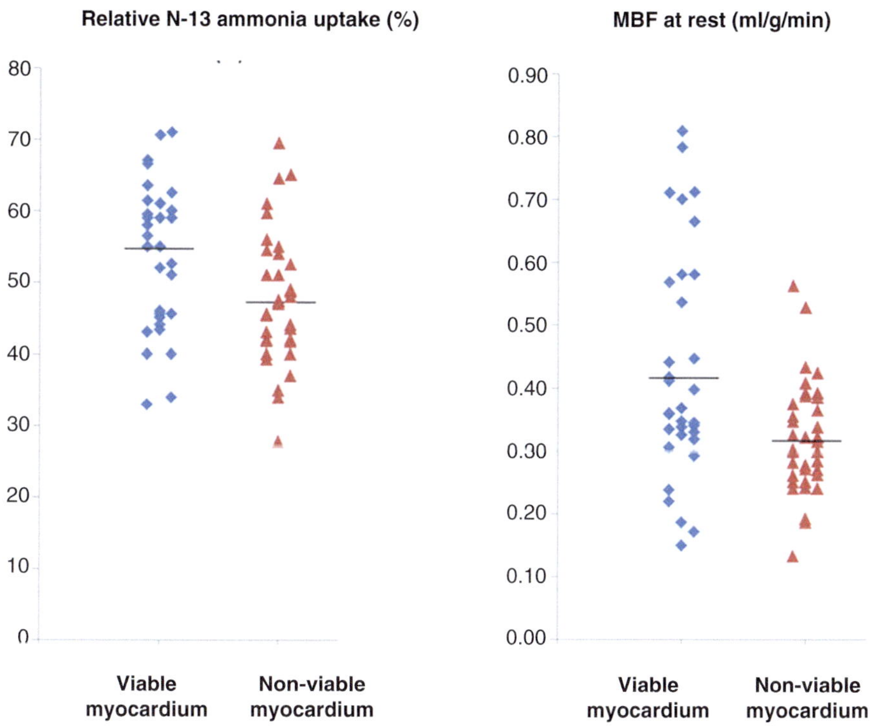

Fig. 6.2 Perfusion and myocardial blood flow (MBF) in viable and nonviable myocardium. Relative reductions in perfusion and MBF at rest in viable myocardial regions and nonviable myocardial regions. Of note, a considerable overlap of flow values between the two kinds of regions (With kind permission from Ref [15])

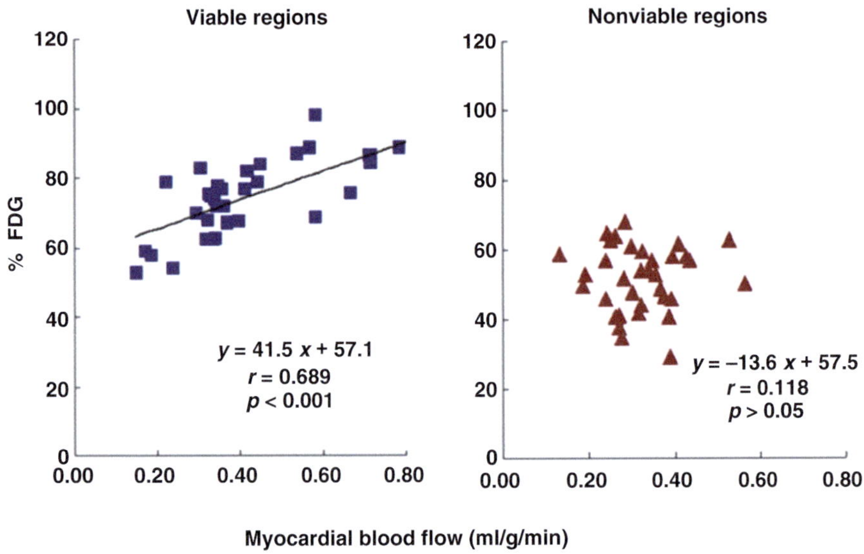

Fig. 6.3 Relative FDG uptake in comparison to regional myocardial blood flow (*MBF*) at rest (% FDG, relative regional FDG uptake). A coupling between FDG uptake and MBF can be appreciated in viable regions, while this is not the case for nonviable regions (With kind permission from Ref. [15])

[22–25]. In this respect, "myocardial viability" *is commonly referred to as impairment in regional myocardial contractile function (akinesia or dyskinesia) that is potentially reversible if revascularized* [26–28]. Although there is a variety of nuclear cardiology techniques for the detection of myocardial viability in ischemic heart failure patients, such as ^{201}thallium (^{210}TI) imaging using a rest-redistribution or stress-rest-reinjection protocols [29], rest-redistribution ^{201}TI imaging as part of a dual-isotope protocol with a technetium-99m perfusion tracer [30], or imaging with a technetium-^{99}m tracer at rest after the administration of nitroglycerin [31], fluorine-18-labeled fluorodeoxyglucose (FDG)-PET has evolved as the standard of reference for the identification of viable myocardium in patients with ischemic cardiomyopathy [6, 21, 28]. Employing FDG-PET for the detection of viable myocardium in cardiomyopathy patients, the mean sensitivity and specificity are reported to be 92 and 63 %, respectively [28, 32]. Viable and ischemic jeopardized myocardium, however, is preferentially identified with PET alone or in concert with SPECT perfusion imaging [21, 28]. The concurrent assessment of myocardial perfusion and viability affords the identification of a "match" (nonviable myocardium: reduced blood flow with concurrent reduction in glucose utilization) and "mismatch" (viable myocardium: reduced blood flow combined with enhanced glucose utilization) patterns (Fig. 6.5a, b) [33]. The latter perfusion-viability "mismatch" pattern is commonly regarded as the hallmark of myocardial hibernation [10, 34].

A pooled analysis of 17 investigations (including SPECT perfusion and FDG-PET) signified an increased diagnostic performance with a positive predictive value of 76 % (range 52–100) and a negative predictive value of 82 %

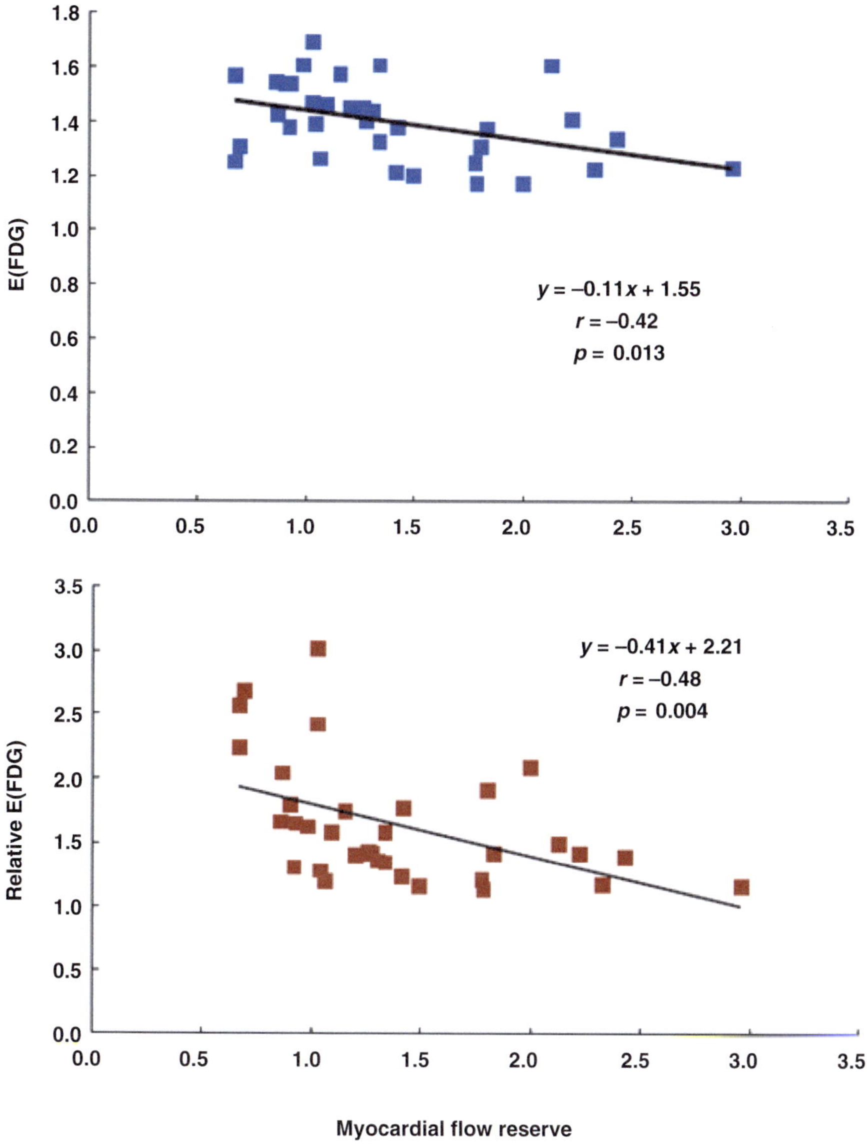

Fig. 6.4 Relationship between myocardial flow reserve (*MFR*) and extraction of FDG in viable regions. E(FDG), index of the regional FDG extraction as the ratio of relative FDG over relative 13N-ammonia tissue concentrations; relative E(FDG) as shown on the ordinate of the figure, FDG extraction in viable myocardium normalized to E(FDG) in remote myocardium. As it can be appreciated, there is an inverse relationship between extraction of FDG and MFR in areas of viable myocardium (With kind permission from Ref. [15])

(range 67–100 %) [32, 35]. The presence and extent of myocardial viability with FDG-PET have been closely related to various clinical outcome parameters [6, 21].

In the clinical scenario, cardiac FDG-PET, or nowadays PET/CT, should be applied in cardiomyopathy patients with a LVEF ≤35 %, who present a stress-rest fixed perfusion defect of ≥4 and akinetic segments of the left ventricle as

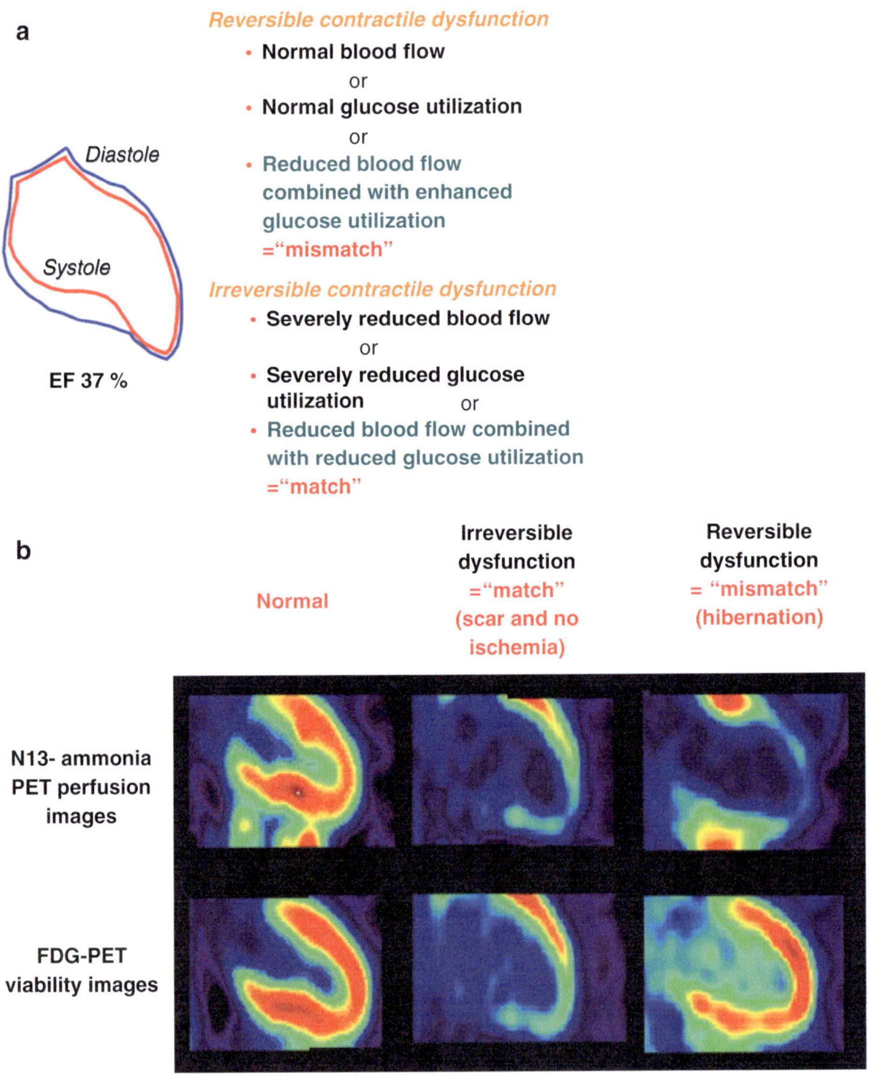

Fig. 6.5 (**a**) Contractile function, flow, and FDG (glucose) uptake. Reversible and irreversible contractile dysfunction in akinetic myocardial segments as defined by SPECT and/or PET assessment of myocardial perfusion and metabolism. (**b**) Reversible and irreversible contractile function. Examples of normal perfusion and FDG uptake (*left panel*), "match" finding with concordant reduction in perfusion and metabolism in the anteroapical and inferior wall, indicative of non-transmural and transmural scar without ischemia (*middle panel*), and "mismatch" finding with reduced resting perfusion anteroapical, apical, and inferoapical and preserved metabolism, suggestive of classical hibernating myocardium (With kind permission from Ref. [33])

determined with SPECT or PET/CT perfusion imaging. Adding FDG-PET/CT may unmask the following four conditions divided into two groups such as:

"Match" findings between perfusion and viability assessment, indicative for:

(a) Transmural necrosis
(b) Non-transmural necrosis and no ischemic component

Or "*mismatch*" findings, denoting:

(c) Non-transmural necrosis with viable but ischemic compromised myocardium
(d) Complete viable and ischemic compromised myocardium

In about 20–40 % of these patients [32, 36], FDG-PET/CT is likely to detect sufficient amount of viable myocardium unmasking viable but ischemic compromised myocardium (c and d). This so-called hibernating-stunning myocardium, if large enough (≥4 segments), principally may benefit from restoration of myocardial flow or perfusion in terms of recovery of left-ventricular function and clinical outcome (Fig. 6.6a–c) [6, 23, 32]. If such patient presents also suitable coronary anatomy and clinical condition, he is commonly referred for coronary revascularization (Fig. 6.7). Conversely, in the absence of hibernating-stunning myocardium, the patient will undergo optimal medical heart failure treatment. If over time, however, a further worsening of left-ventricular function despite optimal medical heart failure treatment ensues, heart transplantation may be considered.

Regarding the functional recovery of ischemic compromised myocardium in heart failure patients, observational investigations have demonstrated an improvement of regional and global left-ventricular ejection fraction (LVEF) after successful revascularization of viable myocardial segments as identified by FDG-PET [10, 21, 32, 37, 38]. In particular, the preoperative extent of a flow-metabolism mismatch was closely related to the magnitude of improvement in post-revascularization heart failure symptoms ($r=0.65$, $p<0.001$) (Fig. 6.8) [38].

Receiver operating curve (ROC) analysis signified that a viability extent of ≥18 %, associated with a sensitivity of 76 % and a specificity of 78 %, had the greatest clinical benefit in improvement of functional status [38]. While the minimum required amount of viable myocardium necessary for a functional recovery after coronary revascularization remains controversial [6], the term "functionally" significant amount of viable myocardium commonly signifies more than 20 % (≥4 out of 17 segments) of the left ventricle. This amount of viable but ischemic jeopardized myocardium is commonly regarded as "functionally" significant, which may recover contractile function after restoration of coronary blood flow [39]. When applying this threshold of 20 % of viable myocardium, functionally significant viability can be anticipated in 25 % of patients with ischemic CMP, who might benefit from coronary revascularization [36]. Apart that restoration of coronary flow to areas of a sufficient amount viable myocardium may improve regional left-ventricular function in areas, it also beneficially affects the remodeling process of the left ventricle [6, 17, 28].

Conversely, when dysfunctional but viable myocardium of less than 20 % of the left-ventricular myocardium is identified, then coronary revascularization may still lead to a significant improvement in clinical outcome or prognosis in these ischemic cardiomyopathy patients, while functional recovery is less likely [23]. As reported in two prospective trials [39, 40], even in the presence of a minimum of only 5 or 7.6 % of viable myocardium, respectively, an improved clinical outcome after revascularization may ensue. This is in agreement with a more recently *post hoc analysis* of the prospective randomized trial, PET and

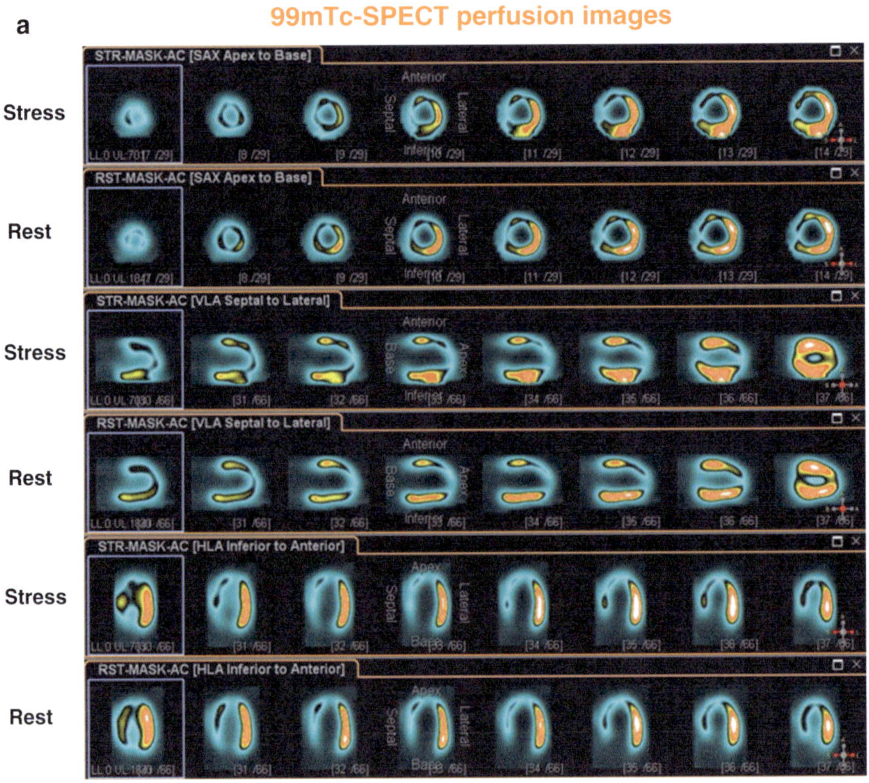

Fig. 6.6 ^{99m}Tc-SPECT/CT perfusion images in a 56-year-old man presenting with recent non-ST-elevation myocardial infarction and stable coronary artery disease. Short, vertical, and horizontal long axis demonstrate a widely fixed and extended perfusion defect in the anterior, septal, apical, and infero-septal wall (**a**), corresponding polar map and three-dimensional display of ^{99m}Tc-SPECT/CT perfusion images (**b**), with a "mismatch" (widely preserved although diminished FDG uptake on PET/CT images) (**c**), consistent with hibernating myocardium in the LAD and RCA territory. Invasive coronary angiography demonstrated two proximal LAD lesions with ≈ 90 %, LCx with ≈ 40–50 %, and RCA with ≈ 90 % stenosis diameter. The patient underwent a percutaneous coronary intervention with dilation of stenosis and stent implantation in LAD and RCA lesions. Echocardiographic follow-up examination after 3 months demonstrated a marked improvement of global left-ventricular ejection fraction from 25 to 40 % (*^{99m}Tc* technetium-99, *CT* computed tomography, *FDG*, fluorine-18-labeled fluorodeoxyglucose, *LCx* left circumflex coronary artery, *LAD* left anterior descending coronary artery, *PET* positron emission tomography, *RCA* right coronary artery, *SPECT* single-photon emission computed tomography) (With kind permission from Ref. [33])

b **Polar map and 3D display**

Stress

Rest

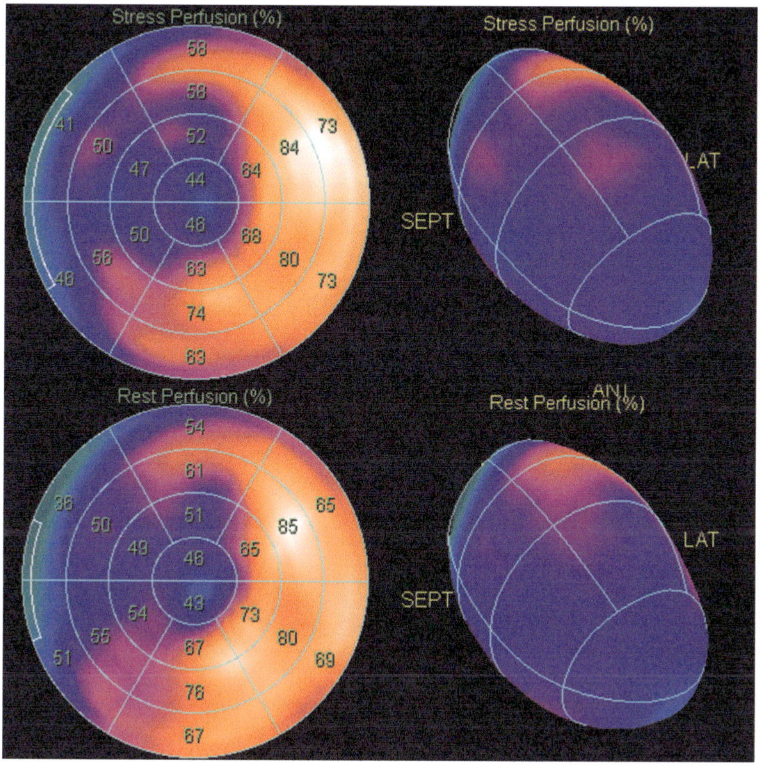

c **Display of FDG-PET/CT Images**

Vertical long axis

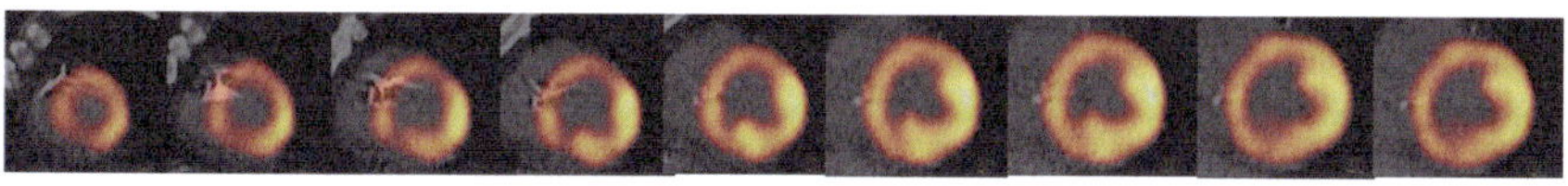

Short axis

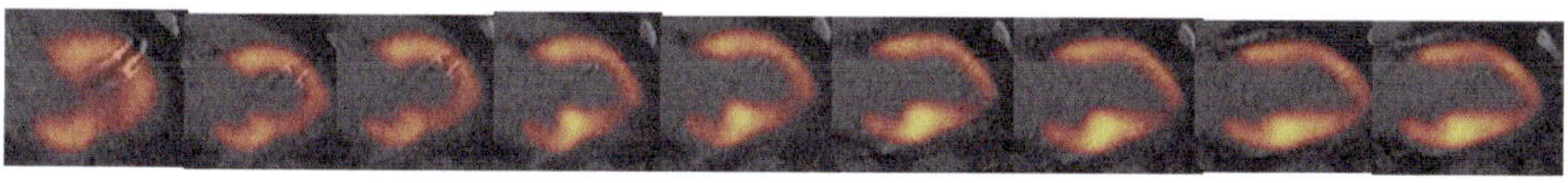

Horizontal long axis

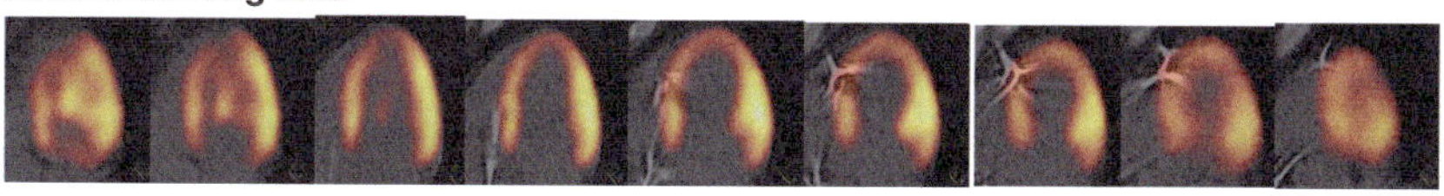

Fig. 6.6 (continued)

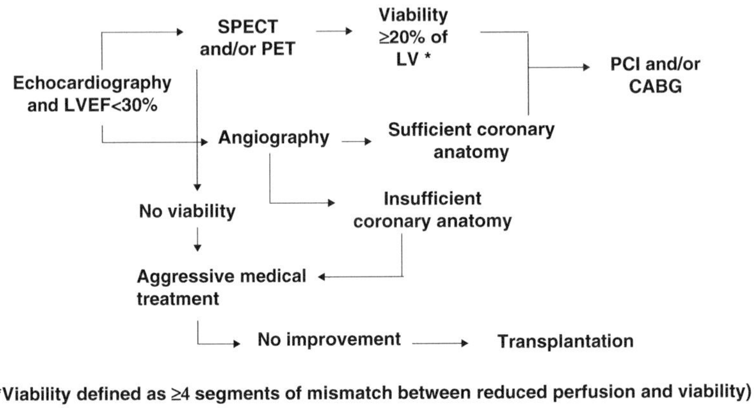

Fig. 6.7 Algorithm to stratify patients with ischemic cardiomyopathy for treatment options. Diagnostic and decision-making process in patients with ischemic cardiomyopathy. (*CABG* coronary artery bypass grafting, *LV* left ventricle, *LVEF* left-ventricular ejection fraction, *PCI* percutaneous coronary intervention, *PET* positron emission tomography, *SPECT* single-photon emission computed tomography) (With kind permission from Ref. [33])

Fig. 6.8 Relationship between the extent of a blood flow-metabolism "mismatch" by PET and the change in the left-ventricular ejection fraction (*LVEF*) after coronary revascularization. As it can be appreciated the extent of the blood flow-metabolism mismatch is paralleled by the increase in LVEF after revascularization (With kind permission from Ref. [38])

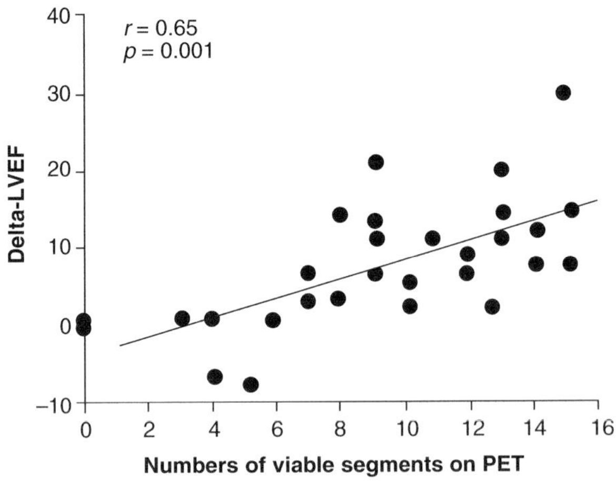

Recovery Following Revascularization-2 (PARR-2) trial. It was reported [41] that a cutoff of ≥ 7 % perfusion-viability mismatch indicated that ischemic cardiomyopathy patients would benefit from coronary revascularization at least prognostically.

Since most clinical investigations assessing the association between revascularization of viable myocardium and improvement in left-ventricular function, symptoms and prognosis in ischemic cardiomyopathy patients were performed prospectively in an observational fashion or in a retrospective analysis, a certain evaluation bias may apply. Notably, it is likely that the decision-making process to perform coronary artery bypass grafting (CABG) and/or percutaneous intervention (PCI) was driven by the results of imaging testing to identify viable myocardium. Further it remains uncertain whether adjustment for pivotal baseline variables was appropriate and whether patients who were not referred for CABG received adequate medical therapy for heart failure. To address these issues, the Canadian PARR-2 trial was conducted in a randomized, controlled design in order to evaluate whether the use of FDG-PET in the clinical decision-making process manifested in a better clinical outcome as compared to standard care where PET was not available [42]. In this multicenter trial, patients with a LVEF ≤35 % and suspected ischemic heart disease, who were being considered for coronary revascularization, transplantation, or heart failure work-up, were included for study purpose. In the FDG-PET arm of this trial, the extent and severity of scar and viable but ischemic compromised myocardium were assessed and evaluated in the context of a previously derived model in the prediction of left-ventricular recovery after revascularization. Employing the results of this model and the interpretation of PET images, the physician and surgeon decided on whether or not to proceed with coronary revascularization procedures. Interestingly, there was a trend for improved clinical outcome and survival using the PET strategy as compared with standard care, but it did not reach statistical significance between the two groups (Figs. 6.9 and 6.10).

When performing a *post hoc analysis* that compared those that adhered to PET recommendations (ADHERE arm), a significantly improved outcome in the PET-guided group than in the one with standard care was noted (Fig. 6.11) [43].

Additionally, it was appreciated that there was a benefit of outcome in experienced centers, in which FDG-PET was routinely used for the decision-making process as regards coronary revascularization or optimal medical treatment of heart failure alone in ischemic cardiomyopathy patients [41]. Taken together, the results of the PARR-2 trial, its sub-studies, and previous observational outcome data support the utility of FDG-PET with the "match" and "mismatch" concept between myocardial perfusion and viability in the identification of high-risk ischemic cardiomyopathy patients, who may benefit from coronary revascularization in terms of recovery of left-ventricular function, associated with improved exercise capacity and reduced symptoms, and clinical outcome.

6.2 Considerations to STICH Trial

More recently, the STICH (Surgical Treatment for Ischemic Heart Failure) trial [44] was performed in a randomized and blinded fashion evaluating whether the proof of viable myocardium as determined with single-photon-emission computed tomography (SPECT), dobutamine echocardiography, or both and restoration of coronary flow improved clinical outcome [44]. Overall, 1,212 ischemic heart failure patients were randomly assigned to receive medical therapy alone or medical therapy plus CABG. In 601 of these patients, information on myocardial viability was available [44]. At first sight, the presence of viable myocardium was associated with a greater likelihood of survival in patients with CAD and

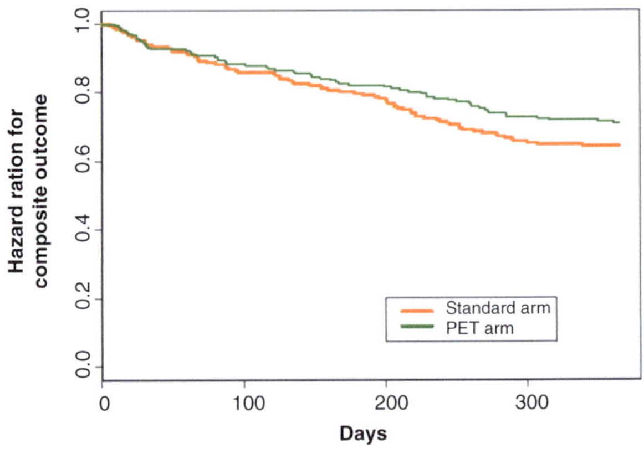

Fig. 6.9 "Survival Curves" (on the Basis of Time to First Occurring Outcome of the Composite Event). Mantel-Haenszel (log-rank) test for differences between 2 survival curves; chi-square =2.1, hazard ratio=0.78, 95 % CI 0.58–1.1, p=0.15 (With kind permission from Ref. [42])

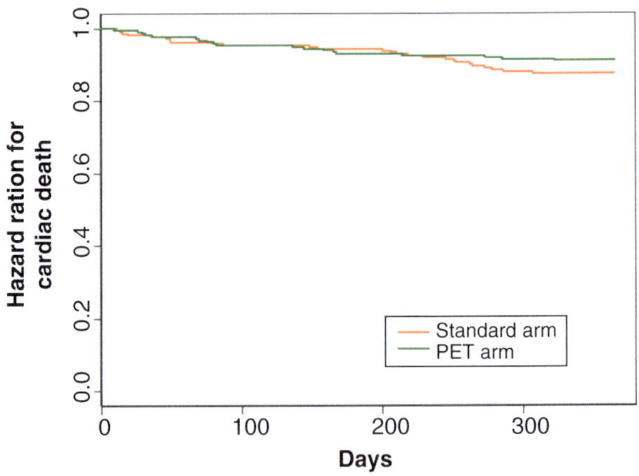

Fig. 6.10 "Survival" Curves (on the Basis of Time to Cardiac Death) for All Individuals. Mantel-Haenszel (log-rank) test for differences between 2 survival curves; chi-square=1.3, hazard ratio=0.72, 95 % CI 0.4–1.3, p=0.25 (With kind permission from Ref. [42])

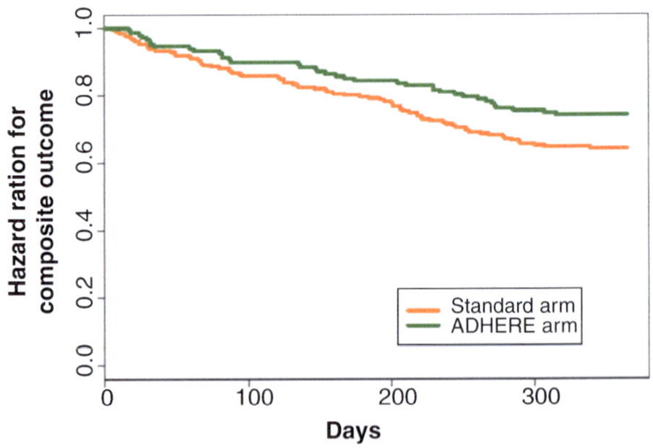

Fig. 6.11 Survival Curves (on the Basis of Time to First Occurring Outcome Out of the Composite Event). The positron emission tomography adherence group versus standard care arm. Mantel-Haenszel (log-rank) test for differences between 2 survival curves; adjusted hazard ratio=0.62, 95 % CI 0.42–0.93, p=0.019 (With kind permission from Ref. [42])

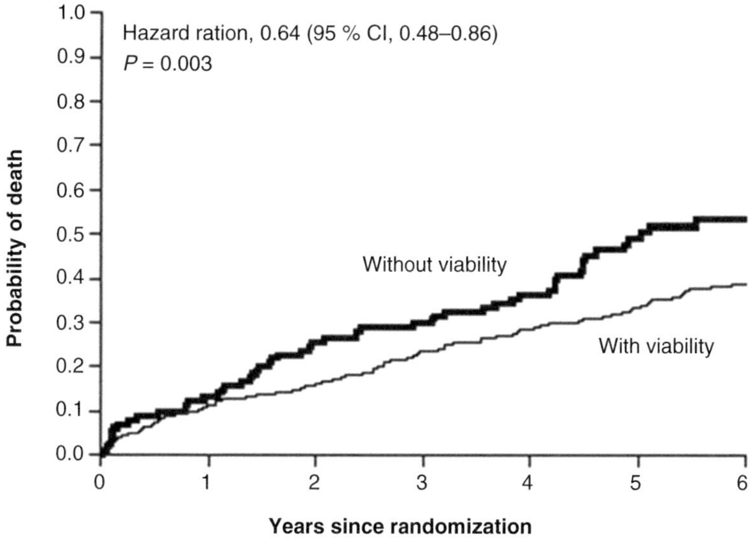

No. at Risk							
Without viability	114	99	85	80	63	36	16
With viability	487	432	409	371	294	188	102

Fig. 6.12 Myocardial Viability and Survival in Ischemic Left-Ventricular Function, the STICH trial. Kaplan-Meier analysis of the probability of death according to the viability status. Comparison not adjusted for other prognostic baseline variables (With kind permission from Ref. [44])

left-ventricular dysfunction (Fig. 6.12). Yet, this relationship did not hold any more after adjustment for other baseline clinical variables (Fig. 6.13). Unexpectedly, the assessment of myocardial viability with SPECT or dobutamine echocardiography did not prove to be superior in identifying those patients who are likely to benefit in respect to survival from CABG as compared to those who received optimal with medical therapy alone [44].

There are certain limitations of the STICH trial worthy of considerations. Patients in the STICH trial had all CAD that was amenable to CABG. Consequently, subgroup analysis of the STICH trial assumes that patients could have been referred either for CABG or medical therapy alone. Given this assumption, many patients with CAD and severely reduced left-ventricular function were not included for study purpose. For example, CAD patients in whom CABG is commonly advised, such as patients with significant left main stem stenosis and/or with severe angina symptoms, were not enrolled. Conversely, patients in whom CABG is commonly denied due to a very high risk of cardiac surgery, limited functional capacity, or reduced likelihood of survival were also not part of the study trial. Another study bias may be seen in a substantial number of patient's crossing over from medical therapy to CABG due to instability (angina symptoms, cardiac decompensation) in the first year after enrollment. In a post hoc subanalysis, it was appreciated that these patients with ischemic

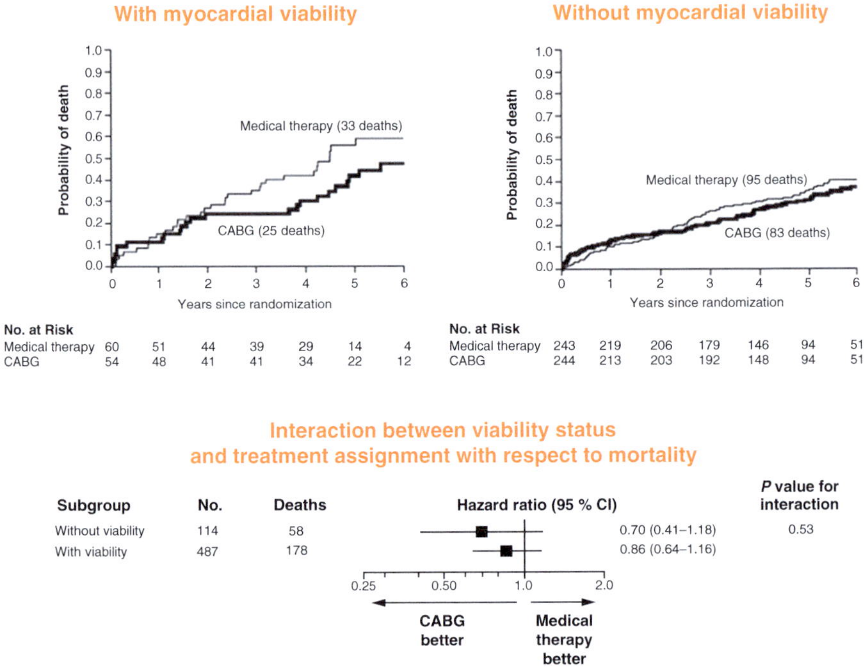

Fig. 6.13 Myocardial Viability and STICH. Kaplan-Meier analysis of survival after adjustment for other prognostic baseline variables such as LVEF, NYHA classification, and renal insufficiency, number of diseased vessels, previous revascularization, and previous myocardial infarction (With kind permission from Ref. [44])

cardiomyopathy, who crossed over to CABG, had a far better outcome than those who had medical therapy alone [45]. Importantly, the observed difference favoring CABG in this subpopulation with clinical instability was independent of the baseline risk of the individual patient. Conversely, there are also a certain number of patients foreseen for CABG that crossed over to medical therapy alone due to patient or family preferences. This may also have confounded the outcome data.

The findings of the STICH trial, however, contrast previous observational investigations or retrospective data analysis in the assessment of myocardial viability in ischemic heart failure patients [6, 9, 10, 21] and thus were not anticipated by many clinicians, which have issued considerable comments and criticism [46–48]. Several factors while several factors, however, may reconcile, at least in part, this controversy in viability assessment, treatment, and clinical outcome of ischemic cardiomyopathy patients, such as (1) the timing of coronary revascularization, (2) absence or presence of ischemic compromised but viable myocardium, (3) stage of myocardial remodeling process, (4) ischemic conditioning, and (5) suboptimal imaging protocols and techniques to determine the presence or absence of ischemic jeopardized but viable myocardium (Table 6.1).

Table 6.1 Factors potentially affecting the effect of flow restoration on viable but dysfunctional myocardium

1. Timing of coronary revascularization
2. Extent and severity of myocardial ischemia in dysfunctional but viable myocardium
3. Myocardial remodeling
4. Left-ventricular dilation

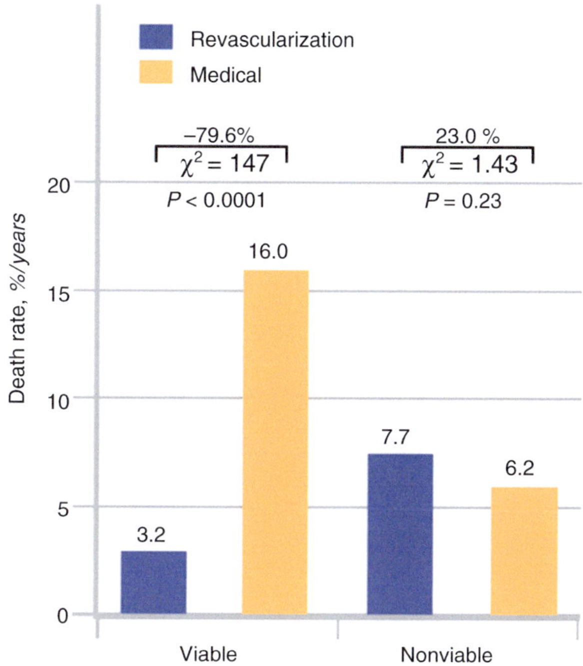

Fig. 6.14 Meta-analysis of pooled data from 24 viability studies. Death rates for patients with and without myocardial viability treated by revascularization or medical therapy (With kind permission from Ref. [21])

6.3 Timing of Coronary Revascularization

A meta-analysis performed by Allman et al. [21] pooled data from 24 viability studies as determined with ^{201}TI-SPECT imaging, FDG-PET, or dobutamine echocardiography. A total of 3,088 cardiomyopathy patients with a mean LVEF of 32 ± 8 % were followed-up for 25 ± 10 months. In patients with defined myocardial viability, annual mortality rate was 16 % in medically treated patients while only 3.2 % in revascularized patients (Fig. 6.14). This again represents 79.6 % relative reduction in risk of death for revascularized patients (Fig. 6.14). Conversely, for patients without proof of viability, annual mortality was not significantly different between the groups with coronary revascularization as compared to those with medical treatment alone (7.7 % versus 6.2 %). Timely revascularization of viable and ischemic compromised myocardium commonly manifests in an improvement in left-ventricular function and prognosis of the patient, which, however, may be less favorable if coronary revascularization is delayed.

Addressing this issue, Tarakji et al. [49] analyzed the survival of 765 consecutive patients (age 64 ± 11 years) with advanced left-ventricular dysfunction (LVEF ≤35 %), who underwent FDG-PET viability study and coronary revascularization over a 5-year follow-up (1997–2002). Early intervention was defined as any cardiac intervention (surgical or percutaneous) within the first 6 months of the PET-FDG study. In the entire study population, 30 % patients ($n = 230$) underwent early intervention, 25 % ($n = 188$) had coronary artery bypass grafting, and 5 % ($n = 42$) had percutaneous revascularization, while 70 % ($n = 535$) were treated medically. Using 39 demographic and FDG-PET variables, 153 of the 230 patients were propensity matched with 153 patients without early coronary revascularization. And indeed, early revascularization was associated with a markedly lower risk of death (3-year mortality rate of 15 % versus 35 %, propensity adjusted hazard ratio 0.52 (95 % CI 0.33–0.81, $p = 0.0004$)) (Fig. 6.15). Interestingly, there was no apparent interaction between survival benefit associated with early cardiac intervention and the amount of viable tissue (ischemic and hibernating tissue) identified by PET.

The exact mechanisms by which early coronary revascularization (<6 months) improved the clinical outcome remain uncertain but may be related to reductions in myocardial ischemia, improved myocardial function, regression of hypertrophy, beneficial effects on myocardial remodeling, and stabilization of arrhythmic substrate. Notably, there was no survival difference until 5–6 months of follow-up, which may be related to a relatively high mortality associated with periprocedural complications among those who underwent surgical intervention. These observations also concur with findings reported from Bax et al. [20] investigating whether a

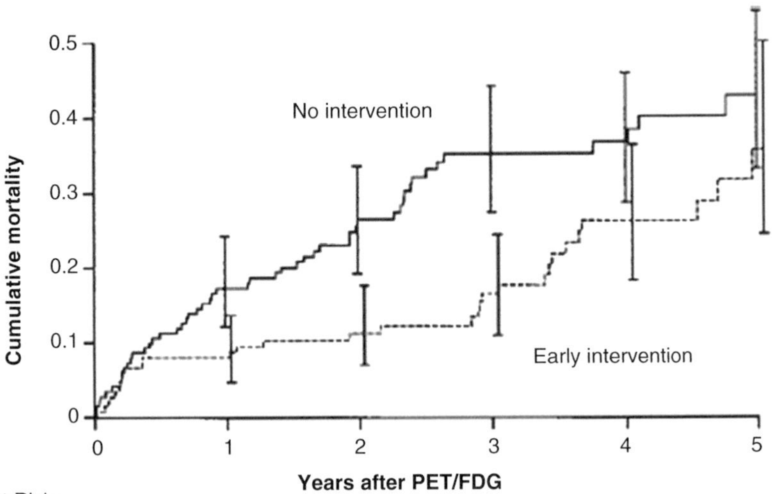

Number at Risk:						
No Intervention	153	125	85	58	38	19
Intervention	153	135	92	75	41	16

Fig. 6.15 Myocardial viability and early revascularization. Propensity-matched patients. Mortality curves of patients treated medically (no intervention) and patients undergoing early intervention (With kind permission from Ref. [49])

delayed coronary revascularization of viable myocardium in ischemic cardiomyopathy patients, as determined with on low-dose dobutamine stress echocardiography (DSE), may less favorably impact clinical outcome. On echocardiography, segmental wall motion was scored according to a 5-point scale: 1 = normal, 2 = mildly hypokinetic, 3 = severely hypokinetic, 4 = akinetic, and 5 = dyskinetic. Subsequently, severely dysfunctional segments (score 3 or more) were evaluated for the presence of viability. The four patterns that were observed in dysfunctional segments during DSE included (1) biphasic response (improvement of wall motion during low dose (5 and 10 μg/kg/min), followed by worsening of wall motion during high-dose dobutamine), (2) sustained improvement (improvement during low- and/or high-dose dobutamine without subsequent deterioration of wall motion), (3) worsening (immediate deterioration of wall motion during dobutamine infusion), and (4) no change (no change in wall motion during DSE). Dysfunctional segments were classified viable when they exhibited any of the patterns except for the "no change" pattern. A patient was considered to have substantial viability in the presence of four or more dysfunctional but viable segments (≥25 % of the left ventricle). Applying these criteria, 85 patients with ischemic cardiomyopathy and substantial viability (≥25 % of the left ventricle) on low-dose dobutamine stress echocardiography were identified as suitable candidates for surgical coronary revascularization. Based on the waiting time for revascularization, patients were divided into two groups: early (≤1 month) and late (>1 month) revascularization. LVEF was assessed before and 9–12 months after revascularization, while follow-up data were acquired up to 2 years after revascularization. As expected [21], early revascularization (20 ± 12 days) of viable myocardium in these patients conferred a high likelihood of an improvement in LVEF (from 28 ± 9 % to 40 ± 12 %) (Fig. 6.16a). Conversely, when coronary revascularization was relatively delayed (85 ± 47 days) in these patients, LVEF virtually remained unchanged (27 ± 10 % to 25 ± 7 %). Notably, delayed coronary revascularization in these patients was associated with a substantial higher mortality rate than in those patients referred for early revascularization of viable myocardium (20 % versus 5 %) (Fig. 6.16b) [20]. As regards the rehospitalization rate for heart failure, it was less in the early – than in the delayed revascularization group (10 % versus 24 %) – although it did not achieve statistical significance (Fig. 6.16b).

Of course, someone may argue that these striking differences of recovery in left-ventricular function and clinical outcome between early and delayed coronary revascularization, respectively, may have been related to the selection criteria in DSE for defining myocardial viability according to the low-dose dobutamine stimulation of contractile function in viable areas. Beanlands et al. [22], therefore, investigated the use of FDG-PET in the assessment of myocardial viability for preoperative risk evaluation. Based on FDG-PET viability imaging, 46 patients with ischemic cardiomyopathy patients and a LVEF of ≤35 % were considered candidates for revascularization, while 35 of these were referred for surgical intervention. According to the median waiting time, patients were divided into two groups: an early group (<35 days; $n = 18$) and a late group (≥35 days; $n = 17$) comparable to the echocardiographic investigation [20]. Preoperative mortality rates were significantly higher in the late than in the early group of revascularization (4 of 17 [24 %]

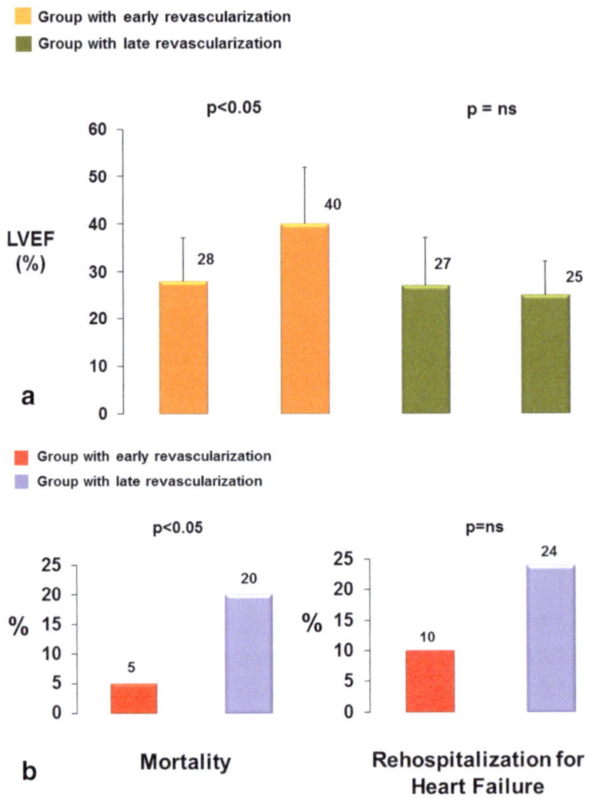

Fig. 6.16 Timing of revascularization, functional recovery, and clinical outcome. Impact of early and late revascularization on left-ventricular ejection fraction (*LVEF*) (**a**) and on mortality and rehospitalization rate, respectively (**b**) (With kind permission from Ref. [20])

versus 0 of 18). During postoperative follow-up (17 ± 7 months), cardiac events were nonsignificantly higher 11 % (2/18) versus 7.8 % (1/13) in the early than in the late group. Conversely, LVEF increased significantly after early revascularization (24 ± 7 % to 29 ± 8 %, $p < 0.001$, baseline versus 3 months) but not in the late group (27 ± 5 % to 28 ± 6 %, $p = \text{ns}$). Preoperative FDG-PET-determined myocardial viability therefore may identify a high-risk group of patients who may benefit from early revascularization. As current available evidence suggests [20, 22, 49], a long waiting time for coronary revascularization of viable myocardium may be associated with a relatively high mortality rate, which favors an early revascularization of hibernating-stunning myocardium, if clinically feasible. Such observations may give rise to a dilemma for the cardiovascular surgeon, who may prefer to perform a CABG as late as possible in order to find optimal heart conditions associated with lower periprocedural and postoperative morbidity and mortality rate [50], which however may be at the expense of a lower gain in left-ventricular function, improved clinical outcome, and prognosis but needing further investigations.

In view of these clinical observations [20, 22, 49], the less impressive findings of the PARR-2 and STICH trial may not be so unexpected [42, 44]. In these two randomized viability and revascularization trials, patients with acute coronary syndrome (ACS) within 4 weeks or 3 months, respectively, were not included for study purpose. The targeted study populations comprised patients with stable and mostly known ischemic cardiomyopathy. For example, in both the PARR-2 and STICH trial, 80 % of heart failure patients had had previous myocardial infarction, while all patients presented different stages of angina symptoms or dyspnea according to the Canadian Cardiovascular Society Angina and NYHA classification, respectively. Most of these patients therefore can be assumed to have had already relatively long-standing ischemic heart disease with advanced cardiac remodeling and interstitial fibrosis [17, 18, 51], which may have prevented or impaired the recovery of left-ventricular function and improvement in cardiovascular prognosis after delayed rather than early CABG. Furthermore, in both the PARR-2 and STICH trial, no detailed information on the time interval between viability assessment and coronary revascularization is provided, respectively. As regards the STICH trial [44], ischemic cardiomyopathy patients were recruited for study analysis if a viability study had been done within 90 days. This again would suggest that also cardiomyopathy patients were included, in whom viability assessment was done 2–3 months before coronary revascularization. Thus, coronary revascularization was rather performed in a delayed fashion lowering the likelihood of functional recovery of viable myocardium and improvement in clinical outcome in these cardiomyopathy patients. Considering this, it may be no surprise that both the PARR-2 and STICH trial [42, 44] did not report a significant reduction in cardiac events in patients with ischemic left-ventricular dysfunction, when viability assessment with various imaging techniques was compared to standard medical care of heart failure, as coronary revascularization was delayed. Thus, the failure of viability assessment to identify those patients with a survival benefit from interventional or surgical revascularization procedures as compared to medical treatment of heart failure in two randomized trials [42, 44] is likely to be related, at least in part, to a relatively delayed coronary revascularization in ischemic cardiomyopathy patients as several investigations suggest [20, 49, 52].

6.4 Extent and Severity of Myocardial Ischemia

As regards the STICH trial, the extent of viable but ischemic jeopardized dysfunctional (hibernating) myocardium is not known [44]. Thus, it is equally possible that a certain percentage of patients with prove of ≥11 viable myocardial segments did not have or have only mildly ischemic compromised myocardium at rest and stress (fixed perfusion defect), so-called "hibernating-stunning" myocardium as evidenced by "mismatch" findings between myocardial perfusion and viability assessment with FDG-PET (Fig. 6.6) [10]. Rest and/or stress-induced myocardial ischemia may be prevented or significantly diminished by the induction of collaterals through a myocardial hypoxic stimulus in patients with chronic ischemic cardiomyopathy, which strives to balance reduced flows during times of increased metabolic demand in myocardial regions subtended by high-grade epicardial narrowing or even occluded vessels [53–55]. It also must be considered that any medical therapy which aims and improves the vasodilator capacity of the coronary circulation, such as

HMG-CoA reductase or angiotensin-converting enzyme inhibitors, may in fact prevent or reduce clinically manifest myocardial ischemia in patients with CAD [56]. In some instances, even the absence of myocardial ischemia in patients having suffered non-transmural myocardial infarction in a region subtended to an occluded artery may be noted. The absence of significant amount of a resting perfusion defect or myocardial ischemia in the infarcted territory due to collateral flow with residual viability subtended to an occluded artery might explain, in part, why the interventional reopening of the occluded infarct-related artery did not lead to a significant reduction in the occurrence of death, reinfarction, or hospitalization for class IV heart failure over a 3-year but also over 6-year mean follow-up compared with optimal medical therapy alone, respectively [57, 58]. Thus, it appears that in these high-risk patients with dysfunctional but viable myocardium, the extent and amount of resting perfusion defect or ischemia is critical for the prediction of recovery in left-ventricular function and improvement in clinical outcome after revascularization. This important aspect is implied in the "match" and "mismatch" concept between perfusion and viability assessment with PET as outlined before [33]. While a "match" finding signifies a concordant reduction in perfusion and metabolism without ischemic component, a "mismatch" observations denotes a more pronounced reduction in perfusion or resting ischemia in preserved areas of viable myocardium, which reflects hibernating-stunning myocardium. Only ischemic jeopardized viable or hibernating-stunning myocardium will truly benefit from coronary revascularization both functionally and prognostically (Fig. 6.17) [6, 10, 20, 21, 39, 41, 59].

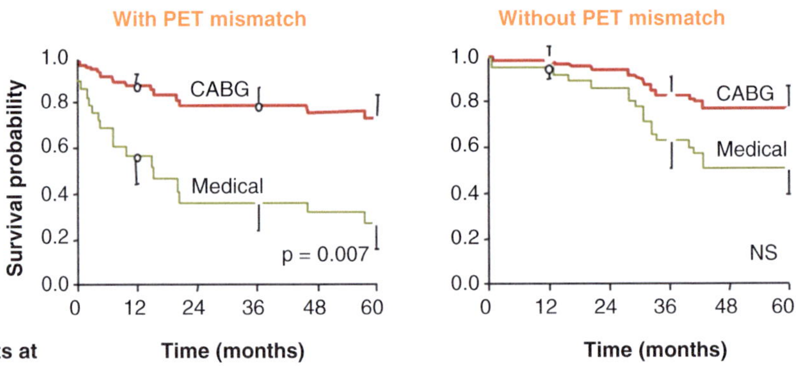

Patients at risk

	0	12	24	36	48	60	0	12	24	36	48	60
CABG	26	22	20	20	19	11	17	16	14	13	8	4
Medical	17	7	3	3	3	3	33	28	25	17	13	7

Fig. 6.17 Survival curves of ischemic cardiomyopathy patients undergoing coronary revascularization. Five-year survival data for patients with ischemic cardiomyopathy according to the proof of blood flow-metabolism mismatches and matches and according to treatment option, respectively. Note the high cardiac mortality in patients with blood flow-metabolism mismatches (*left panel*) on medical treatment and the significantly improved 5-year survival in a comparable group of patients submitted to surgical revascularization (With kind permission from Ref. [38])

This consideration also agrees with previous investigation of Beanlands et al. [60] using ^{201}TI-SPECT for the assessment of perfusion and viability in 23 patients with occluded arteries after myocardial infarction. Also here, the identification and characterization of the extent of resting perfusion defects in dysfunctional but viable myocardium with ^{201}TI myocardial scintigraphy proved to be useful to identify those patients who will most benefit from reopening of the occluded vessel [60]. As in the STICH trial only those patients without acute coronary syndrome within the last 3 months were considered for coronary revascularization, it is equally possible that a certain number of patients with demonstrated myocardial viability on SPECT images or low-dose dobutamine echocardiography did not have advanced ischemic state at rest due to the development of collateral flow and medically improved myocardial flow reserve. Coronary revascularization in these patients without or with only mildly ischemic jeopardized myocardium, therefore, may not have conferred the expected benefit in improvement of left-ventricular function and prognosis as someone might have expected.

6.5 Myocardial Remodeling

Left-ventricular remodeling is clinically characterized as alterations in volume, shape, and/or function of the heart chambers in response to chronically elevated loading conditions, which plays a central role in the clinical course and survival in cardiomyopathy patients. Catecholamine actions [3], the development of interstitial fibrosis [51], energy-depleted hibernating myocardium triggering and maintaining contractile dysfunction [17], continuous tissue degeneration and cardiomyocyte loss due to autophagic cell death and apoptosis [18], and the activation of the myocardial RAS system [5] commonly lead to a maladaptive cellular and molecular response that accompanies left-ventricular remodeling process. An extensive left-ventricular remodeling process, however, may hamper or even prevent a functional recovery of hibernating myocardium after revascularization in cardiomyopathy patients [61, 62]. For example, Bax et al. [52] evaluated 79 patients with ischemic cardiomyopathy, who were referred for surgical revascularization. It was reported that the change in LVEF after revascularization was linearly related to the baseline left-ventricular end-systolic volume (Fig. 6.18a). Higher left-ventricular end-systolic volumes were associated with a low likelihood of improvement in LVEF after revascularization. Thus, even in the presence of a sufficient amount of hibernating myocardium, as detected by a mismatch between FDG-PET and perfusion SPECT, coronary revascularization did not lead to an improvement in LVEF when baseline left-ventricular end-systolic volume was high (Fig. 6.18b) [52]. In those who did not improve LVEF, mean left-ventricular end-systolic volume was 141 ± 31 ml that was markedly increased as to those individuals with increases in LVEF after revascularization (109 ± 46 ml).

These previous observations may also be reflected, at least in part, in the STICH trial, where patients undergoing viability testing were commonly sicker than in those without testing. They had more previous myocardial infarction, a higher prevalence of atrial fibrillation and previous PCI, and, in particular, lower LVEF

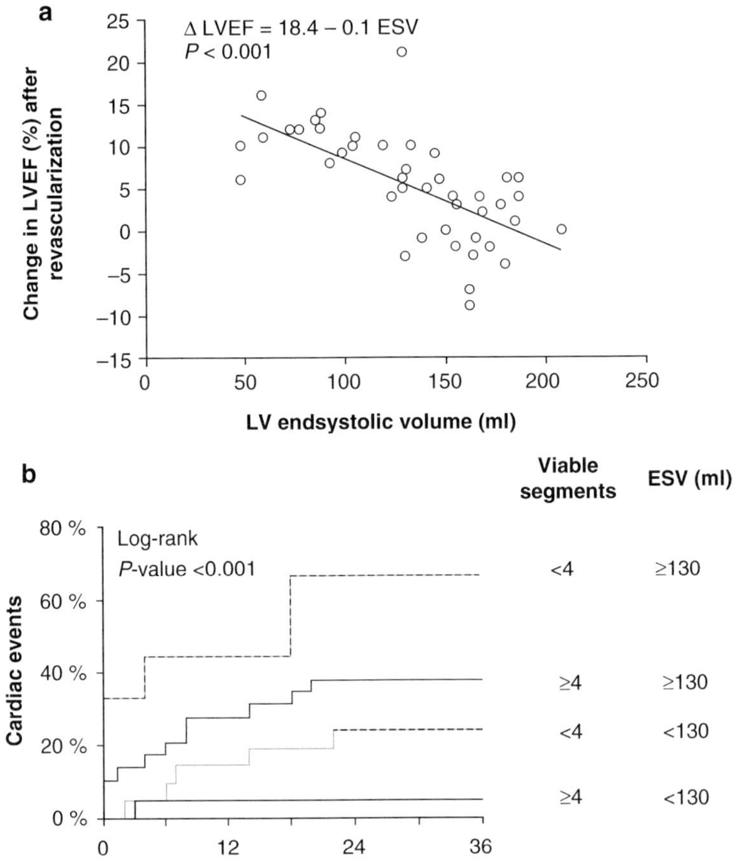

Fig. 6.18 Left-ventricular remodeling, viability, and functional recovery. Relationship between left-ventricular end-systolic volume and change in left-ventricular ejection fraction (*LVEF*) after coronary revascularization (**a**). Cardiac events (cardiac death, myocardial infarction, and hospitalization for heart failure) during 3-year follow-up of different groups according to the amount of viable myocardium and extent of left-ventricular end-systolic volume (LVESV) (**b**) (With kind permission from Ref. [52])

associated with higher LV end-diastolic volume index and LVESVI [44]. An advanced myocardial remodeling process in ischemic heart failure patients, therefore, may be appreciated as a strong negative predictor for recovery of left-ventricular function after revascularization of viable myocardium that needs to be taken into account in the clinical decision-making process.

6.6 Ischemic Conditioning

The observations of the PARR-2 and STICH trial [42, 44] may also be related in part to ischemic conditioning of the heart [63]. Causing brief episodes of ischemia and reperfusion before, during, or even after an episode of sustained and potentially life-threatening myocardial ischemia may substantially decrease myocardial injury. This phenomenon is commonly referred to as ischemic preconditioning, preconditioning, or postconditioning, respectively, depending on the timing of brief ischemic insults. Such observations were first described 1986 by Murry et al. [64]. To the author's surprise, the actual infarct size due to a 40 min occlusion of the left circumflex artery could be reduced by 75 %, if the myocardium had been exposed to four 5 min occlusion of the artery and, in addition, distributed with 5 min period of reperfusion shortly before the infarction. The short periods of ischemia and reperfusion causing the ischemic preconditioning stimulate to distinct time frames of cardioprotection. The classical ischemic preconditioning window occurs immediately after and disappears 2–3 h, while being followed by a second time period of protection that manifests 12–24 h later and may last up to 2–3 days [65]. Thus, an endogenous self-protective program exists that can be stimulated by brief periods of myocardial ischemia-reperfusion. More recently, Waltenberger et al. [66] evaluated the concept of endogenous cardioprotection by pacing postconditioning (PPC) in ST-segment elevation myocardial infarction. Thirty patients with first ST-segment elevation myocardial infarction received either PPC plus percutaneous coronary intervention (PCI) or PCI alone, respectively. PPC constituted of ten time frames of 30 s right-ventricular pacing. Following, contrast-enhanced cardiac magnetic resonance (CMR) was performed 4 days, 4 months, and 12 months after PCI in order to determine the infarct size. The evaluation of the infarct size among the two groups at different time points demonstrated a ≈ 25 % smaller infarct size in the PPC plus PCI than in PCI patients after 4 days ($p = 0.01$), 4 months ($p = 0.02$), and 1 year of PCI ($p = 0.08$). Although the initial area at risk of ischemic jeopardized myocardium due to coronary occlusion was not assessed [67] and determining the infarct size with contrast CMR after 4 days and 4 months may have resulted in a certain overestimation of the myocardial necrosis [68], current data may indeed suggest that PPC is feasible in the clinical scenario of acute myocardial infarction and may confer important cardioprotection during PCI. Conceptually, this concept of endogenous cardioprotection may also apply to hibernating myocardium, as reflected by a mismatch between PET-measured reduced myocardial perfusion at rest and viable myocardium. Hibernating myocardium per se in concert with short and recurrent episodes of stress-induced ischemia may indeed confer cardioprotective effects. The exact mechanisms underlying this endogenous cardioprotection are certainly multifactorial but may be related in part to the reperfusion injury salvage kinase (RISK) pathway [69, 70] that includes a range of antiapoptotic kinases such as Akt and the p42/p44 mitogen-activated protein kinase. Interestingly, a variety of pharmacological substances including G-protein-coupled receptor ligands such as opioids, adenosine and bradykinin; growth factors such as insulin and erythropoietin; natriuretic peptides; adipocytokines; and statins have been demonstrated to stimulate the RISK pathway. The potential role of ischemic conditioning in hibernating-stunning myocardium to confer a certain cardioprotection may be suggested in part by the PARR-2 and STICH trial [42, 44], which, however, awaits further clarification.

6.7 Suboptimal Imaging Protocols for Viability Assessment and Evaluation

Finally, the lack of the STICH trial to demonstrate a survival benefit of ischemic CMP patients with proven myocardial viability after revascularization may also be related in part to suboptimal imaging protocols and techniques to determine the presence or absence of hibernating myocardium. In the STICH trial [44], apart from low-dose dobutamine echocardiography, myocardial viability was assessed predominantly with ^{99m}-technetium (^{99m}Tc)-labeled radiotracers or ^{201}TI-SPECT. Four different SPECT protocols for determining myocardial viability were applied. These included ^{201}TI imaging using a rest-redistribution or stress-rest-reinjection protocols [29], rest-redistribution ^{201}TI imaging as part of a dual-isotope protocol with a technetium-99m perfusion tracer [30], or imaging with a technetium-^{99}m tracer at rest after the administration of nitroglycerin [31]. Based on the regional radiotracer uptake of ^{99}m-Tc or ^{201}TI on SPECT images, viability was signified in those patients demonstrating at least 11 (of 17) viable myocardial segments. A 50 % threshold of radiotracer uptake was used to define viable from nonviable myocardial segments. In addition, the extent of viable myocardium was prespecified with ≥11 viable myocardial segments in order to classify patients in a *binary* fashion as either having or not having a substantial amount of myocardial viability [44]. Such a criterion to define patients with sufficient amount of myocardial viability, however, has not been fully explored in clinical investigations. In addition, the power of SPECT using thresholds of relative radiotracer uptake or viable myocardium in the prediction of recovery of dysfunctional myocardial segments may not be high [23, 71], in particular, when the extent and severity of myocardial ischemia are unknown [21, 39]. Overall, in the STICH trial [44], it is not indicated how many patients were evaluated with echocardiography and how many with SPECT imaging. It is also unclear which specific SPECT methodology was used in how many patients. This then complicates an analysis of the limitations in the assessment of myocardial viability. Yet, assessing only resting myocardial perfusion with SPECT is not evaluating the presence of ischemic compromised but viable myocardium but rather provides information on the extent of scar tissue as there is an inverse relationship between resting myocardial blood flow and the percent scar tissue [23, 71]. As such, the approach is similar to that with late gadolinium-enhanced cardiac magnetic resonance imaging [72]. Accordingly, in the STICH trial [44], we do not know in how many of the 11 segments perfusion were entirely normal and in how many it was reduced. As it was not specified whether the 11 or more myocardial segments required for defining viability were counted only among those segments demonstrating contractile dysfunction in the sense of akinesia and/or dyskinesia or segments with evidence of normal or contractile dysfunction of any degree (hypokinesia, akinesia, and dyskinesia), it remains unknown in how many segments a wall motion abnormality was truly present.

Nuclear cardiac imaging with ^{99m}Tc or ^{201}TI and SPECT or SPECT/CT is state of the art for the detection and characterization of stress-induced myocardial ischemia and necrosis. This may result in several scenarios such as (a) normal stress-rest perfusion, (b) stress-induced ischemia without scar, (c) non-transmural scar with stress-induced periinfarction ischemia, and (d) "fixed" stress-rest perfusion defect, which may suggest transmural scar, non-transmural scar with viable but ischemic compromised myocardium, or in rare instances no scar but with resting ischemia, which does not aggravate during stress testing. The latter scenario may be observed in 20–40 % of ischemic cardiomyopathy patients with LVEF <30 % [32, 36]. Here conventional ^{99m}Tc or ^{201}TI and SPECT approach is limited and necessitates FDG-PET in order to clearly differentiate between the three different conditions in ischemic cardiomyopathy. ^{99m}Tc or ^{201}TI without reinjection protocol and SPECT in the identification of myocardial viability in dysfunctional myocardial segments therefore appears to be suboptimal in ischemic cardiomyopathy. For example, same-day rest/stress ^{99m}Tc-sestamibi SPECT imaging will incorrectly signify 36 % of myocardial regions as being irreversibly impaired and nonviable compared with both ^{201}TI redistribution/reinjection and FDG-PET as the reference standard [73]. ^{201}TI stress-rest and reinjection protocol with SPECT was also compared to FDG-PET imaging in the identification of viable myocardium [25]. In 16 patients with angiographically proven chronic multivessel CAD and left-ventricular dysfunction (LVEF: 27 ± 9 %; ranging from 16 to 47 %), ^{201}TI stress-rest and reinjection protocol with SPECT was compared with FDG-PET [25]. Most irreversible defects with only mild or moderate reduction in ^{201}TI activity reflected viable myocardium as confirmed by FDG uptake. In myocardial regions with severe irreversible ^{201}TI defects on standard exercise-redistribution ^{201}TI imaging, ^{201}TI reinjection identified as viable or nonviable segments quite similar to FDG-PET. Conversely, FDG-PET seems to outperform ^{201}TI-SPECT in the detection of viable myocardium when ^{201}TI stress image acquisition is followed by redistribution imaging after 4 and 24 h without a reinjection protocol, respectively [34]. For example, Brunken et al. [34] investigated in 26 CAD patients with impaired left-ventricular function (LVEF: 32 ± 13 %) and perfusion defects on 24 h ^{201}TI-SPECT images a potential diagnostic value of FDG-PET in viability detection. In 100 fixed, 17 partially reversible, and 12 completely reversible defects on ^{201}TI- SPECT images, PET identified tissue metabolic activity in 51 (51 %) segments with fixed defects (21 PET ischemia, 30 PET normal) and nine (53 %) segments with partially reversible defects (five PET ischemia, four PET normal). When the relative number of segments with fixed ^{201}TI defects and metabolic viability on FDG-PET were displayed as a function of the 24 h ^{201}Tl score, the relative number of segments with metabolic viability declined with increasing severity of ^{201}TI defect or increase in defect score. Conversely, even for defects with severe reductions in 24 h ^{201}TI score (2.61–3.00), there was an approximate one in seven chance that FDG-PET imaging will still identify some viable myocardium. In these ischemic cardiomyopathy patients, however, FDG-PET detected viable myocardium in the majority of fixed 24 h ^{201}TI defects, while very severe 24 h ^{201}TI defects were associated with a relatively low likelihood to demonstrate viable myocardium on FDG-PET images. Similar observations were reported by Akinboboye et al. [74], in which significant metabolic activity by PET was found in 51 % of fixed and severe defects on ^{201}TI-SPECT with various protocols. Thus, ^{201}TI-SPECT may underestimate myocardial viability relative to FDG-PET in patients with severely reduced left-ventricular dysfunction, when only 4 and 24 h redistribution ^{201}TI images without ^{201}TI reinjection protocol are evaluated [34, 74–76]. The exact cause of this underestimation of myocardial viability with ^{201}TI-SPECT on 4 or 24 h redistribution images in ischemic CMP patients remains unknown. Potential explanations include impaired sarcolemma function, attenuation of low-energy photons of ^{201}TI in dilated ventricles, and severe hypoperfusion limiting ^{201}TI delivery. From these investigations, it appears advisable that FDG-PET [34, 74–76] or ^{201}TI-SPECT with reinjection protocol [25, 29, 77, 78] should be added in the clinical evaluation of ischemic cardiomyopathy patients with persistent ^{201}TI defects on redistribution images in whom coronary revascularization is a viable option.

6.8 Role of Echocardiography in Viability Assessment

In clinical routine, a rough differentiation between viable and nonviable myocardium can be performed by assessment of left-ventricular wall thickness with echocardiography [28]. A left-ventricular end-diastolic wall thickness (EDWT) >6 mm is commonly used as threshold to indicate viable myocardium. It appears that an EDWT of less than 6 mm rarely demonstrate contractile reserve during dobutamine stress echocardiography [28]. Conversely, in myocardial segments with an EDWT equal to 6 mm, the response to dobutamine stress echocardiography may vary considerably. Approximately, 60 % of these myocardial segments were identified as viable on dobutamine stress echocardiography, while the remaining 40 % were appreciated as nonviable. Such observations put forth that myocardial segments with an EDWT of less than 6 mm may widely reflect scarred and/or fibrotic tissue less likely to improve function after coronary revascularization. In the clinical scenario, dysfunctional myocardial segments with an EDWT <6 mm may be signified as nonviable, and no further diagnostic work-up may be needed. On the other hand, myocardial segments with an EDWT ≥6 mm should be referred for dobutamine stress echocardiography to further differentiate between viable and nonviable myocardium according to the contractile reserve pattern [28, 79]. In order to measure the contractile reserve, echocardiographic images of the left-ventricle are acquired at rest and with increasing doses of dobutamine infusion starting at 5 μcg/kg body weight/min and increasing until 20 μcg/kg body weight/min for viability assessment (low-dose dobutamine) or 40 μcg/kg body weight/min (high-dose dobutamine) for concurrent ischemia identification, respectively [32]. For concurrent ischemia detection, a target heart rate of 85 % of the predicted maximal heart rate is envisioned with atropine added if necessary.

In dysfunctional regions at baseline, the response to dobutamines is defined as "biphasic" (improvement at low-dose dobutamine and worsening at peak stress), "sustained" improvement (improvement at low-dose dobutamine without further deterioration at peak stress), or "worsening" (worsening of contractile function without improvement at any stage). The biphasic response is commonly regarded as an initial inotropic response at low-dose dobutamine in the hibernating myocardial segment and a subsequent aggravation of left-ventricular function at higher doses of dobutamine owing to stress-induced myocardial ischemia or stunning [32]. Conversely, patients with a sustained contractile response can be deemed to have enough coronary flow even at very high metabolic or oxygen demand and, thus, are less likely to benefit from coronary revascularization [80]. Aggravation of left-ventricular function with dobutamine likely reflects significant scar and/or fibrosis that does not reveal contractile reserve and therefore is unlikely to regain myocardial function after revascularization.

Dobutamine stress echocardiography is a widespread imaging modality for the detection of viable myocardium in patients with ischemic cardiomyopathy. Data from a pooled analysis of 41 studies reported sensitivity and specificity for detection of myocardial viability and prediction of recovery of regional function following coronary revascularization [28]. The mean sensitivity and specificity, respectively, of 80 % and 78 %, with a positive predictive value (PPV) and negative predictive value (NPP) of 75 and 83 % were reported. In addition, data from a pooled analysis of six studies for the prediction of recovery of global left-ventricular function signified a mean sensitivity and specificity of 57 % and 73 %, respectively, with a PPV and NPV of 63 % and 68 %. As regards the prognostic value of viability assessment employing dobutamine stress echocardiography, it was investigated in 11 studies that included 1,753 ischemic cardiomyopathy patients. It was observed that patients with proof of viable myocardium had a low annual mortality rate of 3 % as compared to those with viable myocardium but without revascularization and medical treatment only with a 12 % annual mortality rate [28]. In patients without myocardial viability, the annual mortality rate was virtually the same as in those with viable myocardium and medical treatment only (12 % vs. 12 %), while an intermediate annual mortality rate of 7 % was noted in patients without viable myocardium but with coronary revascularization.

Advantages of echocardiography may be seen in its wide availability, relatively low costs, and absence of radiation burden [32]. Yet, image quality can be limited due to technically difficult and small acoustic echocardiographic window. A high degree of interobserver variability during the interpretation of stress echocardiography needs to be mentioned. For example, an interobserver agreement of <55 % has been reported for dobutamine echocardiography [81]. In addition, it was noted that a substantial number of 37 % of patients had an echocardiographic exam where three or more myocardial segments were insufficiently visualized. In this regard, the use of contrast is certainly of help to improve image quality and interobserver agreement [82]. Another problem of dobutamine stress echocardiography may be seen in the difficulty to accurately identify alterations in contractile function in the presence of severe contractile dysfunction in several segments, which is frequently the case in ischemic cardiomyopathy patients. Novel and more sophisticated echocardiographic techniques, such as contrast echocardiography, strain and strain rate imaging, and 3D contrast echocardiography, are at present under investigation, while their clinical value needs to be awaited [32, 83, 84].

6.9 Emerging Role of Cardiac MRI

Cardiac magnetic resonance imaging (MRI) is an evolving imaging modality and increasingly applied for the assessment of myocardial viability. Similarly to echocardiography, myocardial segments with an end-diastolic wall thickness less than 6 mm are commonly regarded as nonviable myocardium with scar tissue and fibrotic state. Such segments are deemed unlikely to recover contractile function after coronary revascularization. Most centers using cardiac MRI for viability assessment, however, apply late gadolinium enhancement (LGE) imaging with MRI (LGE-MRI) in order to visualize in the infarcted area, while the extent of myocardial viability is estimated by denoting the non-LGE myocardial area. Gadolinium (Gd) is a contrast agent that distributes on its first pass in the myocardium and can be used to determine myocardial perfusion at rest and during pharmacologic vasodilator stress. The first pass extraction of Gd from the intravascular into the myocardial space is reported between 20 and 40 % [85]. In myocardial territories with scar tissue and/or fibrosis, the interstitial space is enlarged, Gd may concentrate, and its washout, as compared to the normal myocardium, is delayed. Since Gd differs in its magnetic properties to the blood and myocardium, the increased Gd content in areas of scar and/or fibrosis becomes enhanced when specific T1-weighted pulse sequences are employed. This technique is a so-called delayed contrast-enhanced imaging [86]. The Gd contrast accumulates in the scar and/or fibrotic tissue, and on T1-weighted images, these myocardial regions demonstrate as hyperenhanced (bright) which are on the MR images. Late Gd imaging with MRI therefore quantifies the spatial extent of myocardial necrosis with a high diagnostic accuracy as demonstrated experimentally in a dog model [87]. Notably, the high spatial resolution of cardiac MRI (often as good as 1.5–1.5 mm in plane resolution) provides the reader with the ability to determine the transmural thickness of the scar. The advantages of Gd delayed-enhancement cardiac MRI renders it highly sensitive for the detection of very small subendocardial infarctions [88]. Due to the excellent spatial resolution, Gd delayed-enhancement cardiac MRI appears to be more sensitive in the identification of small subendocardial, necrotic areas than conventional SPECT or PET in patients with CAD and left-ventricular dysfunction [89, 90]. In clinical routine, the extent of myocardial scarring in the LV wall is commonly expressed as 1–25 %, 26–50 %, 51–75 %, and 76–100 %. In a seminal investigation, Kim et al. [72] assessed the predictive ability of transmural scar to predict recovery following coronary revascularization. As it was observed, of akinetic and dyskinetic segments with no evidence of scar, 100 % had recovery of function, similar segments with 1–25 % transmural scar showed 82 % recovery of function, segments with 26–50 % transmural scar had a 45 % recovery, segments with 51–75 % transmural scar had 7 % recovery, and similar segments with 76–100 % scar had 0 % recovery.

Conversely, the diagnostic accuracy of LGE-MRI in myocardial regions with 1–75 % transmural scar may be limited in part [91]. Wellnhofer et al. [91] investigated 29 ischemic cardiomyopathy patients employing a dual protocol with low-dose dobutamine testing and LGE-MRI. As it was observed, the evaluation of the contractile reserve response to low-dose dobutamine with MRI was superior to LGE-MRI in the prediction of functional recovery after coronary revascularization for range of transmural scar between 1 and 74 % on LGE-MRI. In addition, low-dose dobutamine and conventional LGE-MRI did not differ in predicting functional recovery in patients without evidence of scar or those with a transmural infarction ≥75 %. Overall, adding dobutamine MRI to LGE-MRI enhances the specificity of MRI from 62 to 82 % in the prediction of myocardial viability in akinetic or dyskinetic segments [32]. The lower accuracy of LGE-MRI may be related to gadolinium accumulation not only in the necrotic area but also in surrounding myocardial edema in particular in patients with acute myocardial infarction [92–95]. Such edema may last between 4 weeks and 6 months as recent investigations suggest [68]. LGE-MRI was employed in 30 patients with ST-elevation myocardial infarction (STEMI) treated by primary percutaneous coronary intervention at each of 4 time points: 12–48 h, 5–7 days, 14–17 days, and 6 months. All patients demonstrated edema at 24 h. The mean volume of edema (% left ventricle) was 37 ± 16 at 24 h, increased slightly to 39 ± 17 at 1 week, while a marked reduction to 24 ± 13 was noted after 2 weeks ($p<0.01$) (Fig. 6.19a, b). Notably, the volume of LGE at 24 h demonstrated a 50 % resolution at repeated exam at 6 months follow-up. In myocardial segments with the observed resolution in LGE after 6 months, 65 % also revealed recovery in wall motion. This is also expressed by the myocardial salvage index that markedly increased in the mean of 26 ± 21 % at 24 h to 42 ± 23 % at 6 months ($p=0.02$).

Overall, T2-weighted MRI identified that in STEMI patients, myocardial edema is maximal and constant over the first week, which provides a stable window for the retrospective evaluation of area at risk. In the acute setting of myocardial infarction, however, myocardial regions with high signal intensity in LGE images may resolve over time paralleled with corresponding recovery in regional function. These observations signify that acutely detected LGE does not necessarily reflect irreversible injury and may substantially underestimate salvaged myocardium. Although T2-weighted MRI images may clearly denote periinfarction edema, the subtraction T2-weighted (edema) from T1-weighted (necrosis) LGE-MRI images appears to be suboptimal to accurately define the extent of myocardial infarction in the acute setting [68]. Further progress and refinement in MRI technology for a more accurate identification of myocardial necrosis in the acute phase of myocardial infarction is expected and warrants further validation studies.

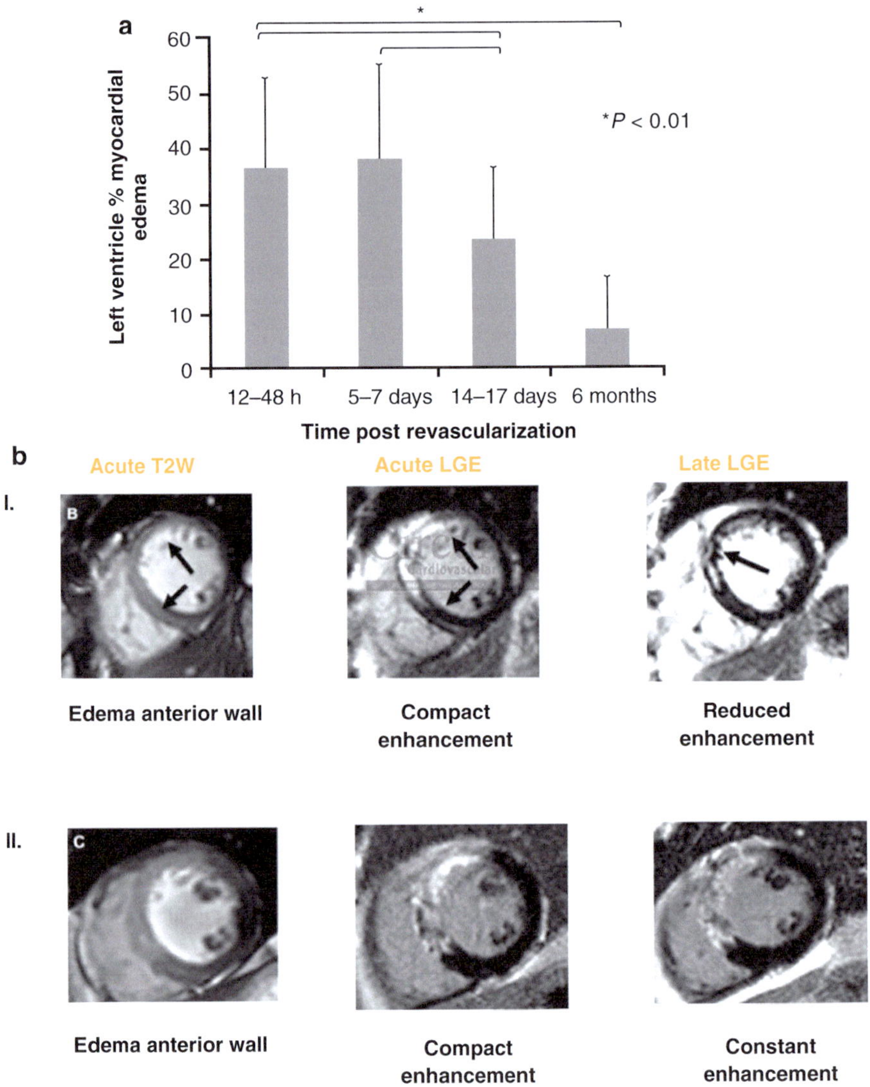

Fig. 6.19 (**a**) Myocardial infarction and time course of edema. Mean percentage of left-ventricular volume positive for myocardial edema at each time point. The volume of edema remained stable in the first week after the event with a significant decrease at 15–17 days with near resolution by 6 months (With kind permission from Ref. [68]). (**b**) Representative cardiac magnetic resonance images (MRI). In the upper row, T2-weighted image (*on the left*) shows edema in the anterior wall; the acute LGE shows compact enhancement (*middle*), which is reduced in size by 6 months (*image on the right*) (*I*). In another example (*bottom row*), edema imaging confirms acute injury. LGE present in the acute phase persists without significant alteration to the 6-month time point (*II*) (With kind permission from Ref. [68])

6.10 Comparison of Cardiac MRI to Scintigraphic Techniques

When comparing conventional cardiac LGE-MRI with FDG-PET/CT, both techniques are highly concordant and reliable for diagnosis and prediction of functional recovery of viable but dysfunctional myocardial segments in ischemic cardiomyopathy patients. There are only a few head-to-head investigations between these two imaging modalities [96–98]. Overall, it appears that FDG-PET/CT is more sensitive, in particular in the intermediate range, for the detection of myocardial viability [96, 97], while LGE-MRI can be regarded as more specific in the prediction of recovery of segmental left-ventricular function following coronary revascularization (Fig. 6.20) [78, 98].

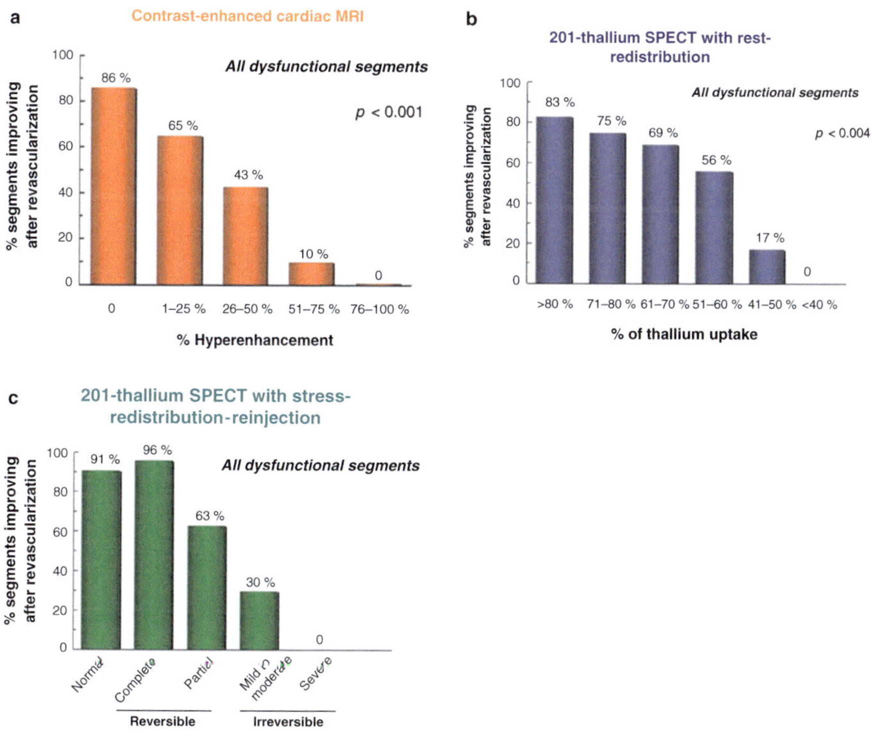

Fig. 6.20 Viability detection with cardiac magnetic resonance imaging (MRI), ^{201}thallium-SPECT, and functional recovery. Relationships between recovery of function after revascularization with contrast-enhanced MRI (**a**) and two ^{201}thallium protocols optimized for viability detection: rest-redistribution (**b**) and stress-redistribution-reinjection (**c**) imaging. Irrespective of the imaging modality applied, the data suggest that recovery of function after revascularization is a continuum and is coupled to the ratio of viable to scarred myocardium within dysfunctional myocardial segments. The extent of infarct size on contrast-enhanced MRI or percent thallium defect on SPECT correlated with decreasing likelihood of functional recovery after revascularization (With kind permission from Ref. [78])

Roes et al. [96] investigated 60 patients with ischemic cardiomyopathy who underwent contrast-enhanced MRI, ^{99m}Tc-tetrofosmin, and FDG-SPECT. A high agreement (91 %) for viability assessment between contrast-enhanced MRI and nuclear imaging was observed in segments without scar tissue on contrast-enhanced MRI as well as in segments with transmural scar tissue (83 %). Yet, disagreement was noted in myocardial segments with subendocardial delayed enhancement on MRI. In myocardial segments with subendocardial scar tissue on contrast-enhanced MRI, the various viability patterns assessed with nuclear imaging were evenly distributed. This suggests that segments with subendocardial scar tissue on contrast-enhanced MRI may have normal perfusion/FDG uptake, perfusion/FDG mismatch, mild perfusion/FDG match, or severe perfusion/ FDG match. Wu et al. [97] again compared contrast-enhanced MRI with FDG-PET/^{201}Tl-SPECT for myocardial viability and prediction of early functional outcome in 41 patients with chronic CAD. Of 252 dysfunctional segments that were successfully revascularized, the sensitivity, specificity, positive predictive value, and negative predictive value of PET/SPECT were 60.2, 98.7, 76.6, and 96.7 % and of MRI were 92.2, 44.9, 72.4, and 78.6 % using the cutoff value of 50 % delayed enhancement on MRI, without significant differences in overall accuracies. When patients were categorized according to the presence of delayed enhancement ≤50 % and >50 %, respectively, the agreement for viability detection between viability as defined by FDG-PET/^{201}Tl-SPECT (mismatch between decreased resting on ^{201}Tl-SPECT and FDG uptake on PET) and DE ≤ 50 % on MRI was high. When the binary threshold of delayed enhancement >50 % on MRI, however, was used, then FDG-PET/^{201}Tl-SPECT still identified 28 out of 71 segments as viable (Fig. 6.21).

When looking in more detail (Table 6.2), then it can be appreciated that in the range of 51–75 % and 76–100 % of transmural delayed enhancement, FDG-PET/^{201}Tl-SPECT still signified 18 out of 40 (45 %) and 10 out of 21 (48 %) dysfunctional segments as viable. Regarding the functional outcome after surgical revascularization, myocardial segments identified as viable on PET/SPECT reliably predicted a functional improvement, while the threshold of 50 % delayed enhancement on MRI did not prove to be a good discriminator of early functional outcome (Fig. 6.22). Patients without any delayed enhancement on MRI, however, were

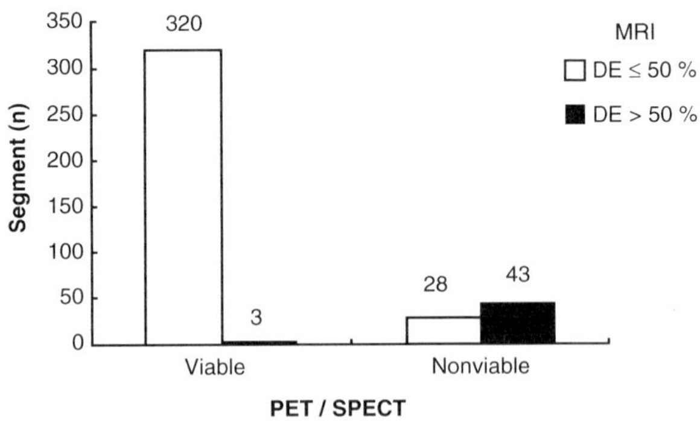

Fig. 6.21 Comparison of MRI and ^{18}F-FDG-PET/^{201}Tl-SPECT in viability detection. Segmental extent of DE by MRI categorized according to ^{18}F-FDG-PET/^{201}Tl-SPECT in dysfunctional myocardium ($n = 394$) (With kind permission from Ref. [97])

prone to recover left-ventricular function and reverse left-ventricular remodeling early after coronary revascularization, while the absence of substantial viable myocardium as defined by and detected on PET/SPECT was always associated with a poor global functional outcome (Fig. 6.22).

Another important evolution in cardiac MRI is the potential to assess the myocardial matrix expansion with T1-weighted sequences [99–101] that can be assumed to reflect, at least in part, adverse myocardial remodeling and interstitial fibrosis [102]. Not surprisingly, the assessment of increased extracellular volume (ECV) fraction with T1-weighted MRI predicted mortality and heart failure-related events in an independent fashion in a general cardiovascular risk cohort but also in a

Table 6.2 Transmurality of delayed enhancement in dysfunctional myocardium ($n = 394$)

Extent of transmurality on cardiac MRI					
PET/SPECT	None	1–25 %	26–50 %	51–75 %	76–100 %
Viable	258	24	38	18	10
Nonviable	0	0	3	22	21

PET positron emission tomography, *SPECT* single-photon emission computed tomography, *MRI* magnetic resonance imaging

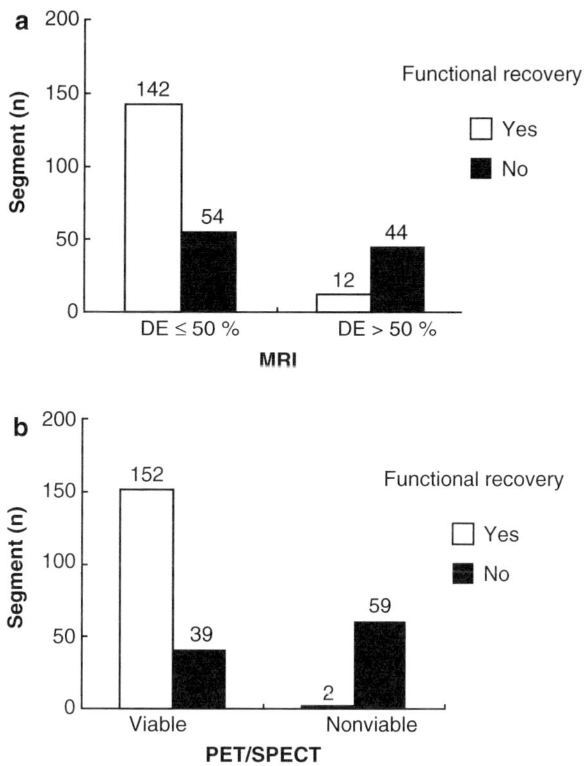

Fig. 6.22 Relationship between myocardial viability, revascularization, and functional recovery. Segmental viability status by MRI categorization (**a**) and 18 F-FDG-PET/201TI-SPECT (**b**) and early functional outcome after surgical revascularization ($n = 252$) (With kind permission from Ref. [97])

specific population of patients with type 2 diabetes mellitus [99, 100]. Determining the ECV with MRI, as a surrogate marker for interstitial fibrosis, may also be of interest in patients with ischemic cardiomyopathy. Such a specific marker of adverse negative remodeling of the failing heart could provide important predictive information on functional and prognostic outcome after coronary revascularization of hibernating-stunning myocardium. For example, this diagnostic approach could be helpful to identify those individuals having hibernating-stunning myocardium on PET images but yet unlikely to recover function despite coronary revascularization as the adverse remodeling process may have advanced beyond a point of no return in the hibernating-stunning but also in the remote myocardium [52] that remains to be evaluated clinically. Overall, the concurrent assessment of metabolism and structural alterations of the myocardium with PET/MRI [86, 103, 104] may emerge as novel hybrid approach in optimizing the prediction of left-ventricular functional recovery after coronary revascularization in patients with ischemic cardiomyopathy.

6.11 Summary

Despite the PARR-2 [42] and the STICH trials [44], the identification of ischemic compromised but viable myocardium in myocardial areas with severe hypokinesis, akinesis, or dyskinesia is critical for the clinical decision-making process in regard to treatment options. Conversely, clinical determinants such as a timely revascularization of ischemic, jeopardized but viable myocardium, effects of advanced stages of myocardial remodeling, ischemic conditioning, and the extent of left-ventricular dilation need to be given considerations. Further refinement of diagnostic and clinical criteria is warranted in order to signify those ischemic cardiomyopathy patients who are likely to benefit most from coronary revascularization procedures.

Acknowledgement Some sections of the manuscript may be similar to sections of an extensive review of cardiac PET by Valenta et al. [33]

References

1. Ezekowitz JA, Kaul P, Bakal JA, Armstrong PW, Welsh RC, McAlister FA. Declining in-hospital mortality and increasing heart failure incidence in elderly patients with first myocardial infarction. J Am Coll Cardiol. 2009;53(1):13–20.
2. Hunt SA, Abraham WT, Chin MH, et al. 2009 Focused update incorporated into the ACC/AHA 2005 Guidelines for the Diagnosis and Management of Heart Failure in Adults A Report of the American College of Cardiology Foundation/American Heart Association Task Force on Practice Guidelines Developed in Collaboration With the International Society for Heart and Lung Transplantation. J Am Coll Cardiol. 2009;53(15):e1–90.
3. Owens AT, Jessup M. The year in heart failure. J Am Coll Cardiol. 2012;60(5):359–68.
4. Sahul ZH, Mukherjee R, Song J, et al. Targeted imaging of the spatial and temporal variation of matrix metalloproteinase activity in a porcine model of postinfarct remodeling: relationship to myocardial dysfunction. Circ Cardiovasc Imaging. 2011;4(4):381–91.

5. Shirani J, Dilsizian V. Imaging left ventricular remodeling: targeting the neurohumoral axis. Nat Clin Pract Cardiovasc Med. 2008;5 Suppl 2:S57–62.
6. Ghosh N, Rimoldi OE, Beanlands RS, Camici PG. Assessment of myocardial ischaemia and viability: role of positron emission tomography. Eur Heart J. 2010;31(24):2984–95.
7. Barnes E, Hall RJ, Dutka DP, Camici PG. Absolute blood flow and oxygen consumption in stunned myocardium in patients with coronary artery disease. J Am Coll Cardiol. 2002;39(3):420–7.
8. Diamond GA, Forrester JS, deLuz PL, Wyatt HL, Swan HJ. Post-extrasystolic potentiation of ischemic myocardium by atrial stimulation. Am Heart J. 1978;95(2):204–9.
9. Marshall RC, Tillisch JH, Phelps ME, et al. Identification and differentiation of resting myocardial ischemia and infarction in man with positron computed tomography, 18F-labeled fluorodeoxyglucose and N-13 ammonia. Circulation. 1983;67(4):766–78.
10. Tillisch J, Brunken R, Marshall R, et al. Reversibility of cardiac wall-motion abnormalities predicted by positron tomography. N Engl J Med. 1986;314(14):884–8.
11. Rahimtoola SH. A perspective on the three large multicenter randomized clinical trials of coronary bypass surgery for chronic stable angina. Circulation. 1985;72(6 Pt 2):V123–35.
12. Canty Jr JM, Fallavollita JA. Hibernating myocardium. J Nucl Cardiol. 2005;12(1):104–19.
13. Canty Jr JM, Fallavollita JA. Hibernating myocardium represents a primary downregulation of regional myocardial oxygen consumption distal to a critical coronary stenosis. Basic Res Cardiol. 1995;90(1):5–8.
14. Canty Jr JM, Suzuki G. Myocardial perfusion and contraction in acute ischemia and chronic ischemic heart disease. J Mol Cell Cardiol. 2012;52(4):822–31.
15. Zhang X, Schindler TH, Prior JO, et al. Blood flow, flow reserve, and glucose utilization in viable and nonviable myocardium in patients with ischemic cardiomyopathy. Eur J Nucl Med Mol Imaging. 2013;40(4):532–41.
16. Fallavollita JA, Perry BJ, Canty Jr JM. 18F-2-deoxyglucose deposition and regional flow in pigs with chronically dysfunctional myocardium. Evidence for transmural variations in chronic hibernating myocardium. Circulation. 1997;95(7):1900–9.
17. Elsasser A, Muller KD, Skwara W, Bode C, Kubler W, Vogt AM. Severe energy deprivation of human hibernating myocardium as possible common pathomechanism of contractile dysfunction, structural degeneration and cell death. J Am Coll Cardiol. 2002;39(7):1189–98.
18. Elsasser A, Vogt AM, Nef H, et al. Human hibernating myocardium is jeopardized by apoptotic and autophagic cell death. J Am Coll Cardiol. 2004;43(12):2191–9.
19. Elsasser A, Schlepper M, Klovekorn WP, et al. Hibernating myocardium: an incomplete adaptation to ischemia. Circulation. 1997;96(9):2920–31.
20. Bax JJ, Schinkel AF, Boersma E, et al. Early versus delayed revascularization in patients with ischemic cardiomyopathy and substantial viability: impact on outcome. Circulation. 2003;108 Suppl 1:II39–42.
21. Allman KC, Shaw LJ, Hachamovitch R, Udelson JE. Myocardial viability testing and impact of revascularization on prognosis in patients with coronary artery disease and left ventricular dysfunction: a meta-analysis. J Am Coll Cardiol. 2002;39(7):1151–8.
22. Beanlands RS, Hendry PJ, Masters RG, deKemp RA, Woodend K, Ruddy TD. Delay in revascularization is associated with increased mortality rate in patients with severe left ventricular dysfunction and viable myocardium on fluorine 18-fluorodeoxyglucose positron emission tomography imaging. Circulation. 1998;98(19 Suppl):II51–6.
23. Camici PG, Prasad SK, Rimoldi OE. Stunning, hibernation, and assessment of myocardial viability. Circulation. 2008;117(1):103–14.
24. Dilsizian V, Rocco TP, Freedman NM, Leon MB, Bonow RO. Enhanced detection of ischemic but viable myocardium by the reinjection of thallium after stress-redistribution imaging. N Engl J Med. 1990;323(3):141–6.
25. Bonow RO, Dilsizian V, Cuocolo A, Bacharach SL. Identification of viable myocardium in patients with chronic coronary artery disease and left ventricular dysfunction. Comparison of thallium scintigraphy with reinjection and PET imaging with 18F-fluorodeoxyglucose. Circulation. 1991;83(1):26–37.

26. Rahimtoola SH. Hibernating myocardium has reduced blood flow at rest that increases with low-dose dobutamine. Circulation. 1996;94(12):3055–61.
27. Rahimtoola SH. Clinical aspects of hibernating myocardium. J Mol Cell Cardiol. 1996;28(12):2397–401.
28. Schinkel AF, Bax JJ, Poldermans D, Elhendy A, Ferrari R, Rahimtoola SH. Hibernating myocardium: diagnosis and patient outcomes. Curr Probl Cardiol. 2007;32(7):375–410.
29. Dilsizian V, Perrone-Filardi P, Arrighi JA, et al. Concordance and discordance between stress-redistribution-reinjection and rest-redistribution thallium imaging for assessing viable myocardium. Comparison with metabolic activity by positron emission tomography. Circulation. 1993;88(3):941–52.
30. Berman DS, Kiat H, Friedman JD, et al. Separate acquisition rest thallium-201/stress technetium-99m sestamibi dual-isotope myocardial perfusion single-photon emission computed tomography: a clinical validation study. J Am Coll Cardiol. 1993;22(5):1455–64.
31. Sciagra R, Bisi G, Santoro GM, et al. Comparison of baseline-nitrate technetium-99m sestamibi with rest-redistribution thallium-201 tomography in detecting viable hibernating myocardium and predicting postrevascularization recovery. J Am Coll Cardiol. 1997;30(2): 384–91.
32. Partington SL, Kwong RY, Dorbala S. Multimodality imaging in the assessment of myocardial viability. Heart Fail Rev. 2011;16(4):381–95.
33. Valenta I, Quercioli A, Ruddy T, Schindler TH. Assessment of myocardial viability after the STICH trial: still viable? Cardiovasc Med. 2013;16(11):289–98.
34. Brunken RC, Mody FV, Hawkins RA, Nienaber C, Phelps ME, Schelbert HR. Positron emission tomography detects metabolic viability in myocardium with persistent 24-hour single-photon emission computed tomography 201Tl defects. Circulation. 1992;86(5):1357–69.
35. Di Carli MF. Myocardial viability assessment with PET and PET/CT. New York: Springer; 2007.
36. Auerbach MA, Schoder H, Hoh C, et al. Prevalence of myocardial viability as detected by positron emission tomography in patients with ischemic cardiomyopathy. Circulation. 1999;99(22):2921–6.
37. Carrel T, Jenni R, Haubold-Reuter S, von Schulthess G, Pasic M, Turina M. Improvement of severely reduced left ventricular function after surgical revascularization in patients with preoperative myocardial infarction. Eur J Cardiothorac Surg. 1992;6(9):479–84.
38. Di Carli MF, Asgarzadie F, Schelbert HR, et al. Quantitative relation between myocardial viability and improvement in heart failure symptoms after revascularization in patients with ischemic cardiomyopathy. Circulation. 1995;92(12):3436–44.
39. Di Carli MF, Davidson M, Little R, et al. Value of metabolic imaging with positron emission tomography for evaluating prognosis in patients with coronary artery disease and left ventricular dysfunction. Am J Cardiol. 1994;73(8):527–33.
40. Lee KS, Marwick TH, Cook SA, et al. Prognosis of patients with left ventricular dysfunction, with and without viable myocardium after myocardial infarction. Relative efficacy of medical therapy and revascularization. Circulation. 1994;90(6):2687–94.
41. D'Egidio G, Nichol G, Williams KA, et al. Increasing benefit from revascularization is associated with increasing amounts of myocardial hibernation: a substudy of the PARR-2 trial. JACC Cardiovasc Imaging. 2009;2(9):1060–8.
42. Beanlands RS, Nichol G, Huszti E, et al. F-18-fluorodeoxyglucose positron emission tomography imaging-assisted management of patients with severe left ventricular dysfunction and suspected coronary disease: a randomized, controlled trial (PARR-2). J Am Coll Cardiol. 2007;50(20):2002–12.
43. Abraham A, Nichol G, Williams KA, et al. 18F-FDG PET imaging of myocardial viability in an experienced center with access to 18F-FDG and integration with clinical management teams: the Ottawa-FIVE substudy of the PARR 2 trial. J Nucl Med. 2010;51(4):567–74.
44. Bonow RO, Maurer G, Lee KL, et al. Myocardial viability and survival in ischemic left ventricular dysfunction. N Engl J Med. 2011;364(17):1617–25.

45. Rouleau JL, Bonow RO. An approach to the rational use of revascularization in heart failure patients. Can J Cardiol. 2014;30(3):281–7.
46. Chareonthaitawee P, Gersh BJ, Panza JA. Is viability imaging still relevant in 2012? JACC Cardiovasc Imaging. 2012;5(5):550–8.
47. Velazquez EJ. Does imaging-guided selection of patients with ischemic heart failure for high risk revascularization improve identification of those with the highest clinical benefit?: Myocardial imaging should not exclude patients with ischemic heart failure from coronary revascularization. Circ Cardiovasc Imaging. 2012;5(2):271–9; discussion 9.
48. Mielniczuk LM, Beanlands RS. Does imaging-guided selection of patients with ischemic heart failure for high risk revascularization improve identification of those with the highest clinical benefit?: Imaging-guided selection of patients with ischemic heart failure for high-risk revascularization improves identification of those with the highest clinical benefit. Circ Cardiovasc Imaging. 2012;5(2):262–70; discussion 70.
49. Tarakji KG, Brunken R, McCarthy PM, et al. Myocardial viability testing and the effect of early intervention in patients with advanced left ventricular systolic dysfunction. Circulation. 2006;113(2):230–7.
50. Maruskova M, Gregor P, Bartunek J, Tintera J, Penicka M. Myocardial viability and cardiac dyssynchrony as strong predictors of perioperative mortality in high-risk patients with ischemic cardiomyopathy having coronary artery bypass surgery. J Thorac Cardiovasc Surg. 2009;138(1):62–8.
51. Schwarz ER, Schoendube FA, Kostin S, et al. Prolonged myocardial hibernation exacerbates cardiomyocyte degeneration and impairs recovery of function after revascularization. J Am Coll Cardiol. 1998;31(5):1018–26.
52. Bax JJ, Schinkel AF, Boersma E, et al. Extensive left ventricular remodeling does not allow viable myocardium to improve in left ventricular ejection fraction after revascularization and is associated with worse long-term prognosis. Circulation. 2004;110(11 Suppl 1): II18–22.
53. Vanoverschelde JL, Wijns W, Depre C, et al. Mechanisms of chronic regional postischemic dysfunction in humans. New insights from the study of noninfarcted collateral-dependent myocardium. Circulation. 1993;87(5):1513–23.
54. Bonow RO. Contractile reserve and coronary blood flow reserve in collateral-dependent myocardium. J Am Coll Cardiol. 1999;33(3):705–7.
55. Meier P, Gloekler S, Zbinden R, et al. Beneficial effect of recruitable collaterals: a 10-year follow-up study in patients with stable coronary artery disease undergoing quantitative collateral measurements. Circulation. 2007;116(9):975–83.
56. Schindler TH, Schelbert HR, Quercioli A, Dilsizian V. Cardiac PET imaging for the detection and monitoring of coronary artery disease and microvascular health. JACC Cardiovasc Imaging. 2010;3(6):623–40.
57. Hochman JS, Lamas GA, Buller CE, et al. Coronary intervention for persistent occlusion after myocardial infarction. N Engl J Med. 2006;355(23):2395–407.
58. Hochman JS, Reynolds HR, Dzavik V, et al. Long-term effects of percutaneous coronary intervention of the totally occluded infarct-related artery in the subacute phase after myocardial infarction. Circulation. 2011;124(21):2320–8.
59. Desideri A, Cortigiani L, Christen AI, et al. The extent of perfusion-F18-fluorodeoxyglucose positron emission tomography mismatch determines mortality in medically treated patients with chronic ischemic left ventricular dysfunction. J Am Coll Cardiol. 2005;46(7):1264–9.
60. Beanlands RS, Labinaz M, Ruddy TD, et al. Establishing an approach for patients with recent coronary occlusion: identification of viable myocardium. J Nucl Cardiol. 1999;6(3): 298–305.
61. Louie HW, Laks H, Milgalter E, et al. Ischemic cardiomyopathy. Criteria for coronary revascularization and cardiac transplantation. Circulation. 1991;84(5 Suppl):III290–5.
62. Yamaguchi A, Ino T, Adachi H, et al. Left ventricular volume predicts postoperative course in patients with ischemic cardiomyopathy. Ann Thorac Surg. 1998;65(2):434–8.

63. Heusch G, Libby P, Gersh B, et al. Cardiovascular remodelling in coronary artery disease and heart failure. Lancet. 2014;383(9932):1933–43.
64. Murry CE, Jennings RB, Reimer KA. Preconditioning with ischemia: a delay of lethal cell injury in ischemic myocardium. Circulation. 1986;74(5):1124–36.
65. Yellon DM, Downey JM. Preconditioning the myocardium: from cellular physiology to clinical cardiology. Physiol Rev. 2003;83(4):1113–51.
66. Waltenberger J, Gelissen M, Bekkers SC, et al. Clinical pacing post-conditioning during revascularization after AMI. JACC Cardiovasc Imaging. 2014;7(6):620–6.
67. Ndrepepa G, Kastrati A, Schwaiger M, et al. Relationship between residual blood flow in the infarct-related artery and scintigraphic infarct size, myocardial salvage, and functional recovery in patients with acute myocardial infarction. J Nucl Med. 2005;46(11):1782–8.
68. Dall'Armellina E, Karia N, Lindsay AC, et al. Dynamic changes of edema and late gadolinium enhancement after acute myocardial infarction and their relationship to functional recovery and salvage index. Circ Cardiovasc Imaging. 2011;4(3):228–36.
69. Schulman D, Latchman DS, Yellon DM. Urocortin protects the heart from reperfusion injury via upregulation of p42/p44 MAPK signaling pathway. Am J Physiol Heart Circ Physiol. 2002;283(4):H1481–8.
70. Hausenloy DJ, Yellon DM. New directions for protecting the heart against ischaemia-reperfusion injury: targeting the Reperfusion Injury Salvage Kinase (RISK)-pathway. Cardiovasc Res. 2004;61(3):448–60.
71. Perrone-Filardi P, Pinto FJ. Looking for myocardial viability after a STICH trial: not enough to close the door. J Nucl Med. 2012;53(3):349–52.
72. Kim RJ, Wu E, Rafael A, et al. The use of contrast-enhanced magnetic resonance imaging to identify reversible myocardial dysfunction. N Engl J Med. 2000;343(20):1445–53.
73. Dilsizian V, Arrighi JA, Diodati JG, et al. Myocardial viability in patients with chronic coronary artery disease. Comparison of 99mTc-sestamibi with thallium reinjection and [18F]fluorodeoxyglucose. Circulation. 1994;89(2):578–87.
74. Akinboboye OO, Idris O, Cannon PJ, Bergmann SR. Usefulness of positron emission tomography in defining myocardial viability in patients referred for cardiac transplantation. Am J Cardiol. 1999;83(8):1271–4, A9.
75. Tamaki N, Kawamoto M, Takahashi N, et al. Prognostic value of an increase in fluorine-18 deoxyglucose uptake in patients with myocardial infarction: comparison with stress thallium imaging. J Am Coll Cardiol. 1993;22(6):1621–7.
76. Dreyfus GD, Duboc D, Blasco A, et al. Myocardial viability assessment in ischemic cardiomyopathy: benefits of coronary revascularization. Ann Thorac Surg. 1994;57(6):1402–7; discussion 7–8.
77. Marin-Neto JA, Dilsizian V, Arrighi JA, et al. Thallium reinjection demonstrates viable myocardium in regions with reverse redistribution. Circulation. 1993;88(4 Pt 1):1736–45.
78. Dilsizian V. Cardiac magnetic resonance versus SPECT: are all noninfarct myocardial regions created equal? J Nucl Cardiol. 2007;14(1):9–14.
79. Balcells E, Powers ER, Lepper W, et al. Detection of myocardial viability by contrast echocardiography in acute infarction predicts recovery of resting function and contractile reserve. J Am Coll Cardiol. 2003;41(5):827–33.
80. La Canna G, Alfieri O, Giubbini R, Gargano M, Ferrari R, Visioli O. Echocardiography during infusion of dobutamine for identification of reversibly dysfunction in patients with chronic coronary artery disease. J Am Coll Cardiol. 1994;23(3):617–26.
81. Hoffmann R, Lethen H, Marwick T, et al. Analysis of interinstitutional observer agreement in interpretation of dobutamine stress echocardiograms. J Am Coll Cardiol. 1996;27(2):330–6.
82. Plana JC, Mikati IA, Dokainish H, et al. A randomized cross-over study for evaluation of the effect of image optimization with contrast on the diagnostic accuracy of dobutamine echocardiography in coronary artery disease The OPTIMIZE Trial. JACC Cardiovasc Imaging. 2008;1(2):145–52.

83. Hoffmann R, Altiok E, Nowak B, et al. Strain rate analysis allows detection of differences in diastolic function between viable and nonviable myocardial segments. J Am Soc Echocardiogr. 2005;18(4):330–5.
84. Chatzizisis YS, Murthy VL, Solomon SD. Echocardiographic evaluation of coronary artery disease. Coron Artery Dis. 2013;24(7):613–23.
85. Brasch RC. New directions in the development of MR imaging contrast media. Radiology. 1992;183(1):1–11.
86. Adenaw N, Salerno M. PET/MRI: current state of the art and future potential for cardiovascular applications. J Nucl Cardiol. 2013;20(6):976–89.
87. Kim RJ, Fieno DS, Parrish TB, et al. Relationship of MRI delayed contrast enhancement to irreversible injury, infarct age, and contractile function. Circulation. 1999;100(19): 1992–2002.
88. Ricciardi MJ, Wu E, Davidson CJ, et al. Visualization of discrete microinfarction after percutaneous coronary intervention associated with mild creatine kinase-MB elevation. Circulation. 2001;103(23):2780–3.
89. Hadamitzky M, Langhans B, Hausleiter J, et al. Prognostic value of late gadolinium enhancement in cardiovascular magnetic resonance imaging after acute ST-elevation myocardial infarction in comparison with single-photon emission tomography using Tc99m-Sestamibi. Eur Heart J Cardiovasc Imaging. 2014;15(2):216–25.
90. Klein C, Nekolla SG, Bengel FM, et al. Assessment of myocardial viability with contrast-enhanced magnetic resonance imaging: comparison with positron emission tomography. Circulation. 2002;105(2):162–7.
91. Wellnhofer E, Olariu A, Klein C, et al. Magnetic resonance low-dose dobutamine test is superior to SCAR quantification for the prediction of functional recovery. Circulation. 2004;109(18):2172–4.
92. Rogers Jr WJ, Kramer CM, Geskin G, et al. Early contrast-enhanced MRI predicts late functional recovery after reperfused myocardial infarction. Circulation. 1999;99(6):744–50.
93. Kramer CM, Rogers Jr WJ, Mankad S, Theobald TM, Pakstis DL, Hu YL. Contractile reserve and contrast uptake pattern by magnetic resonance imaging and functional recovery after reperfused myocardial infarction. J Am Coll Cardiol. 2000;36(6):1835–40.
94. Choi CJ, Haji-Momenian S, Dimaria JM, et al. Infarct involution and improved function during healing of acute myocardial infarction: the role of microvascular obstruction. J Cardiovasc Magn Reson. 2004;6(4):917–25.
95. Petersen SE, Voigtlander T, Kreitner KF, et al. Late improvement of regional wall motion after the subacute phase of myocardial infarction treated by acute PTCA in a 6-month follow-up. J Cardiovasc Magn Reson. 2003;5(3):487–95.
96. Roes SD, Kaandorp TA, Marsan NA, et al. Agreement and disagreement between contrast-enhanced magnetic resonance imaging and nuclear imaging for assessment of myocardial viability. Eur J Nucl Med Mol Imaging. 2009;36(4):594–601.
97. Wu YW, Tadamura E, Yamamuro M, et al. Comparison of contrast-enhanced MRI with (18) F-FDG PET/201Tl SPECT in dysfunctional myocardium: relation to early functional outcome after surgical revascularization in chronic ischemic heart disease. J Nucl Med. 2007;48(7):1096–103.
98. Knuesel PR, Nanz D, Wyss C, et al. Characterization of dysfunctional myocardium by positron emission tomography and magnetic resonance: relation to functional outcome after revascularization. Circulation. 2003;108(9):1095–100.
99. Wong TC, Piehler K, Meier CG, et al. Association between extracellular matrix expansion quantified by cardiovascular magnetic resonance and short-term mortality. Circulation. 2012;126(10):1206–16.
100. Wong TC, Piehler KM, Kang IA, et al. Myocardial extracellular volume fraction quantified by cardiovascular magnetic resonance is increased in diabetes and associated with mortality and incident heart failure admission. Eur Heart J. 2014;35(10):657–64.

101. Schindler TH, Lima JA. Assessment of myocardial matrix expansion with cardiac magnetic resonance: entering a new area of cardiac risk stratification in type 2 diabetes mellitus? Eur Heart J. 2014;35(10):608–11.
102. Di Carli MF, Kwong RY, Jerosch-Herold M. Insights into left ventricular remodeling through noninvasive measures of myocardial matrix expansion with cardiovascular magnetic resonance. Circulation. 2012;126(10):1179–81.
103. Nensa F, Poeppel TD, Beiderwellen K, et al. Hybrid PET/MR imaging of the heart: feasibility and initial results. Radiology. 2013;268(2):366–73.
104. Rischpler C, Nekolla SG, Dregely I, Schwaiger M. Hybrid PET/MR imaging of the heart: potential, initial experiences, and future prospects. J Nucl Med. 2013;54(3):402–15.

Adding T1 Mapping and Extracellular Volume Fraction for Myocardial Fibrosis Assessment: Implications for Cardiovascular Risk Assessment

7

Erik B. Schelbert and Timothy C. Wong

7.1 Introduction

"T1 mapping" and "ECV mapping" techniques offer clinicians and researchers new opportunities to quantify important changes in the human myocardium such as myocardial fibrosis. These cardiovascular magnetic resonance (CMR) techniques employ "native T1" (i.e., without administration of contrast) and "extracellular volume fraction (ECV) measures." These novel parameters can facilitate *diagnosis of disease* as well as associated *prognosis* since these quantitative measures depict the disease severity spectrum beyond its mere presence or absence. As such, these tools may enable the clinician to *identify vulnerable patients* and potentially improve outcomes by *individualizing therapy* and thus match the right treatment to the right patient. Clinicians now can possess new tools to detect *focal* and *diffuse* derangements in *myocardial structure* occurring in cardiac disease that can be otherwise difficult to detect. Fundamentally, increased ECV generally reflects expansion of the interstitial compartment (which includes the myocardial vasculature), whereas native T1 alterations may occur with processes affecting the myocyte or interstitium or both. These measurements complement the traditional functional and geometric surrogates of vulnerability such as left ventricular ejection fraction and volumes and mass [1]. Increased understanding of the role of the interstitium in pathophysiology may facilitate new paradigms of cardiac vulnerability [2]. Various aspects of T1 mapping and ECV have been reviewed in several previous publications [2–15].

E.B. Schelbert, MD, MS (✉) • T.C. Wong, MD, MS
Division of Cardiology, Department of Medicine, University of Pittsburgh
Pittsburgh, PA, USA
e-mail: schelberteb@upmc.edu; wongtc@upmc.edu

T.H. Schindler et al. (eds.), *Molecular and Multimodality Imaging in Cardiovascular Disease*, DOI 10.1007/978-3-319-19611-4_7

7.2 Increased Native T1

T1 is the time constant of the exponential governing magnetization recovery after perturbation by a radiofrequency pulse. Different tissues have varying T1 values which are physical properties of matter. Native T1 measurements (without the use of gadolinium (Gd) contrast) as well as post-contrast T1 measurements are expressed in units of time, e.g., milliseconds. T1 maps can be created whereby each pixel encodes the non-contrast T1 value of the corresponding tissue region. These values can be visualized either with gray-scale images or in color images with a scale bar typically on the T1 map image (Fig. 7.1). T1 maps are usually derived from a pixel-wise parametric fit of a series of images acquired after one or more radiofrequency pulses. Image quality depends heavily on image coregistration and many other factors that have been reviewed previously [5]. If reference values are carefully established for the particular protocol by which T1 is measured, the "parametric" nature of T1 mapping then allows one to detect *focal* and *diffuse* disease processes, whether intracellular or interstitial, acute or chronic. Since T1 parameters can vary significantly with methodology as well as the make and model of the scanner, it is important to define the normal range for each cardiovascular magnetic resonance (CMR) unit. Nonetheless, the ability to detect *diffuse* disease is an important advantage of T1 mapping, because T1 *weighted* images depend on focality (i.e., spatial heterogeneity) to detect changes, and they are inherently insensitive for the detection of diffuse disease processes [16].

If the clinical context is known, native T1 mapping may provide potentially useful information about the presence or absence of disease. Native T1 generally increases in conditions that increase total myocardial water. These may include *focal* myocardial insults such as acute myocardial infarction [17, 18], myocarditis

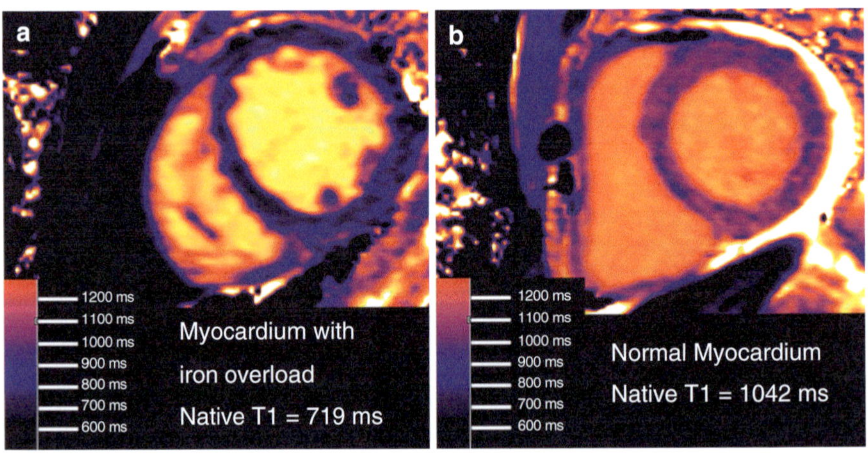

Fig. 7.1 Iron overload in the myocardium decreases native T1 [30]. Native T1 maps from a patient with hemochromatosis and iron overload are shown with a remarkably low myocardial T1 (panel **a**). The native T1 maps in hemochromatosis and iron overload contrast with those from a patient with normal myocardial T1 who also had a small pericardial effusion (panel **b**)

[16, 19], or stress cardiomyopathy [20]. Diffuse and acute myocardial insults also can increase native T1 including global myocarditis [16] and even hyperemia associated with vasodilator stress [21]. Chronic diffuse disease also increases native T1 including diffuse fibrosis [22] in cardiomyopathy [23, 24], amyloidosis [25–27], and even systemic capillary leak syndrome [3]. Importantly, the extent of myocardial native T1 elevations has been shown to relate to prognosis in systemic light-chain amyloidosis [27].

Just like a multitude of other cardiac parameters (e.g., ejection fraction), abnormalities in native T1 need to be interpreted within the clinical context. Edema, increased blood volume, fibrosis, and amyloidosis can all increase native T1 values. Yet, the clinical context is usually known (e.g., a chest pain syndrome or a new cardiomyopathy), so T1 mapping remains as important and promising tool for the clinician and researcher. Investigations into the diagnostic and prognostic performance of native T1 remain an active area of research by many centers.

7.3 Decreased Native T1

Initial work suggests that *low T1* appears sensitive and specific for detecting (a) myocardial *glycosphyngolipid* accumulation in Anderson-Fabry disease [28, 29] or (b) *iron overload* [30] in hemochromatosis (Fig. 7.1), thalassemia, or other disease associated with excess iron. T1 mapping therefore introduces an important CMR tool to detect these important but uncommon conditions that may have immediate diagnostic implications for patients and their physicians. Because T1 mapping appears highly reproducible [31], native T1 mapping may allow one to track response to therapy in these conditions given their ability to quantify disease burden, but such data have not yet been published.

T1 mapping could follow the precedent set by T2* (star) myocardial iron quantification measures whereby *CMR-based care improved outcomes*. Myocardial T2*-guided chelation therapy and clinical care appear to have culminated in dramatically lower cardiac mortality for thalassemia patients. T2* CMR measures can allow one to adjust iron chelation treatment based on myocardial siderosis quantification and match intensity of therapy with disease severity. Mortality rates from cardiac iron overload appear to have improved coincident with the introduction of this capability to clinicians [32]. This scenario of measuring important myocardial tissue changes with CMR parameters illustrates vividly a case where the fundamental promise of CMR, i.e., to match the right treatment to the right patient, appears to have been realized. T1 mapping might have the potential to deliver similar results in the future.

7.4 Extracellular Volume Fraction (ECV) Mapping

The extracellular volume fraction (ECV) quantifies the interstitial space (including the myocardial blood volume contained within the myocardial vasculature estimated to be ~4.5 % [33]) by using Gd contrast as an extracellular space marker [34–36]. ECV measures assume that Gd contrast is not bound to intravascular proteins (e.g., albumin) which would prevent the free distribution of Gd contrast throughout extracellular (plasma and interstitial) fluid. When nonprotein-bound contrast agents are used, ECV maps [3, 37, 38] image the interstitial space and are typically expressed as a percentage or a decimal that is encoded in the signal intensity of each pixel (Fig. 7.2). Clinical ECV mapping images are usually derived from a pixelwise parametric fit of a series of images acquired after one or more radiofrequency pulses for T1 mapping *pre- and post-contrast*. Since ECV mapping is an extension of T1 mapping, coregistration remains an important requirement for image quality.

Conceptually, the ECV technique simply measures the myocardial uptake of Gd relative to plasma, assuming equilibration of Gd contrast between extracellular extravascular and intravascular compartments (without any intravascular protein binding that would prevent free dispersion of contrast). The proportional uptake of myocardium is then a direct measurement of the extracellular space. The ratio of the relative concentrations in the myocardium and whole blood is measured by their specific changes in relaxivity (i.e., $\Delta R1 = 1/T1_{\text{postcontrast}} - 1/T1_{\text{precontrast}}$) to yield the partition coefficient, $\lambda = \Delta R1_{\text{myocardium}}/\Delta R1_{\text{blood}}$. The Gd concentration in myocardial interstitial fluid is in a dynamic equilibrium with *plasma* (not whole blood) during renal clearance, which is relatively slow compared to the dispersion of Gd. Due to the displacement of Gd contrast by erythrocytes in whole blood T1 measurements, one must multiply λ by (1-hematocrit) to yield ECV, which is expressed as a volume percent: $\text{ECV} = \lambda \cdot (1\text{-hematocrit})$. Water exchange effects may introduce some time dependence which is likely a concentration dependence especially at high Gd concentrations or early (i.e., <10 min) after contrast administration [39–43], but these effects do not appear to represent major barriers to its clinical utility as an important imaging biomarker with significant prognostic potential [27, 44–48].

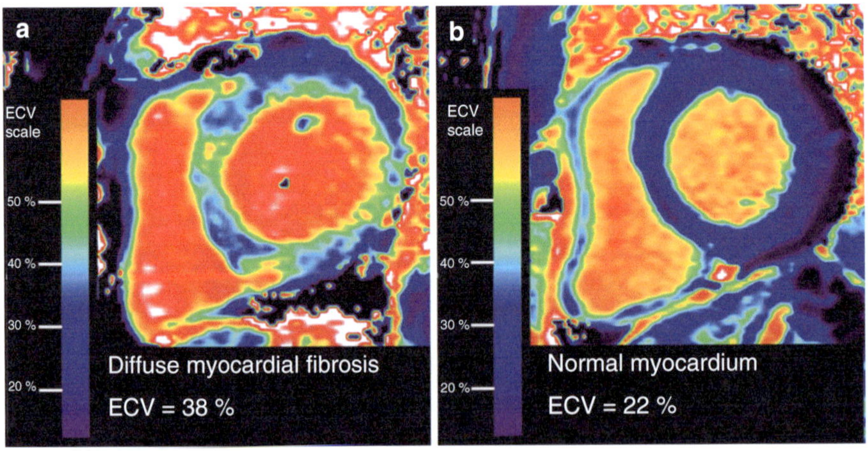

Fig. 7.2 ECV mapping quantifies diffuse fibrosis in a patient with nonischemic cardiomyopathy (panel **a**), in contrast to a patient without fibrosis who demonstrates normal ECV measures (panel **b**)

ECV has been shown to be a robust measure of myocardial fibrosis assuming that myocardial edema or amyloidosis is absent. Although significant distortions in myocardial tissue can occur with tissue processing, multiple studies have still shown high agreement between ECV and histologic measures of myocardial *collagen* content such as the collagen volume fraction (CVF) [40, 49–52]. ECV is also *reproducible* [39, 43, 50, 53–55] although a small amount of Gd dose dependence has been observed as well as cross vendor issues [39–41, 43]. Nonetheless, R^2 values for correlation of myocardial fibrosis between ECV and histologic CVF measures are high [40, 49–52] and range between 0.69 and 0.90 [36, 40, 42, 43, 47]. The R^2 values for ECV compare favorably to significantly lower R^2 ranges of 0.32–0.61 between *isolated post-contrast T1 measures* and CVF measures, where *isolated post-contrast T1 measures* are a surrogate for ECV [56–58]. Isolated post-contrast T1 values are likely confounded by variation-related weight-based gadolinium contrast dosing, renal clearance, time elapsed between contrast bolus and T1 measurement, and displacement of contrast by the hematocrit. Thus, gender, obesity, renal disease, technologist practice, and anemia would be expected to exert greater influence on isolated post-contrast T1 measures than ECV. Notably, large prognostic studies across multiple centers have chosen to report associations between ECV and outcomes rather than *isolated post-contrast T1 measures* [44, 45, 47, 48], suggesting that ECV is the more robust measurement to demonstrate relationships between myocardial fibrosis and outcomes.

7.5 Initial ECV Results

ECV introduces a new concept in cardiology practice and permits one to dichotomize the myocardium into its cellular compartment (mostly myocytes, i.e., 100 %-ECV) and interstitial compartment (i.e., ECV, mostly collagen, but also amyloid protein or edema depending on the clinical setting). The heart may be like other organs (e.g., the lung with pulmonary fibrosis, liver with cirrhosis, or kidney with glomerular fibrosis) where disruption of its architecture through interstitial expansion from myocardial fibrosis leads to organ dysfunction and vulnerability [2, 59]. Importantly, myocardial fibrosis exhibits a high degree of plasticity [60] and has been shown to be a modifiable "intermediate phenotype" of pathologic remodeling [59, 61–64] and "interstitial heart disease" [65] that are fundamentally treatable [66–69]. Myocardial fibrosis may be an important modifiable therapeutic target for both contemporary and emerging treatments. Indeed, myocardial fibrosis can be a common disease pathway from a variety of potential insults [2, 60].

Myocardial fibrosis also indicates vulnerability to adverse outcomes [44–47, 70, 71]. Preliminary outcome data using ECV measures of myocardial fibrosis [44, 45, 48] or amyloidosis [27] suggest that ECV can improve risk stratification [47] as well as identify therapeutic targets for therapy with conventional or newer antifibrotic agents [2]. Even after accounting for common clinical conditions that relate to outcomes in multivariable Cox regression models, ECV may improve the *classification of individual patients at risk* and provided *added prognostic value* beyond age, gender, renal function, myocardial infarction size, ejection fraction, hospitalization status, and heart failure stage using contemporary statistical metrics [47]. Initial outcome data show that increased ECV is associated specifically with mortality or hospitalization for heart failure.

Notably, "antifibrotic" treatment with conventional medications such as lisinopril, losartan, and spironolactone has been shown to reverse fibrosis and improve diastolic function and perfusion reserve [66–69]. These same agents also have improved patient outcomes in several large-scale trials in select populations [71–78], regardless of blood pressure lowering effects [79, 80], even in the absence of clinical heart failure [80]. As one may expect from these data, ECV detects lower myocardial fibrosis in patients receiving renin-angiotensin-aldosterone antagonists, although the extent of the reduction appears modest [44]. Detection of the expected clinical changes in ECV with "antifibrotic treatment" by ECV suggests that ECV is indeed a robust clinical measurement.

Illustrating the importance of quantifying *structural disease in the myocardium*, these associations between ECV and outcomes appear stronger than more traditional risk stratifiers such as ejection fraction or a disease exposure category (e.g., hypertension or diabetes) [44, 45, 47]. Furthermore, myocardial ECV may predict outcomes better than left ventricular mass [46] suggesting that *left ventricular myocardial "quality" may be more important than its "quantity."* Myocardial fibrosis measured by ECV in humans correlates positively with LV mass [44, 45, 81], reflecting prior pathologic observations [70, 82–85]. These findings whereby myocardial mass is *increased* in the setting of myocardial fibrosis suggest that "replacement" is not the solitary mechanism leading to myocardial fibrosis, a situation where one would expect to encounter *decreased* myocardial mass. On this issue, further work is needed to understand complex relationships between the myocyte compartment and the fibroblast in interstitial compartment. In addition, further work is also needed to understand how interstitial expansion from myocardial fibrosis or even amyloid may impact myocyte energetics regardless of the etiology [63, 86]. Interestingly, cardiac amyloidosis yields typically higher values of ECV than myocardial fibrosis which renders it a promising *diagnostic* tool and *prognostic* tool for cardiac amyloidosis [27, 51, 87–90].

7.6 Comparison of ECV Versus Late Gadolinium Enhancement (LGE) to Quantify Interstitial Expansion

Quantifying interstitial expansion *in the noninfarcted myocardium* from fibrosis or amyloidosis is an important endeavor based on the relationship between interstitial expansion, diagnoses, and adverse outcomes [27, 44, 45, 48]. Late gadolinium enhancement (LGE) imaging is the traditional method employing Gd contrast to image regions of higher extracellular space *relative* to the myocardium with less extracellular space. On the other hand, ECV quantifies the full spectrum of interstitial expansion *in the noninfarcted myocardium* regardless of whether LGE is apparent.

Unlike LGE, ECV is inherently quantitative and remains the metric of choice to understand the biology of interstitial expansion in noninfarcted myocardium. ECV is the better metric for this purpose compared to LGE based on (a) robust ECV validation, with high correlations with myocardial CVF measurements [36, 40, 42, 43, 47], (b) excellent ECV reproducibility across separate CMR scans rendering ECV suitable for evaluating serial changes in myocardial fibrosis [39, 43, 50, 53–55], and (c) superior ECV associations with outcomes [44]. In contrast, interscan reproducibility data for use of LGE as a quantitative metric interstitial expansion *in the noninfarcted myocardium* are lacking. *Validation data* for use of LGE as a *quantitative* metric of fibrosis in the noninfarcted myocardium as defined by the collagen volume fraction are also lacking.

In principle, significant limitations related to LGE should not be allowed to bias fully quantitative validated ECV measures of interstitial expansion (e.g., fibrosis) in the noninfarcted myocardium. Spatial variation of interstitial expansion is the key feature that renders it detectable by LGE. There is no biologic rationale to permit spatial variation of myocardial fibrosis (or any interstitial expansion) apparent on LGE images to influence quantification by ECV. Excluding foci of apparent LGE from ECV measurements will arbitrarily bias ECV measures downward to an unpredictable degree based on the same issues that limit LGE as a quantitative metric for myocardial fibrosis in the noninfarcted myocardium. LGE should not be used as an arbiter to gauge the extent of fibrosis in noninfarcted myocardium.

Employing LGE as a *quantitative* measure of fibrosis in the noninfarcted myocardium to capture the full range of fibrosis may be a futile endeavor. There remains a persistent inability to identify a *generalizable* threshold between the normal myocardium and fibrosis in the noninfarcted myocardium over the past 16 years since the initial description of LGE [91]. While most clinicians can agree on the presence of dense foci of "nonischemic" LGE, ascertaining a threshold between lesser degrees of nonischemic LGE and unenhanced myocardium is subjective, remains unresolved, and is not generalizable across centers. Fundamentally, one never knows whether foci of LGE in the noninfarcted myocardium are truly isolated or represent the focal "tip of the iceberg" of a more widespread, diffuse process. One can never discern the extent of fibrosis contained within the nulled, unenhanced myocardium on LGE images. LGE may erroneously portray a "non-enhanced" myocardium as normal [3, 37, 39, 45, 49, 92, 93].

This lack of agreement on an LGE threshold between "normal" and "abnormal" is expected when one considers how patient characteristics and acquisition parameters influence the appearance of fibrosis in the noninfarcted myocardium on LGE images. *These limitations culminate in an inability to identify a threshold that is robust and generalizable.* The appearance of fibrosis in the noninfarcted myocardium on an LGE image varies with the extent of fibrosis contained within the nulled "reference" myocardium that does *not* appear enhanced on LGE images. In addition, the appearance the "threshold" between "normal" and "abnormal" is influenced by pulse sequence and several other parameters (e.g., 2D vs. 3D, phase-sensitive reconstruction, surface coil intensity correction, slice thickness and spatial resolution, inversion time, contrast agent and dose, extent renal clearance, signal-to-noise ratios, patient body habitus such as obesity, segmented versus "single-shot" acquisition, breathholding adequacy, arrhythmia, temporal resolution and heart rate, coil design, parallel imaging acceleration, factor, and other factors). LGE signal intensity is expressed in arbitrary units, and the relationship between LGE signal intensity and Gd concentration is nonlinear.

While LGE is not robust for quantifying fibrosis in noninfarcted myocardium, it is important to recognize that *LGE is the clinical gold standard to quantify myocardial infarction.* LGE is exceedingly well validated for this purpose of detecting and quantifying myocardial infarction [91, 94, 95], whether recognized or not [96–98]. Separating infarcted from noninfarcted myocardium is usually straightforward with LGE given the tremendous difference in signal intensity between infarcted and noninfarcted myocardium. Myocardial infarction typically occurs in spatially constrained patterns (e.g., endocardial involvement, coronary distribution, etc.) which facilitate its identification further [99]. So myocardial infarction is simple to distinguish from the noninfarcted myocardium and quantify its extent.

7.7 Overlap of T1 or ECV Across Patient Groups for Diagnosis Versus Prognosis

While initial results of T1 and ECV data are promising, concern may arise when the distributions of ECV or other T1 data overlap according to a disease classification scheme (e.g., dilated cardiomyopathy [23, 52]) or some disease "exposure variable" such as aortic stenosis [53, 81], diabetes [44], heart failure with or without preserved ejection fraction [100, 101], etc. When native T1 and ECV are used as *diagnostic tools to detect that condition or disease classification scheme*, this concern is valid. Overlapping distributions of T1 and ECV may pose limitations for their use as a diagnostic tool *specifically for that the classification scheme or disease is "exposure variable."* Yet, it is important to put this concern into a biological context. It is expected that the myocardial "response" to a given stimulus or disease state measured by T1 mapping would overlap across disease categories. For example, the spectrum of myocardial fibrosis in the noninfarcted myocardium *measured by histology* is known to vary across individuals [40, 52, 81, 102] and also reflected in the robust histologic validation data for ECV where one encounters a spectrum of disease [40, 49–52]. Determinants of myocardial fibrosis [2] or amyloidosis in the noninfarcted myocardium remain incompletely understood.

The goal of native T1 or ECV *for prognostic purposes*, however, is to measure the myocardial "response" to a given stimulus from a disease state or classification scheme. This "response" or "nonresponse" may be more prognostically relevant than the clinical disease state or classification scheme. It is important to recognize that *outcome data are the final arbiter of what constitutes eventual vulnerability to the patient* among the various parameters that can be measured in the genesis of various disease states. Ascertainment of subsequent event rates therefore represents the gold standard for vulnerability. Therefore, any overlap of ECV data (or other T1 data) between disease categories does not limit their clinical assessment of *vulnerability* nor does any overlap of myocardial fibrosis across disease categories relegates its status as a biologically and prognostically meaningful measurement. Indeed, ECV has robust histological validation data [40, 49–52] and has been shown to have high reproducibility [39, 43, 50, 53–55]. In fact, ECV measures of myocardial fibrosis may be the critical determinant of vulnerability rather than a patient's disease category or classification (e.g., diabetes [44]).

Outcome data are necessary to compare T1 or ECV measures with more traditional disease states of classification schemes for prognostic purposes. Such data are important because they inform paradigms of disease. In general, the stronger the association with outcomes, the more likely the specific measurement is biologically important. Trials that modify the measurement under investigation can then discern whether the measurement is a risk marker or a risk factor that is causal. Notably, despite any overlap in disease category or classification scheme, preliminary data demonstrate that ECV may improve the *classification of individual patients at risk* and provide *added prognostic value* beyond age, gender, renal function, myocardial infarction size, ejection fraction, and heart failure stage [47, 48]. Additional outcome data regarding T1 mapping and ECV mapping to advance our understanding of myocardial fibrosis are accruing.

7.8 ECV and T1 Mapping Limitations

ECV detects subclinical changes [3, 37], but native T1 mapping algorithms are not yet standardized, remaining center dependent and vendor dependent [5]. Normalization to some reference standard may be a potential solution to correct for site-specific difference and still retain the ability to stratify patient cohorts. Optimization of T1 maps and ECV maps is ongoing. Systematic biases in T1 measurements are likely to cancel one another for ECV measurements since ECV is a ratio. This situation is analogous to ejection fraction measurements whereby systematic biases in estimated volumes also cancel one another to a large extent. Indeed, most centers consistently report similar normal ECV reference ranges of <29 % [10, 33, 37, 39, 52–54, 87, 103, 104].

ECV and T1 mapping also remain limited by partial volume effects constrained by their limited spatial resolution, whereby relatively large pixels can straddle tissue borders. As such, T1 mapping and ECV are not yet well suited for quantitative measurements of the right ventricle or left atrium given the thinness of these tissues [5, 105]. ECV also cannot assess the precise composition and structural modifications of the myocardial fibrosis, such as extent of cross-linking and the accumulation of advanced glycation end products. Despite these limitations, T1 mapping and ECV mapping are yielding novel insights into myocardial disease and showing promise as risk stratifiers.

7.9 Summary

T1 and ECV mappings introduce new opportunities to understand disease in the human myocardium. T1 is sensitive to myocardial processes that affect the myocardium globally, i.e., disease specific to the myocyte, the interstitial compartment, or both. Conversely, ECV detects abnormalities limited to expansion of the *extracellular* compartment, typically fibrosis but also amyloidosis and edema (depending on the clinical context). Emerging work suggests that T1 mapping and ECV mapping have the potential to improve the diagnosis of disease as well as the burden of disease. Recent work also suggests that T1 mapping and ECV mapping might refine risk stratification. Ultimately, T1 mapping and ECV mapping promise to improve care by matching the right therapy to each patient, but further work is needed to realize this promise.

References

1. Friedrich MG. There is more than shape and function. J Am Coll Cardiol. 2008;52:1581–3.
2. Schelbert EB, Fonarow GC, Bonow RO, Butler J, Gheorghiade M. Therapeutic targets in heart failure: refocusing on the myocardial interstitium. J Am Coll Cardiol. 2014;63:2188–98.
3. Kellman P, Wilson JR, Xue H, et al. Extracellular volume fraction mapping in the myocardium, part 2: initial clinical experience. J Cardiovasc Magn Reson. 2012;14:64.
4. Treibel TA, White SK, Moon JC. Myocardial tissue characterization: histological and pathophysiological correlation. Curr Cardiovasc Imaging Rep. 2014;7:9254.
5. Moon JC, Messroghli DR, Kellman P, et al. Myocardial T1 mapping and extracellular volume quantification: a Society for Cardiovascular Magnetic Resonance (SCMR) and CMR Working Group of the European Society of Cardiology consensus statement. J Cardiovasc Magn Reson. 2013;15:92.
6. Salerno M, Kramer CM. Advances in parametric mapping with CMR imaging. JACC Cardiovasc Imaging. 2013;6:806–22.
7. Ambale-Venkatesh B, Lima JA. Cardiac MRI: a central prognostic tool in myocardial fibrosis. Nat Rev Cardiol. 2014;12(1):18–29.
8. Maestrini V, Treibel TA, White SK, Fontana M, Moon JC. T1 mapping for characterization of intracellular and extracellular myocardial diseases in heart failure. Curr Cardiovasc Imaging Rep. 2014;7:9287.
9. Jellis CL, Kwon DH. Myocardial T1 mapping: modalities and clinical applications. Cardiovasc Diagn Ther. 2014;4:126–37.
10. Sado DM, Flett AS, Banypersad SM, et al. Cardiovascular magnetic resonance measurement of myocardial extracellular volume in health and disease. Heart. 2012;98:1436–41.
11. Rogers T, Yap ML, Puntmann VO. Myocardial T1 mapping: a non-invasive alternative to tissue diagnosis? Eur Heart J Cardiovasc Imaging. 2014;16(1):108–9.
12. Messroghli DM, Schelbert EB. Clinical Applications of Cardiac T1 Mapping. Radiology. 2015;in press.
13. Mewton N, Liu CY, Croisille P, Bluemke D, Lima JA. Assessment of myocardial fibrosis with cardiovascular magnetic resonance. J Am Coll Cardiol. 2011;57:891–903.
14. h-Ici DO, Jeuthe S, Al-Wakeel N, et al. T1 mapping in ischaemic heart disease. Eur Heart J Cardiovasc Imaging. 2014;15:597–602.
15. Wong TC. Cardiovascular magnetic resonance imaging of myocardial interstitial expansion in hypertrophic cardiomyopathy. Curr Cardiovasc Imaging Rep. 2014;7:9267.

16. Ferreira VM, Piechnik SK, Dall'Armellina E, et al. Native T1-mapping detects the location, extent and patterns of acute myocarditis without the need for gadolinium contrast agents. J Cardiovasc Magn Reson. 2014;16:36.
17. Ugander M, Bagi PS, Oki AJ, et al. Myocardial edema as detected by pre-contrast T1 and T2 CMR delineates area at risk associated with acute myocardial infarction. JACC Cardiovasc Imaging. 2012;5:596–603.
18. Messroghli DR, Niendorf T, Schulz-Menger J, Dietz R, Friedrich MG. T1 mapping in patients with acute myocardial infarction. J Cardiovasc Magn Reson. 2003;5:353–9.
19. Ferreira VM, Piechnik SK, Dall'armellina E, et al. T1-mapping for the diagnosis of acute myocarditis using CMR: comparison to T2-weighted and late gadolinium enhanced imaging. JACC Cardiovasc Imaging. 2013;6(10):1048–58.
20. Ferreira VM, Piechnik SK, Dall'Armellina E, et al. Non-contrast T1-mapping detects acute myocardial edema with high diagnostic accuracy: a comparison to T2-weighted cardiovascular magnetic resonance. J Cardiovasc Magn Reson. 2012;14:42.
21. Mahmod M, Piechnik SK, Levelt E, et al. Adenosine stress native T1 mapping in severe aortic stenosis: evidence for a role of the intravascular compartment on myocardial T1 values. J Cardiovasc Magn Reson. 2014;16:92.
22. Bull S, White SK, Piechnik SK, et al. Human non-contrast T1 values and correlation with histology in diffuse fibrosis. Heart. 2013;99:932–7.
23. Puntmann VO, Voigt T, Chen Z, et al. Native T1 mapping in differentiation of normal myocardium from diffuse disease in hypertrophic and dilated cardiomyopathy. JACC Cardiovasc Imaging. 2013;6:475–84.
24. Puntmann VO, D'Cruz D, Smith Z, et al. Native myocardial T1 mapping by cardiovascular magnetic resonance imaging in subclinical cardiomyopathy in patients with systemic lupus erythematosus. Circ Cardiovasc Imaging. 2013;6:295–301.
25. Fontana M, Banypersad SM, Treibel TA, et al. Native T1 mapping in transthyretin amyloidosis. JACC Cardiovasc Imaging. 2014;7(2):157–65.
26. Karamitsos TD, Piechnik SK, Banypersad SM, et al. Noncontrast T1 mapping for the diagnosis of cardiac amyloidosis. JACC Cardiovasc Imaging. 2013;6:488–97.
27. Banypersad SM, Fontana M, Maestrini V, et al. T1 mapping and survival in systemic light-chain amyloidosis. Eur Heart J. 2014;36(4):244–51.
28. Thompson RB, Chow K, Khan A, et al. T1 mapping with CMR is highly sensitive for Fabry disease independent of hypertrophy and gender. Circ Cardiovasc Imaging. 2013;6(3):392–8.
29. Thompson RB, Chow K, Khan A, et al. T1 mapping with CMR is highly sensitive for Fabry disease independent of hypertrophy and gender. Circ Cardiovasc Imaging. 2013;6(5):637–45.
30. Sado DM, Maestrini V, Piechnik SK, et al. Noncontrast myocardial T mapping using cardiovascular magnetic resonance for iron overload. J Magn Reson Imaging. 2014. doi:10.1002/jmri.24727.
31. Rogers T, Dabir D, Mahmoud I, et al. Standardization of T1 measurements with MOLLI in differentiation between health and disease–the ConSept study. J Cardiovasc Magn Reson. 2013;15:78.
32. Modell B, Khan M, Darlison M, Westwood MA, Ingram D, Pennell DJ. Improved survival of thalassaemia major in the UK and relation to T2* cardiovascular magnetic resonance. J Cardiovasc Magn Reson. 2008;10:42.
33. Jerosch-Herold M, Sheridan DC, Kushner JD, et al. Cardiac magnetic resonance imaging of myocardial contrast uptake and blood flow in patients affected with idiopathic or familial dilated cardiomyopathy. Am J Physiol Heart Circ Physiol. 2008;295:H1234–42.
34. Arheden H, Saeed M, Higgins CB, et al. Measurement of the distribution volume of gadopentetate dimeglumine at echo-planar MR imaging to quantify myocardial infarction: comparison with 99mTc-DTPA autoradiography in rats. Radiology. 1999;211:698–708.
35. Poole-Wilson PA. The intracellular pH, potassium and electrolyte content of heart muscle in acidosis and alkalosis. London: University of Cambridge; 1975.

36. Brading AF, Jones AW. Distribution and kinetics of CoEDTA in smooth muscle, and its use as an extracellular marker. J Physiol. 1969;200:387–401.
37. Ugander M, Oki AJ, Hsu LY, et al. Extracellular volume imaging by magnetic resonance imaging provides insights into overt and sub-clinical myocardial pathology. Eur Heart J. 2012;33:1268–78.
38. Kellman P, Wilson JR, Xue H, Ugander M, Arai AE. Extracellular volume fraction mapping in the myocardium, part 1: evaluation of an automated method. J Cardiovasc Magn Reson. 2012;14:63.
39. Schelbert EB, Testa SM, Meier CG, et al. Myocardial extravascular extracellular volume fraction measurement by gadolinium cardiovascular magnetic resonance in humans: slow infusion versus bolus. J Cardiovasc Magn Reson. 2011;13:16.
40. Miller CA, Naish J, Bishop P, et al. Comprehensive validation of cardiovascular magnetic resonance techniques for the assessment of myocardial extracellular volume. Circ Cardiovasc Imaging. 2013;6(3):373–83.
41. Dabir D, Child N, Kalra A, et al. Reference values for healthy human myocardium using a T1 mapping methodology: results from the international T1 multicenter cardiovascular magnetic resonance study. J Cardiovasc Magn Reson. 2014;16:69.
42. Coelho-Filho OR, Mongeon FP, Mitchell R, et al. The role of transcytolemmal water exchange in magnetic resonance measurements of diffuse myocardial fibrosis in hypertensive heart disease. Circ Cardiovasc Imaging. 2012;6(1):134–41.
43. Kawel N, Nacif M, Zavodni A, et al. T1 mapping of the myocardium: intra-individual assessment of post-contrast T1 time evolution and extracellular volume fraction at 3T for Gd-DTPA and Gd-BOPTA. J Cardiovasc Magn Reson. 2012;14:26.
44. Wong TC, Piehler K, Kang IA, et al. Myocardial extracellular volume fraction quantified by cardiovascular magnetic resonance is increased in diabetes and associated with mortality and incident heart failure admission. Eur Heart J. 2014;35:657–64.
45. Wong TC, Piehler K, Meier CG, et al. Association between extracellular matrix expansion quantified by cardiovascular magnetic resonance and short-term mortality. Circulation. 2012;126:1206–16.
46. Wong TC, Piehler KM, Kellman P, Schelbert EB. Extracellular matrix expansion is more strongly associated with cardiovascular outcomes than left ventricular mass. (Abstract). J Am Coll Cardiol. 2014;63:A986.
47. Schelbert EB, Piehler KM, Zareba KM, et al. Extracellular matrix expansion in non-infarcted myocardium is associated with subsequent death, hospitalization for heart failure, or both across the ejection fraction spectrum (Abstract). J Am Coll Cardiol. 2014;63:A1007.
48. Ghosn MG, Pickett S, Brunner G, et al. Association of myocardial extracellular volume and clinical outcome: a cardiac magnetic resonance study (Abstract). J Am Coll Cardiol. 2015;65:A1077.
49. Flett AS, Hayward MP, Ashworth MT, et al. Equilibrium contrast cardiovascular magnetic resonance for the measurement of diffuse myocardial fibrosis: preliminary validation in humans. Circulation. 2010;122:138–44.
50. Fontana M, White SK, Banypersad SM, et al. Comparison of T1 mapping techniques for ECV quantification. Histological validation and reproducibility of ShMOLLI versus multibreath-hold T1 quantification equilibrium contrast CMR. J Cardiovasc Magn Reson. 2012;14:88.
51. White SK, Sado DM, Fontana M, et al. T1 mapping for myocardial extracellular volume measurement by CMR: bolus only versus primed infusion technique. JACC Cardiovasc Imaging. 2013;6:955–62.
52. Aus dem Siepen F, Buss SJ, Messroghli D, et al. T1 mapping in dilated cardiomyopathy with cardiac magnetic resonance: quantification of diffuse myocardial fibrosis and comparison with endomyocardial biopsy. Eur Heart J Cardiovasc Imaging. 2014;16(2):210–6.
53. Chin CW, Semple S, Malley T, et al. Optimization and comparison of myocardial T1 techniques at 3T in patients with aortic stenosis. Eur Heart J Cardiovasc Imaging. 2014;15:556–65.

54. Singh A, Horsfield MA, Bekele S, Khan J, Greiser A, McCann GP. Myocardial T1 and extracellular volume fraction measurement in asymptomatic patients with aortic stenosis: reproducibility and comparison with age-matched controls. Eur Heart J Cardiovasc Imaging. 2015.
55. Liu S, Han J, Nacif MS, et al. Diffuse myocardial fibrosis evaluation using cardiac magnetic resonance T1 mapping: sample size considerations for clinical trials. J Cardiovasc Magn Reson. 2012;14:90.
56. Sibley CT, Noureldin RA, Gai N, et al. T1 Mapping in cardiomyopathy at cardiac MR: comparison with endomyocardial biopsy. Radiology. 2012;265:724–32.
57. Iles LM, Ellims AH, Llewellyn H, Hare JL, Kaye DM, McLean CA, Taylor AJ. Histological validation of cardiac magnetic resonance analysis of regional and diffuse interstitial myocardial fibrosis. Eur Heart J Cardiovasc Imaging. 2014;16(1):14–22.
58. Iles L, Pfluger H, Phrommintikul A, et al. Evaluation of diffuse myocardial fibrosis in heart failure with cardiac magnetic resonance contrast-enhanced T1 mapping. J Am Coll Cardiol. 2008;52:1574–80.
59. Wynn TA, Ramalingam TR. Mechanisms of fibrosis: therapeutic translation for fibrotic disease. Nat Med. 2012;18:1028–40.
60. Rockey DC, Bell PD, Hill JA. Fibrosis–a common pathway to organ injury and failure. N Engl J Med. 2015;372:1138–49.
61. Weber KT, Brilla CG. Pathological hypertrophy and cardiac interstitium. Fibrosis and renin-angiotensin-aldosterone system. Circulation. 1991;83:1849–65.
62. Swynghedauw B. Molecular mechanisms of myocardial remodeling. Physiol Rev. 1999;79:215–62.
63. Mann DL, Barger PM, Burkhoff D. Myocardial recovery and the failing heart: myth, magic, or molecular target? J Am Coll Cardiol. 2012;60:2465–72.
64. Kong P, Christia P, Frangogiannis NG. The pathogenesis of cardiac fibrosis. Cell Mol Life Sci. 2013;71(4):549–74.
65. Weber KT. Cardiac interstitium in health and disease: the fibrillar collagen network. J Am Coll Cardiol. 1989;13:1637–52.
66. Schwartzkopff B, Brehm M, Mundhenke M, Strauer BE. Repair of coronary arterioles after treatment with perindopril in hypertensive heart disease. Hypertension. 2000;36:220–5.
67. Brilla CG, Funck RC, Rupp H. Lisinopril-mediated regression of myocardial fibrosis in patients with hypertensive heart disease. Circulation. 2000;102:1388–93.
68. Diez J, Querejeta R, Lopez B, Gonzalez A, Larman M, Martinez Ubago JL. Losartan-dependent regression of myocardial fibrosis is associated with reduction of left ventricular chamber stiffness in hypertensive patients. Circulation. 2002;105:2512–7.
69. Izawa H, Murohara T, Nagata K, et al. Mineralocorticoid receptor antagonism ameliorates left ventricular diastolic dysfunction and myocardial fibrosis in mildly symptomatic patients with idiopathic dilated cardiomyopathy: a pilot study. Circulation. 2005;112:2940–5.
70. Tamarappoo BK, John BT, Reinier K, et al. Vulnerable myocardial interstitium in patients with isolated left ventricular hypertrophy and sudden cardiac death: a postmortem histological evaluation. J Am Heart Assoc. 2012;1, e001511.
71. Zannad F, Alla F, Dousset B, Perez A, Pitt B. Limitation of excessive extracellular matrix turnover may contribute to survival benefit of spironolactone therapy in patients with congestive heart failure: insights from the randomized aldactone evaluation study (RALES). Rales Investigators. Circulation. 2000;102:2700–6.
72. Yusuf S, Sleight P, Pogue J, Bosch J, Davies R, Dagenais G. Effects of an angiotensin-converting-enzyme inhibitor, ramipril, on cardiovascular events in high-risk patients. The Heart Outcomes Prevention Evaluation Study Investigators. N Engl J Med. 2000;342:145–53.
73. The SOLVD Investigators. Effect of enalapril on survival in patients with reduced left ventricular ejection fractions and congestive heart failure. N Engl J Med. 1991;325:293–302.
74. Pfeffer MA, Braunwald E, Moye LA, et al. Effect of captopril on mortality and morbidity in patients with left ventricular dysfunction after myocardial infarction. Results of the survival and ventricular enlargement trial. The SAVE Investigators. N Engl J Med. 1992; 327:669–77.

75. Pitt B, Zannad F, Remme WJ, et al. The effect of spironolactone on morbidity and mortality in patients with severe heart failure. Randomized Aldactone Evaluation Study Investigators. N Engl J Med. 1999;341:709–17.
76. Pitt B, Remme W, Zannad F, et al. Eplerenone, a selective aldosterone blocker, in patients with left ventricular dysfunction after myocardial infarction. N Engl J Med. 2003;348:1309–21.
77. Pfeffer MA, McMurray JJ, Velazquez EJ, et al. Valsartan, captopril, or both in myocardial infarction complicated by heart failure, left ventricular dysfunction, or both. N Engl J Med. 2003;349:1893–906.
78. Pfeffer MA, Claggett B, Assmann SF, et al. Regional variation in patients and outcomes in the treatment of preserved cardiac function heart failure with an aldosterone antagonist (TOPCAT) trial. Circulation. 2015;131:34–42.
79. Patel A, MacMahon S, Chalmers J, et al. Effects of a fixed combination of perindopril and indapamide on macrovascular and microvascular outcomes in patients with type 2 diabetes mellitus (the ADVANCE trial): a randomised controlled trial. Lancet. 2007;370:829–40.
80. Heart Outcomes Prevention Evaluation Study Investigators. Effects of ramipril on cardiovascular and microvascular outcomes in people with diabetes mellitus: results of the HOPE study and MICRO-HOPE substudy. Lancet. 2000;355:253–9.
81. Flett AS, Sado DM, Quarta G, et al. Diffuse myocardial fibrosis in severe aortic stenosis: an equilibrium contrast cardiovascular magnetic resonance study. Eur Heart J Cardiovasc Imaging. 2012;13:819–26.
82. van Hoeven KH, Factor SM. A comparison of the pathological spectrum of hypertensive, diabetic, and hypertensive-diabetic heart disease. Circulation. 1990;82:848–55.
83. Tanaka M, Fujiwara H, Onodera T, et al. Quantitative analysis of myocardial fibrosis in normals, hypertensive hearts, and hypertrophic cardiomyopathy. Br Heart J. 1986;55:575–81.
84. Beltrami CA, Finato N, Rocco M, et al. The cellular basis of dilated cardiomyopathy in humans. J Mol Cell Cardiol. 1995;27:291–305.
85. Rossi MA. Pathologic fibrosis and connective tissue matrix in left ventricular hypertrophy due to chronic arterial hypertension in humans. J Hypertens. 1998;16:1031–41.
86. Schaper J, Mollnau H, Hein S, Scholz D, Münkel B, Devaux B. Interactions between cardiomyocytes and extracellular matrix in the failing human heart. Z Kardiol. 1995;84:33–8.
87. Mongeon FP, Jerosch-Herold M, Coelho-Filho OR, Blankstein R, Falk RH, Kwong RY. Quantification of extracellular matrix expansion by CMR in infiltrative heart disease. JACC Cardiovasc Imaging. 2012;5:897–907.
88. Robbers LF, Baars EN, Brouwer WP, et al. T1 mapping shows increased extracellular matrix size in the myocardium due to amyloid depositions. Circ Cardiovasc Imaging. 2012;5:423–6.
89. Banypersad SM, Sado DM, Flett AS, et al. Quantification of myocardial extracellular volume fraction in systemic AL amyloidosis: an equilibrium contrast cardiovascular magnetic resonance study. Circ Cardiovasc Imaging. 2012;6:34–9.
90. Barison A, Aquaro GD, Pugliese NR, et al. Measurement of myocardial amyloid deposition in systemic amyloidosis: insights from cardiovascular magnetic resonance imaging. J Intern Med. 2014;277(5):605–14.
91. Kim RJ, Fieno DS, Parrish TB, et al. Relationship of MRI delayed contrast enhancement to irreversible injury, infarct age, and contractile function. Circulation. 1999;100:1992–2002.
92. Broberg CS, Chugh SS, Conklin C, Sahn DJ, Jerosch-Herold M. Quantification of diffuse myocardial fibrosis and its association with myocardial dysfunction in congenital heart disease. Circ Cardiovasc Imaging. 2010;3:727–34.
93. Schalla S, Bekkers SC, Dennert R, et al. Replacement and reactive myocardial fibrosis in idiopathic dilated cardiomyopathy: comparison of magnetic resonance imaging with right ventricular biopsy. Eur J Heart Fail. 2010;12:227–31.
94. Kim RJ, Albert TS, Wible JH, et al. Performance of delayed-enhancement magnetic resonance imaging with gadoversetamide contrast for the detection and assessment of myocardial infarction: an international, multicenter, double-blinded, randomized trial. Circulation. 2008;117:629–37.

95. Schelbert EB, Hsu LY, Anderson SA, et al. Late gadolinium-enhancement cardiac magnetic resonance identifies postinfarction myocardial fibrosis and the border zone at the near cellular level in ex vivo rat heart. Circ Cardiovasc Imaging. 2010;3:743–52.
96. Kwong RY, Sattar H, Wu H, et al. Incidence and prognostic implication of unrecognized myocardial scar characterized by cardiac magnetic resonance in diabetic patients without clinical evidence of myocardial infarction. Circulation. 2008;118:1011–20.
97. Kwong RY, Chan AK, Brown KA, et al. Impact of unrecognized myocardial scar detected by cardiac magnetic resonance imaging on event-free survival in patients presenting with signs or symptoms of coronary artery disease. Circulation. 2006;113:2733–43.
98. Schelbert EB, Cao JJ, Sigurdsson S, et al. Prevalence and prognosis of unrecognized myocardial infarction determined by cardiac magnetic resonance in older adults. JAMA. 2012;308:890–6.
99. Hunold P, Schlosser T, Vogt FM, et al. Myocardial late enhancement in contrast-enhanced cardiac MRI: distinction between infarction scar and non-infarction-related disease. AJR Am J Roentgenol. 2005;184:1420–6.
100. Su MY, Lin LY, Tseng YH, et al. CMR-verified diffuse myocardial fibrosis is associated with diastolic dysfunction in HFpEF. JACC Cardiovasc Imaging. 2014;7:991–7.
101. Mascherbauer J, Marzluf BA, Tufaro C, et al. Cardiac magnetic resonance postcontrast T1 time is associated with outcome in patients with heart failure and preserved ejection fraction. Circ Cardiovasc Imaging. 2013;6:1056–65.
102. van Heerebeek L, Borbely A, Niessen HW, et al. Myocardial structure and function differ in systolic and diastolic heart failure. Circulation. 2006;113:1966–73.
103. Liu CY, Chang Liu Y, Wu C, et al. Evaluation of age related interstitial myocardial fibrosis with cardiac magnetic resonance contrast-enhanced T mapping in the multi-ethnic study of atherosclerosis (MESA). J Am Coll Cardiol. 2013;62(14):1280–7.
104. Lee JJ, Liu S, Nacif MS, et al. Myocardial T1 and extracellular volume fraction mapping at 3 tesla. J Cardiovasc Magn Reson. 2011;13:75.
105. Kellman P, Hansen MS. T1-mapping in the heart: accuracy and precision. J Cardiovasc Magn Reson. 2014;16:2.

Role of Multimodality Imaging in Atherosclerotic Plaque Burden and Metabolism

8

Nikhil Vilas Joshi, David E. Newby, and Marc R. Dweck

8.1 Introduction

Cardiovascular diseases are the leading cause of death and illness worldwide [1, 2]. Atherosclerosis – a progressive disease characterised by the accumulation of lipids and fibrous elements in the large arteries – constitutes the single most important contributor to this burden and has been intensely studied over the past century. Indeed, our understanding of the pathophysiology underlying this important disease has evolved substantively over this period. Previously it was considered to be a bland lipid storage disorder, with passive deposition of lipid encapsulated within the intima and separated from the vessel lumen by a capsule of smooth muscle cells. More recently, substantial advances in basic and translational science have highlighted the role of inflammation, lipid oxidisation, cell death, matrix metalloproteinase activity, calcification and angiogenesis [3–6]. In particular compelling evidence has emerged with respect to the importance of inflammation at both the basic and clinical levels, indicating that better understanding the link between inflammation and atherosclerosis might yield predictive and prognostic information of considerable clinical utility [7–10].

Atherosclerosis has origins in childhood and by middle age subclinical atheroma is almost ubiquitous [11–14]. Indeed, atherosclerosis has one of the longest incubation periods amongst human disease, offering the tantalising opportunity to prevent clinical events via timely detection and treatment of subclinical disease. Whilst anti-atherosclerotic agents of increasing efficacy are evolving constantly, identification of those in need of preventive therapy remains a real challenge.

N.V. Joshi, MD (✉) • D.E. Newby, MD PhD • M.R. Dweck, MD PhD
Centre for Cardiovascular Science, University of Edinburgh, Edinburgh, UK

Clinical Research Imaging Centre, University of Edinburgh, Edinburgh, UK

Heart Centre, Edinburgh, UK
e-mail: nikhil.joshi@ed.ac.uk; marcdweck@hotmail.com

T.H. Schindler et al. (eds.), *Molecular and Multimodality Imaging in Cardiovascular Disease*, DOI 10.1007/978-3-319-19611-4_8

Atherosclerosis is a true systemic disease characterised by widespread development of its localised manifestation: the atherosclerotic plaque. Atherosclerosis has a particular predilection for medium- and large-sized arteries, with the coronary arteries, carotid arteries, iliofemoral arteries and aorta being particularly susceptible. The location of the plaque and its stability largely determines the clinical manifestation of the disease process. These manifestations can be diverse. At one end of the spectrum, fixed obstructive stenoses result in demand ischemia leading to classical symptoms of exertional angina and leg claudication [15–17]. However, the most dreaded consequences of atherosclerotic disease – stroke and myocardial infarction – instead occur as a result of abrupt atherosclerotic plaque rupture and subsequent thrombosis. Whilst angiographic techniques can identify lesions likely to cause angina, we lack the ability to identify high-risk atherosclerotic plaques at risk of rupture and causing myocardial infarction. This is seen as a major goal in cardiology because if these plaques could be identified and subsequent rupture and thrombosis averted, then atherosclerosis would be rendered a much more benign disease.

In this chapter we will first discuss the underlying pathophysiological mechanism leading to plaque vulnerability and rupture. Each of these processes and stages provides a non-invasive imaging target, and we will then discuss how modern techniques might use these targets to identify high-risk vulnerable plaques in vivo. Finally, we will focus on the utility of metabolic imaging using positron emission tomography in vascular biology and the recent exciting developments in this field.

8.2 Pathology of Atherosclerotic Disease

Atherosclerotic lesions are focal thickenings of the innermost arterial layer, the intima. The content of these lesions typically consists of connective tissue, lipids and inflammatory and smooth muscle cells [18]. This chronic inflammatory process preferentially occurs at sites of disturbed laminar flow, such as branch points and bifurcations, most likely due to the effects of reduced shear stress [19]. Endothelial cells in these regions appear to be more permeable due to their polygonal shape, allowing large molecules such as low-density lipoproteins (LDL) to accumulate beneath the endothelium [20]. This accumulation appears to be greatest in cases of hypercholesterolemia as a result of excess levels of circulating LDL. Indeed, the earliest stages of lesion development are characterised by subendothelial accumulation and retention of apolipoprotein B-containing lipoproteins (apoB-LPs) [21]. LDL retained within the vessel wall undergoes a series of oxidative and enzymatic modifications including oxidation, lipolysis, proteolysis and aggregation [22, 23]. Initially this results in the formation of minimally oxidised LDL which has a stimulatory effect on the endothelial cells to produce a variety of growth factors, chemotactic proteins and adhesion molecules. These pro-inflammatory molecules allow leukocytes entry into the arterial wall.

Adhesion, the 'rolling' of leukocytes along the endothelial surface, is mediated by selectins, which bind to carbohydrate ligands on leukocytes. Studies of mice deficient in P- and E-selectins or the cell adhesion molecule ICAM have revealed the role of these adhesion molecules in atherosclerosis [24, 25]. In particular, adhesion of monocytes and T cells has been shown to be controlled by the interaction of the integrin VLA-4 with VCAM-1 on the endothelial surface [26]. Following the passage of these monocytes into the vessel wall, the growth factor M-CSF promotes their proliferation and differentiation to macrophages. Normally, LDL is not taken up by macrophages quickly enough to produce heavily lipid-laden foam cells. Further modification of LDL is first required by reactive oxygen species and the enzymes myeloperoxidase, sphingomyelinase and secretory phospholipase 2. This modification process produces a highly oxidised form of LDL, which is rapidly taken up by macrophages, resulting in the generation of foam cells [27, 28]. This process appears to be mediated by a group of receptors which recognise a wide array of ligands. Two such 'scavenger receptors', SR-A and CD-36, are thought to be of particular importance [29, 30]. As the lesion progresses, there is formation of a fibrous cap mainly consisting of smooth muscle cells (SMC) and a proteoglycan-collagen matrix which covers an underlying lipid pool [31]. In time the cells present within this lipid pool undergo apoptosis or necrosis, ultimately leading to the formation of a necrotic core consisting primarily of cellular debris [32].

8.2.1 Stages of Plaque Progression

Atherosclerosis is a dynamic process with multiple stages: intimal thickening, fibrous cap atheroma (fibroatheroma) formation, thin-cap fibroatheroma and plaque rupture [31]. To understand plaque rupture, it is useful to review these different stages of plaque development.

8.2.2 Intimal Thickening and Intimal Xanthomas

The flow-mediated adaptive, intimal thickening is observed at bifurcation points soon after birth. Whilst some plaques may begin as fatty streaks, evidence suggests that the intimal thickening is the likely precursor to symptomatic atherosclerotic disease since these lesions occur in children at similar locations as advanced plaques in adults, although fatty streaks are known to regress [33]. However, considerable debate exists as to whether these lesions should be classified as atherosclerosis per se [34]. Intimal thickening primarily consists of smooth muscle cells and proteoglycan-collagen matrix without significant infiltrating inflammatory cells. Fatty streaks, which are predominantly observed at branch points, correspond to the accumulation of macrophages within the intima and regress with age [35].

8.2.3 Pathological Intimal Thickening

The stage in between intimal thickening/fatty streaks and more advanced lesions known as fibroatheromas is referred to as pathological intimal thickening and is characterised by the presence of lipid pools containing proteoglycans typically

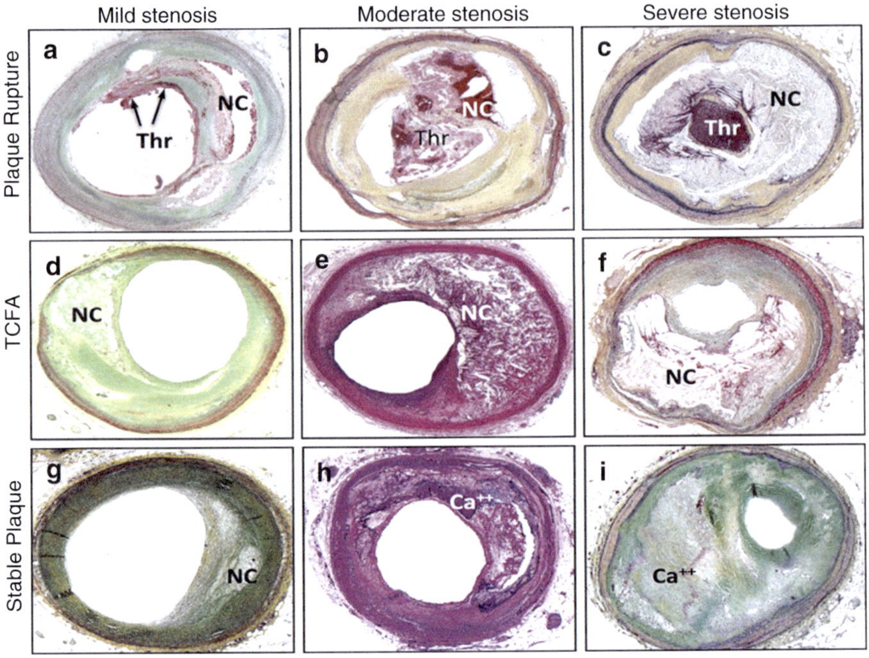

Fig. 8.1 Photomicrographic cross section of human coronary PR, TCFA and FA with varying degrees of luminal stenosis. (**a–c**) Plaque rupture with mild, moderate and severe luminal stenosis, respectively. Non-occlusive thrombus (*Thr*) is observed in the microphotograph A, whereas occlusive thrombus is occupying the lumen in the images **b** and **c**. (**d–f**) TCFA with mild, moderate and severe luminal stenosis, respectively. Necrotic core (*NC*) is covered by a thin fibrous cap, and thrombus is not present in the lumen. (**g–i**) Stable plaque or FA with mild, moderate and severe luminal stenosis, respectively. The size of necrotic core is relatively small when present, and calcification (*Ca++*) is frequently seen (Reprinted from Narula et al. [44] with permission from Elsevier)

without necrosis [31]. The lipid pools are located in the deeper intimal layers near the arterial media, but in contrast the macrophage infiltrates are present in the luminal surface away from the area of accumulated lipid. Early calcification may be seen and likely results from the death of smooth muscle cells and as a healing response to early inflammation [36]. Pathological intimal thickening can be associated with plaque erosion and subsequent acute coronary syndromes.

8.2.4 Fibrous Cap Atheroma

Fibrous cap atheroma or fibroatheromas represents the earliest of the advanced coronary lesions (Fig. 8.1) [31]. Typically, the fibroatheromas consist of lipid-rich necrotic core consisting of macrophage infiltration within lipid pool and encapsulated by fibrous tissue. There is loss of proteoglycans and collagen without much free cholesterol in the early phases. The later phases of fibroatheromas are characterised by increased free cholesterol, cellular debris and an expanding necrotic core.

Such plaques may expand outwardly (positive remodelling) or inwards often due to progressive fibrosis and calcification (negative remodelling). The latter may lead to significant luminal stenosis and the development of anginal symptoms.

The thin-cap fibroatheroma is a subtype of fibroatheromas characterised by a large necrotic core (typically >25 % of total plaque volume) that is separated from the lumen by a thin fibrous cap (typically <65 μm). Usually, the fibrous cap tends to be heavily infiltrated with macrophages [31]. This well-characterised lesion is considered to be the plaque subtype most likely to result in plaque rupture and is therefore a key imaging target for both invasive and non-invasive approaches [31].

8.2.5 What Exactly Defines a High-Risk Plaque?

Two distinct plaque morphologies have been implicated in acute coronary events: plaque rupture and plaque erosion. A few cases (2–7 %) are attributable to a third plaque morphology called calcified nodule [37]. It is believed that 60–75 % of acute coronary syndromes are initiated by plaque rupture [38]. Plaque erosion or denudation of the coronary arterial endothelium with an intact fibrous cap is responsible for acute coronary syndromes in most of the remainder cases and is typically observed in young, female smokers [31].

James Muller first introduced the concept of the vulnerable plaque in 1989. Muller categorised 'hemodynamically insignificant, albeit dangerous lesions as vulnerable plaque' [39]. Subsequent studies have confirmed the notion that most plaques that cause myocardial infarction are non-flow limiting and therefore missed on antecedent coronary arteriography or myocardial stress testing. Traditionally, the term vulnerable plaque has been used for all plaque types that have been associated with luminal thrombosis [37]; however, recently attention has focused in the thin fibrous cap atheroma as the most common precursor of plaque rupture. In particular virtual histology intravascular ultrasound (VH-IVUS) has been used to identify such plaque in the recent Providing Regional Observations to Study Predictors of Events in the Coronary Tree (PROSPECT) and the VH-IVUS in Vulnerable Atherosclerosis (VIVA) studies [40, 41]. Whilst most of the clinical events in these studies were attributable to TCFAs, what was also clear is the vast majority of these lesions are clinically silent.

Pioneering work over the last two decades has established that plaques that go on to rupture demonstrate several histological features that differentiate them over and beyond the classical intact TCFA. These include a larger necrotic core, higher macrophage infiltration of the fibrous cap and plaque microcalcification [37, 42]. This would suggest that there is an intermediate stage between a thin-cap fibroatheroma and a ruptured plaque, which appears characterised by advanced plaque metabolism [43]. In particular by ongoing macrophage infiltration and cell death within the lipid core, that leads to a self-perpetuating cycle of inflammation, hypoxia angiogenesis and further inflammatory cell infiltration.

How then does calcification fit into this model? Calcification as elsewhere in the body is believed to occur as a healing response to intense inflammation within the necrotic core. Although ultimately advanced areas of macroscopic calcification appear to wall off the thrombogenic contents of this core, thereby imparting stability to the plaque, the very earliest stages of microcalcification are instead consistently associated with increased plaque instability and risk of rupture. In part this may reflect the fact that in the early stages of microcalcification, healing has not yet occurred and the inflamed necrotic environment that predisposes to rupture persists. However, recent data suggests that microcalcification might also directly increase vulnerability, acting as a focal point that intensifies mechanical stresses on the surface of the cap. Whatever the mechanism, microcalcification represents an important additional target for the identification of high-risk plaques.

8.3 Imaging Modalities to Identify High-Risk Plaques

8.3.1 Plaque Morphology with Intravascular Ultrasound

Intravascular ultrasound (IVUS) was one of the earliest invasive techniques to allow imaging of the lumen and vessel wall, and despite the development of novel techniques, IVUS still remains the standard method for assessing plaque burden. This technique also allows us to assess many other structural features within the plaques, including positive remodelling, thrombi, plaque length, lumen narrowing, spotty and macroscopic calcification and the presence of a lipid-rich core [45–49]. Moreover, recent advances making use of ultrasound backscatter (VH-IVUS) provide even more information with respect to plaque morphology and characteristics [50]. Various plaque contents such as calcium, fibrous tissue, fibrofatty tissue and necrotic core can be resolved. Moreover, as discussed, VH-IVUS can classify plaque types such as pathological intimal thickening and thick- and thin-cap fibroatheromas with a high degree of accuracy as compared to ex vivo plaques [50].

VH-IVUS has become widely available and has been the subject of intense investigation, having to date been tested in 3 major prospective clinical studies: Providing Regional Observations to Study Predictors of Events in the Coronary Tree (PROSPECT) [41], VH-IVUS in Vulnerable Atherosclerosis (VIVA) [40] and the European Collaborative Project on Inflammation and Vascular Wall Remodelling in Atherosclerosis (ATHEROREMO-IVUS) study [51]. However, the prospects of identifying patients or indeed plaques that will cause future cardiovascular events using radiofrequency IVUS have been rather disappointing. Indeed, amongst 697 patients enrolled in the PROSPECT study, 595 thin-cap fibroatheromas were identified by IVUS across the cohort, only 26 of these plaques were sites of subsequent events at 3 years and the majority of events were related to rehospitalisation for angina rather than myocardial infarction. Plaque burden greater than 70 %, minimal luminal area less than 4 mm^2 and the presence of thin-cap fibroatheromas were thought to be the primary drivers. However, when all these three factors were present in the same lesion, the positive predictive value of an event was only xx%. Consistent with these findings, the VIVA and ATHEROREMO-IVUS studies suggested that whilst identification of thin fibrous cap atheromas identified subsequent MACE, it did not predict future MI per se, and once again the vast majority of these lesions did not result in clinical sequelae.

One of the important limitations of VH-IVUS is its limited axial resolution of 100–150 μm [52], which means that it will tend to overestimate the number of plaques with a thin fibrous cap (traditionally defined by a thickness of <60 μm). This may account for the low event rate associated with VH-IVUS-defined TCFAs.

8.3.2 Assessment of Fibrous Cap Thickness with Optical Coherent Tomography

Optical coherence tomography (OCT) is an imaging modality that provides high-resolution (15–20 μm) tomographic visualisation of the coronary arteries. Although OCT lacks penetration (1–2 mm into the plaque), it is especially good for examining the surface of the plaque, for estimating the thickness of the fibrous cap and for identifying regions of plaque rupture and superimposed thrombus. These high-resolution capabilities make OCT attractive for the identification of high-risk plaques although its poor depth penetration hampers full characterisation of coronary plaque morphology and burden. In particular the potential of OCT to identify TCFAs in vivo is of major potential interest [53], and it has also been suggested that the capability of OCT to measure changes in the fibrous cap thickness could be useful in monitoring the plaque-stabilising effects of statins and other drugs [54, 55]. Future studies investigating whether the identification of plaques with a thin cap on OCT identifies high-risk patients or predicts clinical events are therefore urgently required.

8.3.3 Assessment of Plaque Surface Characteristics with Angioscopy

Angioscopy has demonstrated an association between plaque colour and lipid-rich plaques in patients with MI [56, 57]. Indeed, yellow plaques as defined by quantitative colorimetry have been associated with a large lipid core and a thin fibrous cap. However, the predictive capability of this technology is yet to be defined.

8.3.4 Lipid Core Burden Assessment with Near-Infrared Spectroscopy (NIRS)

NIRS takes advantage of the fact that different organic molecules absorb and scatter NIR light at different degrees and at various wavelengths. The processing of the reflected signal provides information about the chemical composition of different tissues and seems to permit reliable detection of the lipid component. Atherosclerotic plaques, especially lipid-rich plaques, have a specific chemical signature related to cholesterol esters present in lipid cores. Ex vivo studies have demonstrated the feasibility of atherosclerotic lipid-rich plaque detection using near-infrared spectroscopy. A catheter-based NIRS system and a chemometric algorithm for the detection of lipid core plaques were recently developed and prospectively validated in a human coronary artery autopsy study [58]. NIRS data are presented as a 'chemogram' representing the probability that a lipid core plaque is present (yellow for high probability, red for low probability). A first-in-human validation study demonstrated the mathematical and statistical similarity of spectra acquired in vivo compared with those obtained in autopsy specimens [59]; the algorithm identified lipid core plaque in 60 % of imaged segments in patients undergoing PCI for stable angina or ACS. NIRS can collect data with rapid acquisition times, avoiding the need to obstruct blood flow. A limitation of NIRS, however, is that it does not create an image of the vessel wall. Thus, no information is provided as to the depth of lipid core plaque nor can it differentiate thin and thick capped atheroma.

The reliability of this technique has been evaluated in histology-based studies, whereas the SPECTroscopic Assessment of Coronary Lipid (SPECTACL) study was the first report to demonstrate the feasibility of a NIRS catheter in the clinical setting. Recently, NIRS has been used to assess changes in plaque composition with the Reduction in Yellow Plaque by Aggressive Lipid-Lowering Therapy (YELLOW) trial [60] using NIRS to assess the short-term effect of intensive medical treatment with rosuvastatin on both plaque burden and composition. PROSPECT II is a natural history, multicenter study, which will assess the ability of intracoronary NIRS to predict adverse clinical events.

8.3.5 Assessment of Calcific Plaque Disease with Coronary Artery Calcium Score

Ever since Agatston et al. described the calculation of the total calcific burden using coronary artery calcium (CAC) scoring in 1990, this method has become a reliable and reproducible non-invasive technique to quantify coronary atherosclerosis [61]. Total CAC score is derived by multiplying individual areas of calcified plaque by a factor derived from the maximal plaque density (CT attenuation) in Hounsfield units and then adding the values obtained for all coronary plaques identified. Subsequent studies have established CT calcium scoring to be one of the most powerful predictors of future cardiovascular events in asymptomatic individuals irrespective of ethnicity [62–66]. Moreover, risk prediction can be further refined by examining the progression of coronary calcification [67].

CT calcium scoring quantifies macroscopic calcification in the coronary arteries. These plaques are believed to be stable, healed and unlikely to rupture. Indeed, it is well established that calcific fibroatheromas and calcified nodules are very rarely responsible for coronary thrombosis [37]. Why then does calcium scoring predict cardiovascular risk related to rupture? The likely explanation is that it provides a surrogate of plaque burden. The more calcified stable plaques you have, the more unstable non-calcified plaques you are also likely to have in addition [68, 69].

8.3.6 Assessment of Low-Attenuation Plaque, Positive Remodelling and Spotty Calcification with Computed Tomography Coronary Angiography (CTCA)

Due to its wide availability and adoption, one of the most important non-invasive techniques for the evaluation of the coronary vasculature is CTCA. Several studies have reported on the correlation between CTCA plaque features with invasive coronary imaging modalities, such as IVUS, IVUS-VH and OCT. Identification of spotty calcification using CTCA has been associated with high-risk plaque type [70]. Furthermore, Motoyama et al. reported that positive remodelling and low-attenuation plaque on CTCA predict a higher likelihood of future plaque rupture [71]. Others have described features such as the 'napkin ring' or the 'signet ring' sign for identification of plaque vulnerability [72]. However, interpretation of such features on CTCA comes with significant limitations. Suboptimal resolution does not allow precise definition of the vascular boundary, and the extent of positive remodelling may be over- or underestimated. Similarly, low-attenuation plaque is defined based on specific thresholds in the Hounsfield unit measurements which may be influenced by various imaging and technical parameters in regions of non-calcified plaque.

8.3.7 Metabolic Imaging with Positron Emission Tomography-Computed Tomography (PET-CT)

Combined positron emission and computed tomography (PET-CT) is a modern non-invasive imaging technique that combines functional information from PET with the fine anatomical detail provided by CT, allowing the activity of specific pathological processes to be studied within even small structures in the body. This technique has been widely used in the clinical assessment of patients with cancer for many years, resulting in the widespread availability of PET-CT scanners [73]. Recent technological advances including ECG gating alongside improved PET resolution and fusion with detailed CT angiography of the coronary vessels have allowed translation of this technology into the heart. Theoretically any pathological process can be studied dependent on a suitable radiotracer being developed so that in principle any of the above characteristics of high-risk plaque can be targeted. However, to date the most promising studies investigating coronary atherosclerosis have utilised the tracers18F-fluorodeoxyglucose (18F-FDG) as a marker of inflammation and 18F-fluoride as a marker of microcalcification.

8.3.7.1 Targeting Inflammation with 18F-Fluorodeoxyglucose

18F-fluorine-labelled 2-deoxy-2-fluoro-D-glucose (18F-FDG) is used extensively to image metabolically active cells with PET-CT. Indeed, it has been employed very successfully to identify metastases in patients with high-grade poorly differentiated tumours [73]. In cardiovascular disease, several studies have demonstrated a close association between 18F-FDG and tissue macrophage burden in the carotid arteries [74, 75]. Furthermore, 18F-FDG uptake is associated with traditional cardiovascular risk factors including age, male gender and metabolic syndrome as well as inflammatory biomarkers [76, 77]. Moreover, vascular 18F-FDG uptake is elevated in patients infected with human immunodeficiency virus [78] and with rheumatoid arthritis [79], perhaps accounting for the increased cardiovascular events in these patient populations. Indeed, 18F-FDG has become a widely used measure of vascular inflammation and employed to demonstrate the anti-inflammatory effects of statins and other lipid-lowering agents [80, 81]. However, recent data have suggested that the mechanisms underlying vascular 18F-FDG activity may be more complex, implicating hypoxia as an important driver of 18F-FDG uptake by both macrophages and vascular smooth muscle cells [82]. Recent data have also suggested that 18F-FDG preferentially labels M1-type pro-inflammatory macrophages rather than the anti-inflammatory M2 type [83].

Whilst 18F-FDG uptake has been validated in large vessels such as the aorta, carotid, iliac and femoral arteries, attempts to utilise this tracer in the coronary arteries have been less successful. Increased 18F-fluorodeoxyglucose in the coronary arteries has been described in patients with coexisting malignancy [84, 85]. Since then, three prospective studies have examined the feasibility and reproducibility of assessing uptake of this tracer in the coronary vasculature [86–88]. Whilst two early studies [86, 88] suggested that 18F-fluorodeoxyglucose might identify some inflamed plaques in patients with recent myocardial infarction, others have more recently demonstrated that in 50 % of patients with acute myocardial infarction, there was no uptake of 18F-fluorodeoxyglucose in the culprit plaque [88].

We reported the coronary uptake of 18F-FDG in patients with and without aortic stenosis (Fig. 8.2) [87]. The 18F-FDG uptake was difficult to quantify, particularly in the left main stem and circumflex artery. It was not possible to quantify accurately in 49 % of the vessel territories examined in this cohort. This was largely the

Fig. 8.2 18F-fluoride and 18F-FDG uptake in patients with myocardial infarction and stable angina: Focal ^{18}F-fluoride and ^{18}F-fluorodeoxyglucose uptake in patients with myocardial infarction and stable angina. Patient with acute ST segment elevation myocardial infarction with (**a**) proximal occlusion (*red arrow*) of the left anterior descending artery on invasive coronary angiography and (**b**) intense focal ^{18}F-fluoride uptake (*yellow-red*) at the site of the culprit plaque (*red arrow*) on the combined positron emission and computed tomogram (PET-CT). Corresponding ^{18}F-fluorodeoxyglucose PET-CT image (**c**) showing no uptake at the site of the culprit plaque (18F-FDG). Note the significant myocardial uptake overlapping with the coronary artery (*yellow arrow*) and uptake within the oesophagus (*blue arrow*). Patient with anterior non-ST segment elevation myocardial infarction with (**d**) culprit (*red arrow*; left anterior descending artery) and bystander non-culprit (*white arrow*; circumflex artery) lesions on invasive coronary angiography that were both stented during the index admission. Only the culprit lesion had increased ^{18}F-NaF uptake on PET-CT (**e**) after percutaneous coronary intervention. Corresponding ^{18}F-fluorodeoxyglucose PET-CT showing no uptake either at the culprit or the bystander stented lesion. Note intense uptake within the ascending aorta. In a patient with stable angina with previous coronary artery bypass grafting, invasive coronary angiography (**g**) showed non-obstructive disease in the right coronary artery. Corresponding PET-CT scan (**h**) showed a region of increased ^{18}F-NaF activity (positive lesion, *red line*) in the mid-right coronary artery and a region without increased uptake in the proximal vessel (negative lesion, *yellow line*). Radiofrequency intravascular ultrasound shows that the ^{18}F-NaF-negative plaque (**i**) is principally composed of fibrous and fibrofatty tissue (*green*) with confluent calcium (*white* with acoustic shadow) but little evidence of necrosis. On the contrary, the ^{18}F-NaF-positive plaque (**j**) shows high-risk features such as a large necrotic core (*red*) and microcalcification (*white*) (Reprinted from Joshi et al. [89] under CC BY open access) result of myocardial spillover into the coronary arteries, which was observed despite the dietary restrictions imposed in the study. Overall, we did not find any difference in patients within control group and patients with atherosclerosis.

More recently, we have prospectively evaluated 18F-FDG in patients with stable and unstable coronary disease [89]. Again, we failed to demonstrate the utility of this tracer in identifying culprit or high-risk plaques in patients with myocardial infarction or stable angina, primarily due to intense myocardial uptake of this tracer that hampered assessment in the coronary arteries. This was despite stringent dietary recommendations that successfully suppressed myocardial uptake in 70–85 % of

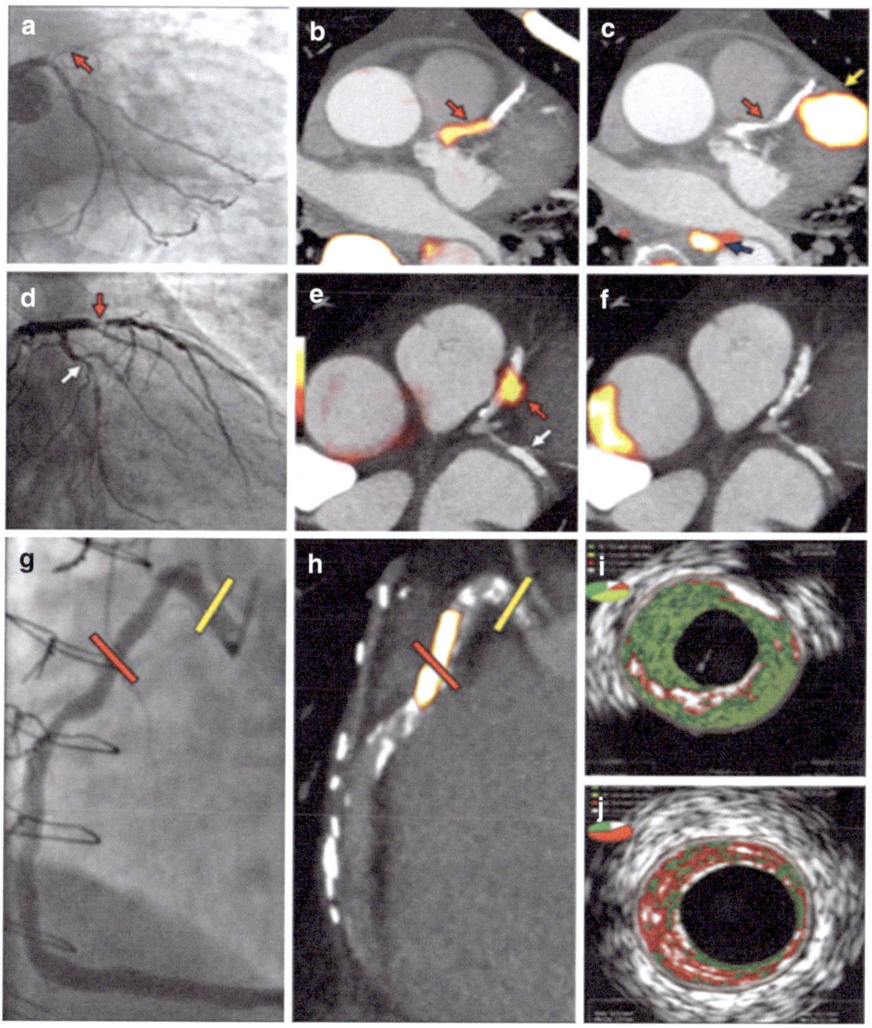

patients, a rate that compares favourably with previous studies (57–84 %) [86, 88]. However, frequently this suppression resulted in a patchy distribution of myocardial uptake that obscured activity in one or more coronary vessels. Given its limitations, we believe that 18F-FDG is unlikely to become sufficiently robust to permit its clinical application to the coronary circulation unless we find a more effective way to suppress myocardial uptake. However, we believe that 18F-FDG uptake remains a very important measure of general vascular inflammation and will remain the principal tracer in assessment of inflammation in large arteries such as the aorta and carotid arteries.

Whilst advances in suppressing myocardial 18F-FDG activity and cardiac motion correction are likely to improve this technique, ultimately we believe that more macrophage-specific tracers will be required. Indeed, the development of such tracers is an active area of research with several agents, including 1C-PK11195 [90] and 18F-fluorodeoxymannose [3], holding real promise. Specifically, 18F-fluorodeoxymannose (FDM) also binds to mannose receptors present on activated anti-inflammatory (M2) macrophages that are associated with plaque features of high risk such as neovascularisation and intra-plaque haemorrhage. By targeting mannose receptor expression in addition to plaque glucose metabolism, 18F-FDM is potentially able to both quantify and characterise plaque inflammation.

8.3.7.2 Targeting Plaque Necrosis and Microcalcification with 18F-Fluoride

18F-fluoride is a PET tracer with favourable pharmacokinetic properties, first introduced by Blau and coworkers in 1962 for study of bone diseases [91–96]. 18F-fluoride uptake is characterised by excellent tissue to background ratios allowing an accurate assessment of tracer activity within the vascular tissue. Specifically, the tracer exchanges with hydroxyl groups in regions of hydroxyapatite at the surface of the bone to form fluorapatite [91–93]. In so doing, 18F-fluoride acts as a marker of bone mineralisation and has been extensively utilised to study various bone-related clinical conditions [14, 97–103], including the detection of malignant bone involvement [104–108].

The mechanisms of 18F-fluoride uptake within the vasculature are similar to those observed in the bone. 18F-fluoride primarily highlights areas of vasculature undergoing active calcification. The degree of 18F-NaF uptake is dependent on the surface area of the hydroxyapatite crystalline structure [109]. As a consequence of this surface area effect, 18F-NaF preferentially binds to regions of this newly developing calcification as opposed to field macroscopic calcification where much of the hydroxyapatite is internalised and not available for binding. Within an atherosclerotic plaque, calcification is believed to occur as a direct response to intense necrotic inflammation similar to that observed in caseating granulomata. Hydroxyapatite crystals are laid out within the areas of necrosis to which 18F-fluoride binds. Indeed, recent unpublished data suggests that 18F-fluoride is a specific marker of calcification activity within atherosclerotic tissue [110].

The vascular uptake of 18F-fluoride has been recently described in large vessels such as the aorta, carotids and femoral vessels. In the latter 18F-fluoride uptake has been shown to correlate with cardiovascular risk factors and plaque burden [111–113]. However, only a fifth of all calcified plaques on CT demonstrated increased 18F-fluoride uptake, highlighting that this tracer provides different information to CT [114]. Furthermore, the distribution of 18F-fluoride and 18F-FDG uptake demonstrated poor co-localisation confirming that these two tracers highlight distinct pathological processes [115].

Coronary 18F-fluoride has been subsequently described in the patients with and without aortic stenosis with excellent reproducibility (Fig. 8.2) [87, 116]. Furthermore, the ability of this tracer to distinguished patients with increased cardiovascular risk scores, prior MACE and patients with higher rates of angina symptoms has been demonstrated [87]. 18F-NaF uptake in the coronary arteries demonstrated a different distribution to the presence of macroscopic calcium detected by computed tomography. Indeed, we observed that 41 % of patients with very high coronary artery calcium scores (above 1000 Agatston units) did not have increased 18F-NaF uptake, suggesting the ability of 18F-fluoride to distinguish between patients with dormant pacified calcific disease and metabolically active ongoing calcification.

Subsequently, 18F-fluoride has been studied in patients with myocardial infarction, stable angina and symptomatic carotid disease [89]. Amongst 40 patients with ST and non-ST elevation myocardial infarction, increased 18F-fluoride uptake was observed at the site of the culprit plaque in 93 % of patients. Indeed, activity was around 30 % higher in the culprit plaque than the maximum activity recorded anywhere else in the coronary vasculature, independent of the effects of coronary artery stenting. In patients with symptomatic carotid disease who had undergone carotid endarterectomy, 18F-fluoride signal co-localised to the site of macroscopic plaque rupture. Histological analysis of these 18F-fluoride-positive regions of atheroma showed increased levels of macrophage infiltration, cell death, necrosis and calcification activity as compared to 18F-fluoride negative areas.

In patients with stable angina, about two-fifths of patients with stable angina had increased fluoride uptake with 18F-fluoride-positive plaques demonstrating multiple features of plaque vulnerability including a higher necrotic core burden, positive remodelling and microcalcification as compared to plaques without uptake.

What then is the explanation for 18F-fluoride identifying ruptured and high-risk coronary atheroma? As in bone, 18F-fluoride is believed to bind to hydroxyapatite proportional to the available surface area of this crystal for binding. This is much higher in regions of nanocrystalline microcalcification than the regions of macroscopic calcium traditionally identified by CT. Indeed, this has been confirmed in recent mechanistic studies and explains the different information provided by these two imaging modalities and the ability of 18F-fluoride PET to identify high-risk lesions with newly developing microcalcification, the latter presumably occurring as a response to intense inflammation within the necrotic core of these plaques.

The next question is whether all plaques with increased 18F-fluoride activity will go on to rupture and cause myocardial infarction. We believe this is highly unlikely. In the first instance, the calcific healing response to intense necrotic inflammation is often likely to prove successful in pacifying the plaque and avoiding rupture.

Moreover, we know that even if the plaque does go on to rupture, this is actually a ubiquitous event that most commonly is subclinical and does not result in myocardial infarction. Nonetheless, we believe that 18F-fluoride will have a role in identifying the vulnerable patient, those subjects with high-risk atheroma that will be at an elevated risk of an event compared to subjects with truly stable coronary artery disease [117]. This issue will be addressed in the ongoing multicentre prospective study PREFFIR which will investigate whether 18F-fluoride PET imaging can prospectively predict plaque rupture events and disease progression in patients with coronary artery disease. The DIAMOND study will then go on to investigate whether such patients might then benefit from aggressive medical therapy.

8.3.7.3 Alternative Novel Radiotracers

The great strength of PET imaging is that tracers can ultimately be developed to target any pathological process of interest and can therefore be directed to any of the features that characterise high-risk plaques. Whilst this is an expensive process, the studies using 18F-fluoride have clearly demonstrated that metabolic plaque imaging in the coronary arteries is now feasible, making an expansion of activity in this area likely.

Given its pathophysiological importance, inflammation would appear to be the prime potential target. As discussed, 18F-FDG, whilst an excellent tracer for measuring inflammation in the aorta and carotids arteries, is of limited use in the coronary arteries, the metabolic activity of which governs the majority of clinical events. There is therefore an urgent need to develop more macrophage-specific tracers that crucially do not demonstrate increased activity in adjacent structures as the myocardium.

Inflammation Imaging with ^{68}Ga-DOTATATE

There has been significant interest in inflammation imaging with 68Ga-DOTATATE, a novel tracer with receptor binding specificity to somatostatin 2. Although primarily overexpressed in malignancies, in particular neuroendocrine tumours, somatostatin receptors are thought to be preferentially expressed in damaged and proliferating endothelium and by activated macrophages [118–120]. Indeed, murine data has shown good correlation between tracer activity and macrophage density in atherosclerotic lesions [121]. Observational data from oncology patients has reported uptake for this tracer in large vessels again demonstrating a good correlation with calcific plaque burden. Interestingly, in this study, 18F-FDG uptake did not co-localise with 68Ga-DOTATATE suggesting labelling of distinct process within vascular inflammation [122]. Furthermore, uptake has been described in the coronaries with modest correlation with calcific plaque burden and previous cardiovascular events [123, 124].

Inflammation Imaging with 11C-PK11195, 18F-FMCH and 11C-Choline

11C-PK11195 is a selective ligand for peripheral benzodiazepine receptors expressed in activated macrophages and is primarily used to image neuroinflammation. It has been recently investigated in atherosclerotic plaque imaging. In preclinical models, 11C-PK11195 localised to areas of vascular inflammation [125] and has also been investigated for the use in atherosclerosis imaging. Indeed, carotid uptake of 11C-PK11195 has been shown to be increased in symptomatic carotid atherosclerosis, with good correlation between the tracer autoradiography and CD68 macrophage expression in ex vivo plaques [126]. Uptake of 11C-PK11195 has also been described in patients with active systemic vasculitis [127].

Other tracers that are thought to bind to activated macrophages include 18F-FMCH and 11C-choline. Primarily used in cancer imaging, the tracers are thought to be incorporated within the cell membrane after phosphorylation by choline kinase [128]. Similar to other tracers, uptake has been described in murine models of atherosclerosis and oncological patients in retrospective analysis [129–132].

Assessment of Hypoxia with 18F-Fluoromisonadazole (FMISO) and Neoangiogenesis with 18F-Galacto and 18F-Fluciclatide

Other important features of plaque vulnerability apart from inflammation include hypoxia and neoangiogenesis, both of which are legitimate atherosclerotic targets. Tissue hypoxia within the plaque increases with the size of the necrotic core and creates a stimulus for new microvessel formation through hypoxia-inducible factor 1α [133]. Newly formed microvessels are fragile and permeable without lack of supporting structures and are prone to intra-plaque haemorrhage [37, 134]. Extravasation of erythrocytes within the plaque is a rich source of free cholesterol and cholesterol ester, which play an important role in plaque progression and vulnerability.

18F-FMISO uptake has been shown to co-localise with regions of hypoxia determined by pimonidazole staining. Histological evidence in murine models of atherosclerosis suggests that its uptake is deep within the necrotic core of the plaque in areas of macrophage infiltration [135]. Prospective studies of this tracer in patients with carotid atherosclerosis comparing its uptake to that of 18F-FDG uptake are currently underway.

New blood cells express the cell surface integrin receptors αvβ3 and αvβ5, which recognise the arginine-glycine-aspartate (RGD) motif. RGD-containing PET tracers such as 18F-galacto and 18F-fluciclatide have therefore been utilised to study angiogenesis [136, 137]. 18F-galacto has recently been reported in patients with significant carotid atherosclerosis and validated as a biomarker for αvβ3 integrin expression [138]. 18F-fluciclatide is currently being evaluated in patients with coronary atherosclerosis.

8.4 Summary

There is a recent interest in the study of atherosclerotic plaque vulnerability, and the race is on for identification of techniques that will improve the prediction of myocardial infarction. Breakthrough transitional research in invasive and non-invasive modalities based on our improved understanding of the underlying pathophysiology has advanced the field of in vivo plaque imaging. In this regard, metabolic imaging using 18F-fluoride PET-CT has shown great promise in identification of high-risk vulnerable atherosclerotic plaques. Prospective studies are now underway to investigate whether this approach can identify patients at increased risk of myocardial infarction so that ultimately these patients can be targeted with aggressive medical therapy aimed at preventing adverse events.

References

1. Lozano R, Naghavi M, Foreman K, et al. Global and regional mortality from 235 causes of death for 20 age groups in 1990 and 2010: a systematic analysis for the Global Burden of Disease Study 2010. Lancet. 2012;380:2095–128.
2. Mozaffarian D, Benjamin EJ, Go AS, et al. Heart disease and stroke statistics-2015 update: a report from the American Heart Association. Circulation. 2015;131(4):e29–322.
3. Tahara N, Mukherjee J, de Haas HJ, et al. 2-deoxy-2-[(18)F]fluoro-d-mannose positron emission tomography imaging in atherosclerosis. Nat Med. 2014;20:215–9.
4. Otsuka F, Sakakura K, Yahagi K, Joner M, Virmani R. Has our understanding of calcification in human coronary atherosclerosis progressed? Arterioscler Thromb Vasc Biol. 2014;34: 724–36.
5. Golestani R, Sadeghi MM. Emergence of molecular imaging of aortic aneurysm: implications for risk stratification and management. J Nucl Cardiol. 2014;21:251–67; quiz 268–70.
6. Thompson RC, Allam AH, Lombardi GP, et al. Atherosclerosis across 4000 years of human history: the Horus study of four ancient populations. Lancet. 2013;381:1211–22.
7. Falk E, Nakano M, Bentzon JF, Finn AV, Virmani R. Update on acute coronary syndromes: the pathologists' view. Eur Heart J. 2013;34:719–28.
8. Budoff MJ, Young R, Lopez VA, et al. Progression of coronary calcium and incident coronary heart disease events: MESA (Multi-Ethnic Study of Atherosclerosis). J Am Coll Cardiol. 2013;61:1231–9.
9. Palombo D, Morbelli S, Spinella G, et al. A positron emission tomography/computed tomography (PET/CT) evaluation of asymptomatic abdominal aortic aneurysms: another point of view. Ann Vasc Surg. 2012;26:491–9.
10. Kataoka Y, Wolski K, Uno K, et al. Spotty calcification as a marker of accelerated progression of coronary atherosclerosis: insights from serial intravascular ultrasound. J Am Coll Cardiol. 2012;59:1592–7.
11. Libby P, DiCarli M, Weissleder R. The vascular biology of atherosclerosis and imaging targets. J Nucl Med. 2010;51 Suppl 1:33S–7.
12. Jaffer FA, Libby P, Weissleder R. Optical and multimodality molecular imaging: insights into atherosclerosis. Arterioscler Thromb Vasc Biol. 2009;29:1017–24.
13. Jaffer FA, Libby P, Weissleder R. Molecular imaging of cardiovascular disease. Circulation. 2007;116:1052–61.
14. Naghavi M, Libby P, Falk E, et al. From vulnerable plaque to vulnerable patient: a call for new definitions and risk assessment strategies: Part I. Circulation. 2003;108:1664–72.
15. Falk E, Shah PK, Fuster V. Coronary plaque disruption. Circulation. 1995;92:657–71.
16. Hackett D, Davies G, Maseri A. Pre-existing coronary stenoses in patients with first myocardial infarction are not necessarily severe. Eur Heart J. 1988;9:1317–23.
17. Ambrose JA, Tannenbaum MA, Alexopoulos D, et al. Angiographic progression of coronary artery disease and the development of myocardial infarction. J Am Coll Cardiol. 1988;12:56–62.
18. Stary HC, Chandler AB, Dinsmore RE, et al. A definition of advanced types of atherosclerotic lesions and a histological classification of atherosclerosis. A report from the Committee on Vascular Lesions of the Council on Arteriosclerosis, American Heart Association. Circulation. 1995;92:1355–74.
19. Moore KJ, Tabas I. Macrophages in the pathogenesis of atherosclerosis. Cell. 2011;145: 341–55.

20. Gimbrone Jr MA. Vascular endothelium, hemodynamic forces, and atherogenesis. Am J Pathol. 1999;155:1–5.
21. Williams KJ, Tabas I. The response-to-retention hypothesis of early atherogenesis. Arterioscler Thromb Vasc Biol. 1995;15:551–61.
22. Skalen K, Gustafsson M, Rydberg EK, et al. Subendothelial retention of atherogenic lipoproteins in early atherosclerosis. Nature. 2002;417:750–4.
23. Goldstein JL, Ho YK, Basu SK, Brown MS. Binding site on macrophages that mediates uptake and degradation of acetylated low density lipoprotein, producing massive cholesterol deposition. Proc Natl Acad Sci U S A. 1979;76:333–7.
24. Dong ZM, Chapman SM, Brown AA, Frenette PS, Hynes RO, Wagner DD. The combined role of P- and E-selectins in atherosclerosis. J Clin Invest. 1998;102:145–52.
25. Collins RG, Velji R, Guevara NV, Hicks MJ, Chan L, Beaudet AL. P-Selectin or intercellular adhesion molecule (ICAM)-1 deficiency substantially protects against atherosclerosis in apolipoprotein E-deficient mice. J Exp Med. 2000;191:189–94.
26. Shih PT, Brennan ML, Vora DK, et al. Blocking very late antigen-4 integrin decreases leukocyte entry and fatty streak formation in mice fed an atherogenic diet. Circ Res. 1999;84: 345–51.
27. Falk E. Pathogenesis of atherosclerosis. J Am Coll Cardiol. 2006;47:C7–12.
28. Hansson GK. Inflammation, atherosclerosis, and coronary artery disease. N Engl J Med. 2005;352:1685–95.
29. Suzuki H, Kurihara Y, Takeya M, et al. A role for macrophage scavenger receptors in atherosclerosis and susceptibility to infection. Nature. 1997;386:292–6.
30. Febbraio M, Podrez EA, Smith JD, et al. Targeted disruption of the class B scavenger receptor CD36 protects against atherosclerotic lesion development in mice. J Clin Invest. 2000;105:1049–56.
31. Virmani R, Kolodgie FD, Burke AP, Farb A, Schwartz SM. Lessons from sudden coronary death: a comprehensive morphological classification scheme for atherosclerotic lesions. Arterioscler Thromb Vasc Biol. 2000;20:1262–75.
32. Littlewood TD, Bennett MR. Apoptotic cell death in atherosclerosis. Curr Opin Lipidol. 2003;14:469–75.
33. Velican C. A dissecting view on the role of the fatty streak in the pathogenesis of human atherosclerosis: culprit or bystander? Med Int. 1981;19:321–37.
34. Getz GS. When is atherosclerosis not atherosclerosis? Arterioscler Thromb Vasc Biol. 2000;20:1694.
35. McGill Jr HC, McMahan CA, Zieske AW, et al. Associations of coronary heart disease risk factors with the intermediate lesion of atherosclerosis in youth. The Pathobiological Determinants of Atherosclerosis in Youth (PDAY) Research Group. Arterioscler Thromb Vasc Biol. 2000;20:1998–2004.
36. Kolodgie FD, Burke AP, Nakazawa G, Virmani R. Is pathologic intimal thickening the key to understanding early plaque progression in human atherosclerotic disease? Arterioscler Thromb Vasc Biol. 2007;27:986–9.
37. Virmani R, Burke AP, Farb A, Kolodgie FD. Pathology of the vulnerable plaque. J Am Coll Cardiol. 2006;47:C13–8.
38. Davies MJ. Anatomic features in victims of sudden coronary death. Coronary artery pathology. Circulation. 1992;85:I19–24.
39. Muller JE, Tofler GH, Stone PH. Circadian variation and triggers of onset of acute cardiovascular disease. Circulation. 1989;79:733–43.
40. Calvert PA, Obaid DR, O'Sullivan M, et al. Association between IVUS findings and adverse outcomes in patients with coronary artery disease: the VIVA (VH-IVUS in Vulnerable Atherosclerosis) Study. JACC Cardiovasc Imaging. 2011;4:894–901.
41. Stone GW, Maehara A, Lansky AJ, et al. A prospective natural-history study of coronary atherosclerosis. N Engl J Med. 2011;364:226–35.

42. Kolodgie FD, Burke AP, Farb A, et al. The thin-cap fibroatheroma: a type of vulnerable plaque: the major precursor lesion to acute coronary syndromes. Curr Opin Cardiol. 2001;16:285–92.
43. Joshi NV, Vesey A, Newby DE, Dweck MR. Will 18F-sodium fluoride PET-CT imaging be the magic bullet for identifying vulnerable coronary atherosclerotic plaques? Curr Cardiol Rep. 2014;16:521.
44. Narula J, Nakano M, Virmani R, et al. Histopathologic characteristics of atherosclerotic coronary disease and implications of the findings for the invasive and noninvasive detection of vulnerable plaques. J Am Coll Cardiol. 2013;61:1041–51.
45. Yamagishi M, Terashima M, Awano K, et al. Morphology of vulnerable coronary plaque: insights from follow-up of patients examined by intravascular ultrasound before an acute coronary syndrome. J Am Coll Cardiol. 2000;35:106–11.
46. Kotani J, Mintz GS, Castagna MT, et al. Intravascular ultrasound analysis of infarct-related and non-infarct-related arteries in patients who presented with an acute myocardial infarction. Circulation. 2003;107:2889–93.
47. Fujii K, Kobayashi Y, Mintz GS, et al. Intravascular ultrasound assessment of ulcerated ruptured plaques: a comparison of culprit and nonculprit lesions of patients with acute coronary syndromes and lesions in patients without acute coronary syndromes. Circulation. 2003;108:2473–8.
48. Ehara S, Kobayashi Y, Yoshiyama M, et al. Spotty calcification typifies the culprit plaque in patients with acute myocardial infarction: an intravascular ultrasound study. Circulation. 2004;110:3424–9.
49. Garcia-Garcia HM, Jang IK, Serruys PW, Kovacic JC, Narula J, Fayad ZA. Imaging plaques to predict and better manage patients with acute coronary events. Circ Res. 2014;114: 1904–17.
50. Garcia-Garcia HM, Mintz GS, Lerman A, et al. Tissue characterisation using intravascular radiofrequency data analysis: recommendations for acquisition, analysis, interpretation and reporting. EuroIntervention. 2009;5:177–89.
51. Cheng JM, Garcia-Garcia HM, de Boer SP, et al. In vivo detection of high-risk coronary plaques by radiofrequency intravascular ultrasound and cardiovascular outcome: results of the ATHEROREMO-IVUS study. Eur Heart J. 2014;35:639–47.
52. Rodriguez-Granillo GA, Garcia-Garcia HM, Mc Fadden EP, et al. In vivo intravascular ultrasound-derived thin-cap fibroatheroma detection using ultrasound radiofrequency data analysis. J Am Coll Cardiol. 2005;46:2038–42.
53. Kume T, Akasaka T, Kawamoto T, et al. Measurement of the thickness of the fibrous cap by optical coherence tomography. Am Heart J. 2006;152:755 e1–4.
54. Chia S, Raffel OC, Takano M, Tearney GJ, Bouma BE, Jang IK. Association of statin therapy with reduced coronary plaque rupture: an optical coherence tomography study. Coron Artery Dis. 2008;19:237–42.
55. Takarada S, Imanishi T, Kubo T, et al. Effect of statin therapy on coronary fibrous-cap thickness in patients with acute coronary syndrome: assessment by optical coherence tomography study. Atherosclerosis. 2009;202:491–7.
56. Ohtani T, Ueda Y, Mizote I, et al. Number of yellow plaques detected in a coronary artery is associated with future risk of acute coronary syndrome: detection of vulnerable patients by angioscopy. J Am Coll Cardiol. 2006;47:2194–200.
57. Ishibashi F, Aziz K, Abela GS, Waxman S. Update on coronary angioscopy: review of a 20-year experience and potential application for detection of vulnerable plaque. J Interv Cardiol. 2006;19:17–25.
58. Gardner CM, Tan H, Hull EL, et al. Detection of lipid core coronary plaques in autopsy specimens with a novel catheter-based near-infrared spectroscopy system. JACC Cardiovasc Imaging. 2008;1:638–48.
59. Waxman S, Dixon SR, L'Allier P, et al. In vivo validation of a catheter-based near-infrared spectroscopy system for detection of lipid core coronary plaques: initial results of the SPECTACL study. JACC Cardiovasc Imaging. 2009;2:858–68.

60. Kini AS, Baber U, Kovacic JC, et al. Changes in plaque lipid content after short-term intensive versus standard statin therapy: the YELLOW trial (reduction in yellow plaque by aggressive lipid-lowering therapy). J Am Coll Cardiol. 2013;62:21–9.
61. Agatston AS, Janowitz WR, Hildner FJ, Zusmer NR, Viamonte Jr M, Detrano R. Quantification of coronary artery calcium using ultrafast computed tomography. J Am Coll Cardiol. 1990;15:827–32.
62. Detrano R, Guerci AD, Carr JJ, et al. Coronary calcium as a predictor of coronary events in four racial or ethnic groups. N Engl J Med. 2008;358:1336–45.
63. Greenland P, LaBree L, Azen SP, et al. Coronary artery calcium score combined with Framingham score for risk prediction in asymptomatic individuals. JAMA. 2004;291:210–5.
64. Budoff MJ, Shaw LJ, Liu ST, et al. Long-term prognosis associated with coronary calcification: observations from a registry of 25,253 patients. J Am Coll Cardiol. 2007;49:1860–70.
65. Arad Y, Goodman KJ, Roth M, Newstein D, Guerci AD. Coronary calcification, coronary disease risk factors, C-reactive protein, and atherosclerotic cardiovascular disease events: the St. Francis Heart Study. J Am Coll Cardiol. 2005;46:158–65.
66. Taylor AJ, Bindeman J, Feuerstein I, Cao F, Brazaitis M, O'Malley PG. Coronary calcium independently predicts incident premature coronary heart disease over measured cardiovascular risk factors: mean three-year outcomes in the Prospective Army Coronary Calcium (PACC) project. J Am Coll Cardiol. 2005;46:807–14.
67. Raggi P, Callister TQ, Shaw LJ. Progression of coronary artery calcium and risk of first myocardial infarction in patients receiving cholesterol-lowering therapy. Arterioscler Thromb Vasc Biol. 2004;24:1272–7.
68. Otsuka F, Finn AV, Virmani R. Do vulnerable and ruptured plaques hide in heavily calcified arteries? Atherosclerosis. 2013;229:34–7.
69. Mauriello A, Servadei F, Zoccai GB, et al. Coronary calcification identifies the vulnerable patient rather than the vulnerable Plaque. Atherosclerosis. 2013;229:124–9.
70. Motoyama S, Kondo T, Sarai M, et al. Multislice computed tomographic characteristics of coronary lesions in acute coronary syndromes. J Am Coll Cardiol. 2007;50:319–26.
71. Motoyama S, Sarai M, Harigaya H, et al. Computed tomographic angiography characteristics of atherosclerotic plaques subsequently resulting in acute coronary syndrome. J Am Coll Cardiol. 2009;54:49–57.
72. Maurovich-Horvat P, Hoffmann U, Vorpahl M, et al. The napkin-ring sign: CT signature of high-risk coronary plaques? JACC Cardiovasc Imaging. 2010;3:440–4.
73. Lardinois D, Weder W, Hany TF, et al. Staging of non-small-cell lung cancer with integrated positron-emission tomography and computed tomography. N Engl J Med. 2003;348:2500–7.
74. Tawakol A, Migrino RQ, Bashian GG, et al. In vivo 18F-fluorodeoxyglucose positron emission tomography imaging provides a noninvasive measure of carotid plaque inflammation in patients. J Am Coll Cardiol. 2006;48:1818–24.
75. Rudd JH, Warburton EA, Fryer TD, et al. Imaging atherosclerotic plaque inflammation with [18F]-fluorodeoxyglucose positron emission tomography. Circulation. 2002;105:2708–11.
76. Yun M, Jang S, Cucchiara A, Newberg AB, Alavi A. 18F FDG uptake in the large arteries: a correlation study with the atherogenic risk factors. Semin Nucl Med. 2002;32:70–6.
77. Tahara N, Kai H, Yamagishi S, Mizoguchi M, et al. Vascular inflammation evaluated by [18F]-fluorodeoxyglucose positron emission tomography is associated with the metabolic syndrome. J Am Coll Cardiol. 2007;49:1533–9.
78. Subramanian S, Tawakol A, Burdo TH, et al. Arterial inflammation in patients with HIV. JAMA. 2012;308:379–86.
79. Maki-Petaja KM, Elkhawad M, Cheriyan J, et al. Anti-tumor necrosis factor-alpha therapy reduces aortic inflammation and stiffness in patients with rheumatoid arthritis. Circulation. 2012;126:2473–80.
80. Tahara N, Kai H, Ishibashi M, et al. Simvastatin attenuates plaque inflammation: evaluation by fluorodeoxyglucose positron emission tomography. J Am Coll Cardiol. 2006;48:1825–31.

81. Fayad ZA, Mani V, Woodward M, et al. Safety and efficacy of dalcetrapib on atherosclerotic disease using novel non-invasive multimodality imaging (dal-PLAQUE): a randomised clinical trial. Lancet. 2011;378:1547–59.
82. Folco EJ, Sheikine Y, Rocha VZ, et al. Hypoxia but not inflammation augments glucose uptake in human macrophages: Implications for imaging atherosclerosis with 18fluorine-labeled 2-deoxy-D-glucose positron emission tomography. J Am Coll Cardiol. 2011;58:603–14.
83. Satomi T, Ogawa M, Mori I, et al. Comparison of contrast agents for atherosclerosis imaging using cultured macrophages: FDG versus ultrasmall superparamagnetic iron oxide. J Nucl Med. 2013;54:999–1004.
84. Dunphy MP, Freiman A, Larson SM, Strauss HW. Association of vascular 18F-FDG uptake with vascular calcification. J Nucl Med. 2005;46:1278–84.
85. Wykrzykowska J, Lehman S, Williams G, et al. Imaging of inflamed and vulnerable plaque in coronary arteries with 18F-FDG PET/CT in patients with suppression of myocardial uptake using a low-carbohydrate, high-fat preparation. J Nucl Med. 2009;50:563–8.
86. Rogers IS, Nasir K, Figueroa AL, et al. Feasibility of FDG imaging of the coronary arteries: comparison between acute coronary syndrome and stable angina. JACC Cardiovasc Imaging. 2010;3:388–97.
87. Dweck MR, Chow MW, Joshi NV, et al. Coronary arterial 18F-sodium fluoride uptake: a novel marker of plaque biology. J Am Coll Cardiol. 2012;59:1539–48.
88. Cheng VY, Slomka PJ, Le Meunier L, et al. Coronary arterial 18F-FDG uptake by fusion of PET and coronary CT angiography at sites of percutaneous stenting for acute myocardial infarction and stable coronary artery disease. J Nucl Med. 2012;53:575–83.
89. Joshi NV, Vesey AT, Williams MC, et al. F-fluoride positron emission tomography for identification of ruptured and high-risk coronary atherosclerotic plaques: a prospective clinical trial. Lancet. 2014;383(9918):705–13.
90. Bird JL, Izquierdo-Garcia D, Davies JR, et al. Evaluation of translocator protein quantification as a tool for characterising macrophage burden in human carotid atherosclerosis. Atherosclerosis. 2010;210:388–91.
91. Blau M, Nagler W, Bender MA. Fluorine-18: a new isotope for bone scanning. J Nucl Med. 1962;3:332–4.
92. Blau M, Ganatra R, Bender MA. 18F-fluoride for bone imaging. Semin Nucl Med. 1972;2:31–7.
93. Hawkins RA, Choi Y, Huang SC, et al. Evaluation of the skeletal kinetics of fluorine-18-fluoride ion with PET. J Nucl Med. 1992;33:633–42.
94. Blake GM, Park-Holohan SJ, Cook GJ, Fogelman I. Quantitative studies of bone with the use of 18F-fluoride and 99mTc-methylene diphosphonate. Semin Nucl Med. 2001;31:28–49.
95. Wootton R, Dore C. The single-passage extraction of 18F in rabbit bone. Clin Phys Physiol Meas. 1986;7:333–43.
96. Hoh CK, Hawkins RA, Dahlbom M, et al. Whole body skeletal imaging with [18F]fluoride ion and PET. J Comput Assist Tomogr. 1993;17:34–41.
97. Cook GJ, Blake GM, Marsden PK, Cronin B, Fogelman I. Quantification of skeletal kinetic indices in Paget's disease using dynamic 18F-fluoride positron emission tomography. J Bone Miner Res. 2002;17:854–9.
98. Installe J, Nzeusseu A, Bol A, Depresseux G, Devogelaer JP, Lonneux M. (18)F-fluoride PET for monitoring therapeutic response in Paget's disease of bone. J Nucl Med. 2005;46:1650–8.
99. Frost ML, Fogelman I, Blake GM, Marsden PK, Cook Jr G. Dissociation between global markers of bone formation and direct measurement of spinal bone formation in osteoporosis. J Bone Miner Res. 2004;19:1797–804.
100. Messa C, Goodman WG, Hoh CK, et al. Bone metabolic activity measured with positron emission tomography and [18F]fluoride ion in renal osteodystrophy: correlation with bone histomorphometry. J Clin Endocrinol Metab. 1993;77:949–55.
101. Brenner W, Vernon C, Conrad EU, Eary JF. Assessment of the metabolic activity of bone grafts with (18)F-fluoride PET. Eur J Nucl Med Mol Imaging. 2004;31:1291–8.

102. Hsu WK, Feeley BT, Krenek L, Stout DB, Chatziioannou AF, Lieberman JR. The use of 18F-fluoride and 18F-FDG PET scans to assess fracture healing in a rat femur model. Eur J Nucl Med Mol Imaging. 2007;34:1291–301.
103. Schiepers C, Broos P, Miserez M, Bormans G, De Roo M. Measurement of skeletal flow with positron emission tomography and 18F-fluoride in femoral head osteonecrosis. Arch Orthop Trauma Surg. 1998;118:131–5.
104. Petren-Mallmin M, Andreasson I, Ljunggren O, et al. Skeletal metastases from breast cancer: uptake of 18F-fluoride measured with positron emission tomography in correlation with CT. Skeletal Radiol. 1998;27:72–6.
105. Schirrmeister H, Guhlmann A, Kotzerke J, et al. Early detection and accurate description of extent of metastatic bone disease in breast cancer with fluoride ion and positron emission tomography. J Clin Oncol. 1999;17:2381–9.
106. Hetzel M, Arslandemir C, Konig HH, et al. F-18 NaF PET for detection of bone metastases in lung cancer: accuracy, cost-effectiveness, and impact on patient management. J Bone Miner Res. 2003;18:2206–14.
107. Even-Sapir E, Metser U, Mishani E, Lievshitz G, Lerman H, Leibovitch I. The detection of bone metastases in patients with high-risk prostate cancer: 99mTc-MDP Planar bone scintigraphy, single- and multi-field-of-view SPECT, 18F-fluoride PET, and 18F-fluoride PET/CT. J Nucl Med. 2006;47:287–97.
108. Beheshti M, Vali R, Waldenberger P, et al. Detection of bone metastases in patients with prostate cancer by 18F fluorocholine and 18F fluoride PET-CT: a comparative study. Eur J Nucl Med Mol Imaging. 2008;35:1766–74.
109. Rey C, Combes C, Drouet C, Glimcher MJ. Bone mineral: update on chemical composition and structure. Osteoporos Int. 2009;20:1013–21.
110. Agnese Irkle JLB, Skepper JN, Dweck MR, et al. 18F-NaF – a specific marker for vascular calcification in atherosclerosis. Circulation. 2013;128, A17385.
111. Janssen T, Bannas P, Herrmann J, et al. Association of linear (18)F-sodium fluoride accumulation in femoral arteries as a measure of diffuse calcification with cardiovascular risk factors: a PET/CT study. J Nucl Cardiol. 2013;20:569–77.
112. Li Y, Berenji GR, Shaba WF, et al. Association of vascular fluoride uptake with vascular calcification and coronary artery disease. Nucl Med Commun. 2012;33:14–20.
113. Beheshti M, Saboury B, Mehta NN, et al. Detection and global quantification of cardiovascular molecular calcification by fluoro18-fluoride positron emission tomography/computed tomography–a novel concept. Hell J Nucl Med. 2011;14:114–20.
114. Derlin T, Richter U, Bannas P, et al. Feasibility of 18F-sodium fluoride PET/CT for imaging of atherosclerotic plaque. J Nucl Med. 2010;51:862–5.
115. Derlin T, Toth Z, Papp L, et al. Correlation of inflammation assessed by 18F-FDG PET, active mineral deposition assessed by 18F-fluoride PET, and vascular calcification in atherosclerotic plaque: a dual-tracer PET/CT study. J Nucl Med. 2011;52:1020–7.
116. Dweck MR, Jones C, Joshi NV, et al. Assessment of valvular calcification and inflammation by positron emission tomography in patients with aortic stenosis. Circulation. 2012;125:76–86.
117. Mann J, Davies MJ. Mechanisms of progression in native coronary artery disease: role of healed plaque disruption. Heart. 1999;82:265–8.
118. Armani C, Catalani E, Balbarini A, Bagnoli P, Cervia D. Expression, pharmacology, and functional role of somatostatin receptor subtypes 1 and 2 in human macrophages. J Leukoc Biol. 2007;81:845–55.
119. Adams RL, Adams IP, Lindow SW, Zhong W, Atkin SL. Somatostatin receptors 2 and 5 are preferentially expressed in proliferating endothelium. Br J Cancer. 2005;92:1493–8.
120. Dalm VA, van Hagen PM, van Koetsveld PM, et al. Expression of somatostatin, cortistatin, and somatostatin receptors in human monocytes, macrophages, and dendritic cells. Am J Physiol Endocrinol Metab. 2003;285:E344–53.
121. Li X, Bauer W, Kreissl MC, et al. Specific somatostatin receptor II expression in arterial plaque: (68)Ga-DOTATATE autoradiographic, immunohistochemical and flow cytometric studies in apoE-deficient mice. Atherosclerosis. 2013;230:33–9.

122. Li X, Samnick S, Lapa C, et al. 68Ga-DOTATATE PET/CT for the detection of inflammation of large arteries: correlation with18F-FDG, calcium burden and risk factors. EJNMMI Res. 2012;2:52.
123. Rominger A, Saam T, Vogl E, et al. In vivo imaging of macrophage activity in the coronary arteries using 68Ga-DOTATATE PET/CT: correlation with coronary calcium burden and risk factors. J Nucl Med. 2010;51:193–7.
124. Mojtahedi A, Alavi A, Thamake S, et al. Assessment of vulnerable atherosclerotic and fibrotic plaques in coronary arteries using (68)Ga-DOTATATE PET/CT. Am J Nucl Med Molec Imaging. 2015;5:65–71.
125. Laitinen I, Marjamaki P, Nagren K, et al. Uptake of inflammatory cell marker [11C]PK11195 into mouse atherosclerotic plaques. Eur J Nucl Med Mol Imaging. 2009;36:73–80.
126. Gaemperli O, Shalhoub J, Owen DR, et al. Imaging intraplaque inflammation in carotid atherosclerosis with 11C-PK11195 positron emission tomography/computed tomography. Eur Heart J. 2012;33:1902–10.
127. Pugliese F, Gaemperli O, Kinderlerer AR, et al. Imaging of vascular inflammation with [11C]-PK11195 and positron emission tomography/computed tomography angiography. J Am Coll Cardiol. 2010;56:653–61.
128. Owen DR, Lindsay AC, Choudhury RP, Fayad ZA. Imaging of atherosclerosis. Annu Rev Med. 2011;62:25–40.
129. Laitinen IE, Luoto P, Nagren K, et al. Uptake of 11C-choline in mouse atherosclerotic plaques. J Nucl Med. 2010;51:798–802.
130. Matter CM, Wyss MT, Meier P, et al. 18F-choline images murine atherosclerotic plaques ex vivo. Arterioscler Thromb Vasc Biol. 2006;26:584–9.
131. Bucerius J, Schmaljohann J, Bohm I, et al. Feasibility of 18F-fluoromethylcholine PET/CT for imaging of vessel wall alterations in humans–first results. Eur J Nucl Med Mol Imaging. 2008;35:815–20.
132. Kato K, Schober O, Ikeda M, et al. Evaluation and comparison of 11C-choline uptake and calcification in aortic and common carotid arterial walls with combined PET/CT. Eur J Nucl Med Mol Imaging. 2009;36:1622–8.
133. Marsch E, Sluimer JC, Daemen MJ. Hypoxia in atherosclerosis and inflammation. Curr Opin Lipidol. 2013;24:393–400.
134. Moreno PR, Purushothaman KR, Fuster V, et al. Plaque neovascularization is increased in ruptured atherosclerotic lesions of human aorta: implications for plaque vulnerability. Circulation. 2004;110:2032–8.
135. Mateo J, Izquierdo-Garcia D, Badimon JJ, Fayad ZA, Fuster V. Noninvasive assessment of hypoxia in rabbit advanced atherosclerosis using (1)(8)F-fluoromisonidazole positron emission tomographic imaging. Circ Cardiovasc Imaging. 2014;7:312–20.
136. Brooks PC, Clark RA, Cheresh DA. Requirement of vascular integrin alpha v beta 3 for angiogenesis. Science. 1994;264:569–71.
137. Beer AJ, Haubner R, Sarbia M, et al. Positron emission tomography using [18F]Galacto-RGD identifies the level of integrin alpha(v)beta3 expression in man. Clin Cancer Res. 2006;12:3942–9.
138. Beer AJ, Pelisek J, Heider P, et al. PET/CT imaging of integrin alphavbeta3 expression in human carotid atherosclerosis. JACC Cardiovasc Imaging. 2014;7:178–87.

Computed Tomography in the Concurrent Assessment of Coronary Morphology and Myocardial Perfusion

9

Ravi K. Sharma, Joao A.C. Lima, and Richard T. George

Abbreviations

CAD	Coronary artery disease
CTA	Coronary computed tomography angiography
CTP	Myocardial computed tomography perfusion
FFR	Fractional flow reserve
ICA	Invasive coronary angiography
MDCT	Multidetector computed tomography
MPI	Myocardial perfusion imaging
NPV	Negative predictive value
PET	Positron emission tomography
PPV	Positive predictive value
SPECT	Single-photon emission computed tomography

R.K. Sharma, MD (✉)
Division of Cardiology, Department of Medicine, Johns Hopkins University, Baltimore, MD, USA
e-mail: rsharm25@jhmi.edu

J.A.C. Lima, MD
Radiology and Epidemiology, Johns Hopkins University, School of Medicine, Cardiology, Baltimore, MD, USA
e-mail: jlima@jhmi.edu

R.T. George, MD
Johns Hopkins University, School of Medicine, Cardiology, Baltimore, MD, USA
e-mail: rgeorge3@jhmi.edu

T.H. Schindler et al. (eds.), *Molecular and Multimodality Imaging in Cardiovascular Disease*, DOI 10.1007/978-3-319-19611-4_9

9.1 Introduction

Rapid advancement in multidetector computed tomography (MDCT) technology has allowed rapid acquisition and assessment of coronary anatomy with high spatial resolution establishing itself as a compelling alternative to invasive coronary angiography (ICA). Coronary MDCT angiography (CTA) is the preferred imaging modality in patients with low- to intermediate-risk probability of coronary artery disease (CAD) given its high sensitivity and negative predictive value in assessment of CAD [1, 2]. However, anatomic imaging does not necessarily implicate that the detected stenosis causes downstream myocardial ischemia [3, 4], a potential therapeutic target using revascularization procedures. Thus, clinical practice guidelines strongly recommend ischemia assessment prior to elective revascularization procedure [5]. The revascularization in patients with concurrent ischemia has been shown to reduce mortality and symptomatic angina. Initial evidence emerges from the Coronary Artery Surgery Study (CASS) registry [6] which reported that patients with multivessel CAD had improved survival with surgical revascularization in the presence of severe ischemia on exercise stress testing, whereas medical therapy was a better approach in patients without significant ischemia. In the nuclear substudy of the COURAGE trial [7], coronary interventions resulted in a reduction in myocardial ischemia burden compared to optimal medical therapy arm, and the reduction of ischemia was associated with mitigation in anginal symptoms and translated into improved prognosis of the patients. The FAME (Fractional Flow Reserve vs. Angiography for Guiding PCI in Patients with Multivessel Coronary Artery Disease) trial [8] demonstrated that fractional flow reserve (FFR)-guided intervention to determine the functional severity of a coronary stenosis resulted in about one-third reduction in mortality and rate of coronary events (myocardial infarctions) compared to anatomic evaluation of stenosis alone.

The relationship between coronary stenosis and myocardial perfusion deficit is complex [3, 4]. The presence and extent of a myocardial perfusion deficit are influenced by multiple factors such as graded severity of stenosis, atherosclerotic burden, microvascular disease, collateral blood flow, as well as endothelial dysfunction [9, 10]. Since the discrepancies occur between the anatomic severity of a lesion and its concurrent hemodynamic effect, functional evaluation of a lesion is essential for clinical decision making, particularly for intermediate severity stenosis. The presence of a hemodynamically significant stenosis confers high risk of future cardiovascular events [11]. From a physician's perspective, it is advantageous to translate these findings into clinical practice in designing preventive or therapeutic interventions for a given patient.

Combination of anatomic and functional imaging offers a solution to the problem with software-based automatic/semiautomatic co-registration of image datasets that is both feasible and reliable. Hybrid imaging systems with CTA as an anatomic arm combined with myocardial perfusion imaging (MPI) in the form of positron emission tomography (PET) or single-photon emission computed tomography (SPECT) allows direct integration of morphologic and functional information. Availability of integrated scanner systems with the capability to perform PET/SPECT imaging in the same setting has made hybrid imaging convenient and logistically feasible. The other alternative is to derive functional information using single imaging platform with either a single-scan acquisition (CT-FFR) or performing stress myocardial CT perfusion (CTP) imaging. Acquisition of images in the same setting by a single imaging platform is advantageous in routine clinical practice. While CTP has been established as an incremental diagnostic predictor of flow-limiting stenosis [12], CT-FFR that provides hemodynamic information about a focal stenosis from a single image acquisition using complex computational fluid dynamic simulations is currently being investigated for broader applicability [13–15]. These modalities are discussed later in the chapter.

9.2 Background Principles

9.2.1 SPECT and PET-CT Myocardial Perfusion Imaging

Myocardial perfusion SPECT imaging is the most widely used and well-established noninvasive method for assessment of myocardial ischemia. Radionuclide myocardial perfusion imaging uses tracers tagged with radioisotopes that have minimal redistribution and high uptake properties; thereby the concentration of tracer is related to the myocardial blood flow and perfusion [16]. The perfusion pattern reflects the myocardial distribution of the tracer at the time of injection (peak stress) which can be qualitatively and/or quantitatively analyzed [17]. The reported sensitivity for SPECT for detecting >50 % angiographic stenosis is 87 % (range, 71–97 %), whereas the average specificity is 73 % (range, 36–100 %) [18]. With the use of attenuation correction methods, specificity improves especially among patients undergoing exercise stress testing [18]. With PET-MPI, the reported average sensitivity for detecting >50 % angiographic stenosis is 91 % (range, 83–100 %), whereas the average specificity is 89 % (range, 73–100 %) [17].

Initially implemented as an investigative imaging tool to evaluate in vivo quantification of myocardial perfusion and metabolism, PET-MPI has been increasingly utilized as a clinical perfusion imaging modality. PET-MPI in comparison to SPECT imaging has better spatial and contrast resolution. Additionally, well-validated attenuation correction limits the artifacts caused by soft tissue attenuation. This results into improved diagnostic accuracy of PET scanning for detecting obstructive CAD with reported sensitivity and specificity above 90 % [17]. Moreover, PET allows absolute quantification of myocardial perfusion (mL/min/g) that is particularly helpful in assessing the extent of CAD and its downstream perfusion abnormalities in multivessel disease (Fig. 9.1) [19–21]. Recent studies have underlined the clinical significance of absolute myocardial perfusion and have shown that quantitative analysis improves the diagnostic power of detecting CAD disease burden [22–24]. A nonuniform photo attenuation of SPECT imaging results in lower specificity, particularly in obese patients and in women where PET has shown to have improved diagnostic accuracy [21, 25].

Radionuclide perfusion imaging provides information about myocardial perfusion; however, it lacks information about coronary anatomy. Hence, nonobstructive stenoses below the threshold of causing an abnormal perfusion deficit cannot be detected. Simultaneous co-registration of perfusion deficit to a coronary stenosis and coronary artery distribution remain a challenge in the absence of information on

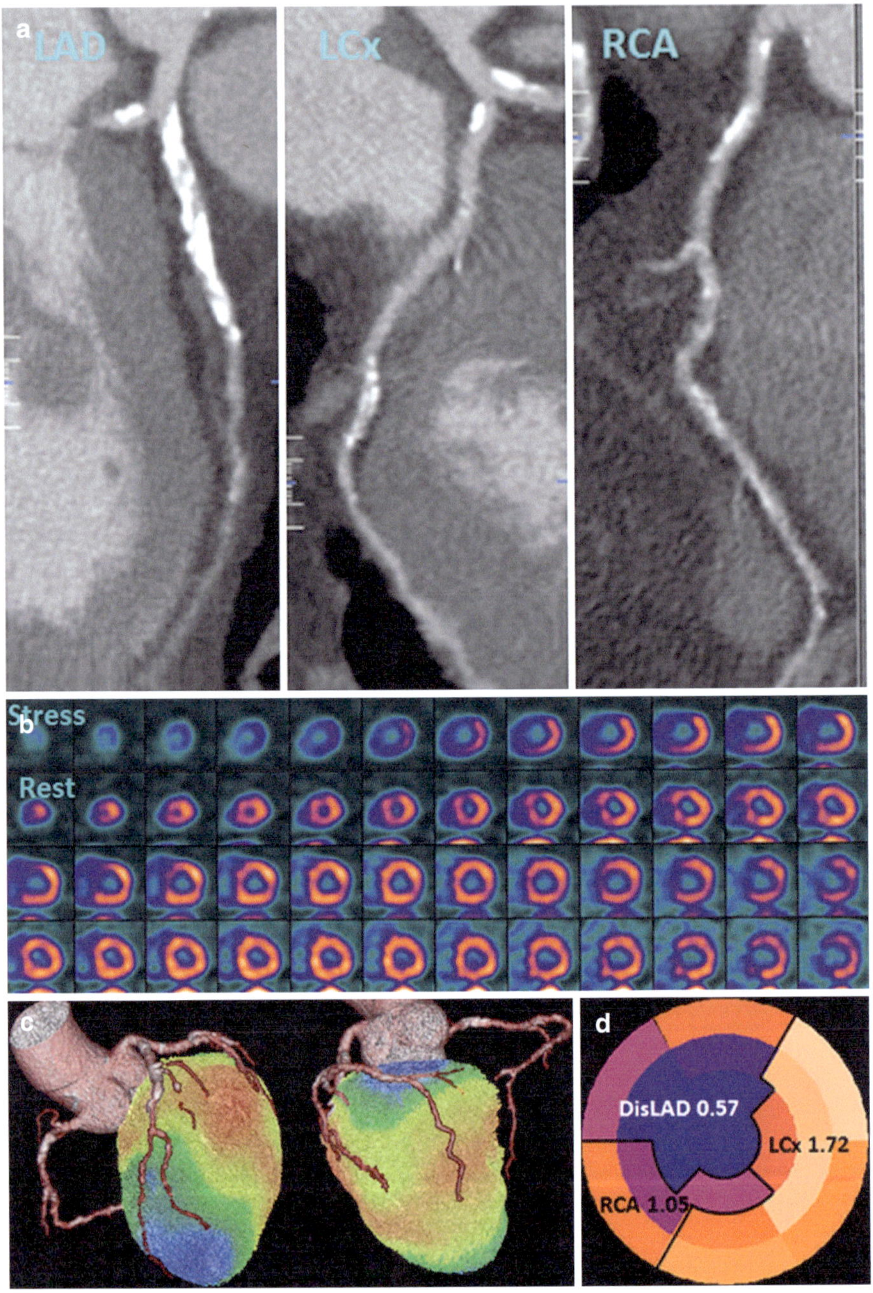
a
LAD
LCx
RCA
Stress
b
Rest
c
d
DisLAD 0.57
LCx 1.72
RCA 1.05

individual coronary anatomy. Standardized allocation of myocardial segment to the individual coronary artery and mental co-registration during scan interpretation may be a simplistic and familiar approach; however, significant anatomic variation exists among standardized vascular "territories" and corresponding coronary segments resulting in disagreement in up to 72 % of the cases [26]. Also, microvascular dysfunction in the absence of epicardial stenosis cannot be ascertained. Thus, accurate spatial localization of myocardial perfusion deficit and designating the individualized coronary artery segment significantly improve the diagnostic value of hybrid imaging and help in devising preventive and therapeutic intervention [17, 27].

9.2.2 Myocardial CTP Imaging

Myocardial CT perfusion imaging was made feasible with the availability of 16-row detector scanner systems [28, 29]. Progression of CT technology to 64-slice scanners allowed the combination of reliable coronary angiogram with stress-induced myocardial CTP technically possible to perform. Previous studies have shown good results with 64-row single-source and dual-source CT scanners [30–33]. However, these systems provide limited coverage of the heart and require cardiac volume acquisitions over several heartbeats, resulting in the more cranial portions of the heart being scanned earlier in time than the more caudal portions causing temporal heterogeneity and making comparisons in signal intensities between the two areas more difficult due to time-related changes in the myocardial contrast concentration [34, 35]. Introduction of wide-coverage (256-row and 320-row) MDCT systems permitted coverage of the entire cardiac volume in a single heartbeat over one gantry rotation. Along with the wide-coverage scan acquisition, prospective cardiac-gated imaging triggered during a specific period of the cardiac cycle (static CTP) mitigated the problem of temporal heterogeneity caused by time attenuation of iodinated contrast concentration in the myocardium. This resulted in significant

Fig. 9.1 Integrated PET/CTA study in a 66-year-old man with obesity, dyslipidemia, and diabetes mellitus. (**a**) Curved multiplanar reconstructions. The proximal LAD shows a long calcified plaque with 85 % stenosis. The LCx artery shows calcified plaques with 47 % stenosis proximally and 77 % stenosis distally. The RCA has a proximal, calcified plaque with 92 % stenosis. The summed stenosis score was 19 in the LAD, 6 in the LCx, and 16 in the RCA. The Duke CAD index was 74. (**b**) Stress and rest myocardial perfusion imaging shows extensive and severe ischemia in LAD territory with transient ischemic dilatation. (**c**) PET/CTA fusion imaging demonstrating that the mid- and basal inferior segments were supplied by a large-dominant LCx in contrast to the standard AHA model. (**d**) $MFR_{regional}$ were 0.57, 1.72, and 1.05 in the in LAD, LCx, and RCA territories, respectively. MFR_{global} was 1.28 (Adapted with permission from Naya et al. [85])

reduction in radiation so as to permit combined coronary CTA and stress myocardial perfusion assessment, providing comprehensive cardiac assessment with acceptable radiation dose. Additionally, faster acquisition has decreased scan times, reducing the amount of contrast material per scan [36].

Contrary to radionuclide myocardial perfusion imaging that uses tracers tagged with radioisotopes, myocardial CTP utilizes iodinated contrast as a perfusion agent. By measuring the concentration over time of the tracer in the myocardium, absolute blood flow in different regions of the myocardium can be estimated [34]. Iodinated contrast has comparable pharmacodynamics properties to gadolinium-based contrast agent used for magnetic resonance perfusion imaging. Iodinated contrast agent is extracted into the extracellular space in a linear relation to time and is excluded from the intracellular space bound by intact cellular membranes [37]. This concentration of iodinated contrast is directly proportional to the measured signal attenuation on a CT image (Hounsfield unit) (Fig. 9.2a, b). It represents a linear relationship between CT-derived metrics and myocardial blood flow and volume, which can be quantitatively analyzed [30, 34]. The extraction fraction of iodinated contrast from intravascular into the extracellular space is paradoxically higher at low blood flow and low at high flows [37]. This is important to consider when quantifying myocardial blood with CT, particularly in regard to correcting for the extraction of iodinated contrast at various flows.

Myocardial rest CT perfusion and delayed enhanced CT are capable of defining myocardial tissue characteristics [38, 39] as well as detecting acute and chronic myocardial infarction and viability [40–42]. However, for the detection of myocardial ischemia, a provocative stress test is necessary to assess for inducible myocardial ischemia. This can be performed by using exercise or dobutamine, both resulting in an increase in heart rate, or using pharmacologic vasodilation with adenosine, dipyridamole, or regadenoson. Since increase in heart rate is not ideal for quality cardiac CT scan acquisition, a vasodilator drug is a preferred stress agent for myocardial CTP with stress images acquired at the time of maximum hyperemia [30, 31, 34]. Adenosine is usually employed as a vasodilator agent and has the advantage of a short half-life that precludes need of reversal agent. However, adenosine administration requires an infusion pump, and side effects include atrioventricular block and bronchospasm [30, 31, 43]. Dipyridamole shares similar pharmacologic properties and side effect with adenosine except having a longer half-life that often requires reversal with aminophylline. Regadenoson is a specific A_{2A} agonist with lower incidence of side effects, primarily in regard to bronchospasm and heart block. Regadenoson's greatest advantage is its ease of administration. It comes in a prefilled syringe with uniform dosing for all patients eliminating drawing up or mixing of drug, infusion pump, and tubing. Regadenoson does cause a slightly higher heart rate than adenosine and dipyridamole [44, 45].

Myocardial stress CTP images can be acquired during a specified time period around the peak of the contrast bolus (static imaging) or serially as the contrast bolus traverses the coronary arteries and myocardial vasculature (dynamic perfusion). For static CTP, images are acquired during the late upslope, peak, and early downslope (Fig. 9.2a) of the contrast bolus and provide data that are qualitative or

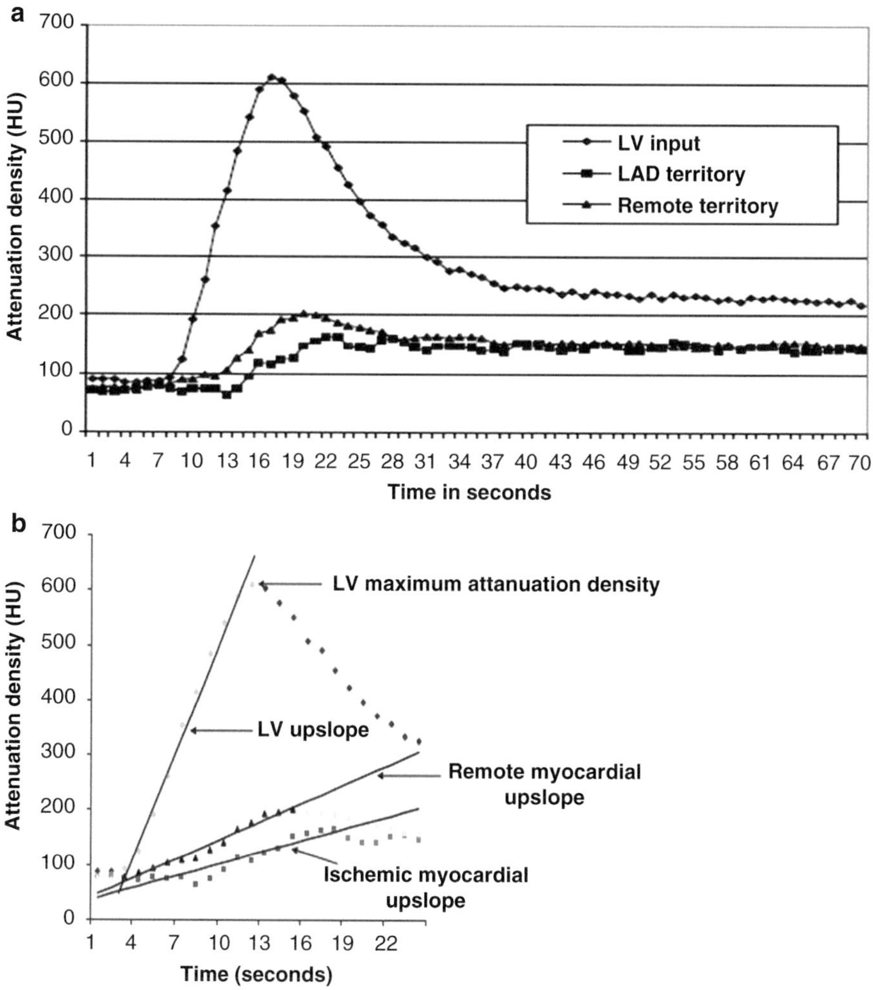

Fig. 9.2 (**a**) Time-attenuation curves for the left ventricle (*LV*), left anterior descending artery (*LAD*), and remote territories. Attenuation densities over time duration are expressed in Hounsfield units (*HU*). Significant differences are noted in the time-attenuation curves between stenosed LAD territory and remote myocardium. Also note that the LAD territory curve has a delay in onset and time to peak contrast enhancement as well as a lower peak myocardial attenuation density. (**b**) Dynamic MDCT parameters used in the upslope analysis methods. Upslopes of the left ventricular (*LV*) blood pool, remote myocardium, and ischemic myocardium were calculated by applying a best-fit linear regression line from the data points when iodinated contrast first enters the LV cavity to the peak contrast enhancement of the region of interest. Myocardial upslopes were normalized to the LV maximum attenuation density (MUS/LVM ratio) and the LV upslope (MUS/LVUS ratio) (Adapted with permission from George et al. [34])

semiquantitative [34]. Dynamic CTP involves construction of time-attenuation curves of the myocardium and the reference artery allowing calculation of myocardial blood flow and flow reserve [34, 46].

9.2.3 Computed Tomography-Fractional Flow Reserve (CT-FFR)

Recent developments in image-based modeling techniques have allowed accurate segmentation of coronary artery tree and application of computational fluid dynamics within the confines of coronary artery system. Mediated by complex algorithms and calculations applied to the simulated boundary conditions, coronary flow and pressure information can be obtained from rest CTA images. These models can also be used to quantify luminal stenosis and perform flow-pressure simulation models to determine the hemodynamic significance of a lesion, without a necessity of additional scan acquisition or administration of a pharmacologic stress agent.

The CT-FFR method involves derivation of fractional flow reserve (FFR) from anatomic CT data. FFR is defined as a ratio of intracoronary pressure distal to a stenosis and aortic pressure. Principally, segmentation algorithms are applied to create an anatomic model of the coronary artery anatomy followed by mathematical representation of coronary physiology derived using cardiac output, aortic pressure, and microcirculatory resistance. Allometric scaling laws, which analyze the relationship of mass of an object to shape, anatomy, and physiology, are used to define the relation of organ size to flow rate [47]. This enables the computation of coronary flow and pressure. Exploiting these principles, myocardial mass and volume extracted from the coronary CTA data are applied to estimate overall coronary flow under resting conditions. Based on consistent relationship between coronary flow and resistance, total coronary resistance can then be calculated using the coronary flow rate. Extending the mathematical relationship between vessel size and flow rate based on Poiseuille's equation ($Q\ f(dk)$, where Q is the flow rate through a blood vessel, d is its diameter, and k is a constant), information on the flow rate and relative resistance of the branches arising from the coronary arteries are obtained (Fig. 9.3).

Image segmentation algorithms define the luminal surface of the major vessels and branches, leading up to the vessel diameter limited by the spatial resolution of CTA. Based on the morphometric law, a unique resistance value is then assigned for each coronary artery and its branch outlets. Finally, maximum hyperemic conditions are simulated to model in the effect of adenosine administration (76 % drop from the resting values with intravenous administration of 140 mg/kg/min adenosine) [48] in decreasing the coronary resistance (Fig. 9.4). CT-FFR can then be determined by solving the equations of blood flow for the velocity and pressure fields and normalizing the mean hyperemic pressure field by the average mean hyperemic pressure in the aorta.

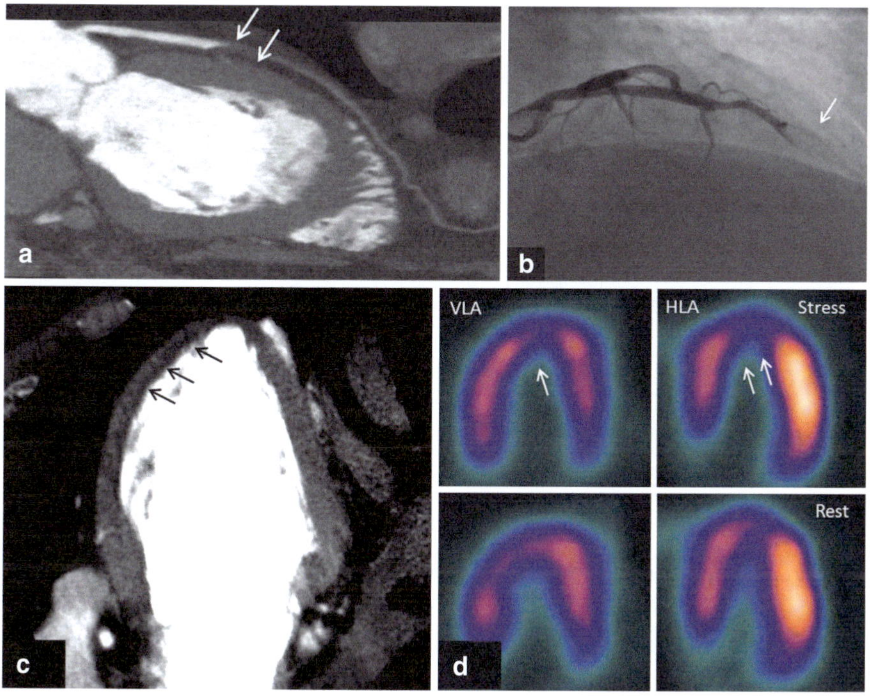

Fig. 9.3 Figures represent combined coronary CTA and myocardial CTP imaging showing flow-limiting stenosis confirmed by invasive coronary angiography and SPECT. CTA (panel-**a**) shows total occlusion of mid-LAD with corresponding CT hypoattenuation (panel-**c**, *black arrows*) involving anterior, anteroseptal, and apical myocardial segments consistent with myocardial CTP deficit. Panel **b** shows complete occlusion (100 % lesion) of mid-LAD on invasive coronary angiography with concurrent SPECT perfusion (panel **d**) defects read in similar myocardial segments as CTP

9.3 Clinical Evidence

9.3.1 Hybrid Imaging

With technical enhancements in image processing software and advent of hybrid scanners, it is possible to perform fusion of the two imaging modalities with simultaneous co-registration of anatomic-physiologic information that enables assigning perfusion territories to a specific stenosis. Clinical data on the diagnostic utility of hybrid imaging is largely restricted to single-center studies. Among intermediate-to high-pretest-likelihood patients, Schaap et al. reported that hybrid SPECT/CTA had a sensitivity of 96 %, specificity 95 %, PPV 96 %, and NPV 95 % [49]. The same group, in a high-risk and known CAD population, also reported that hybrid SPECT/CTA imaging had better diagnostic performance (c-index, 0.96) compared

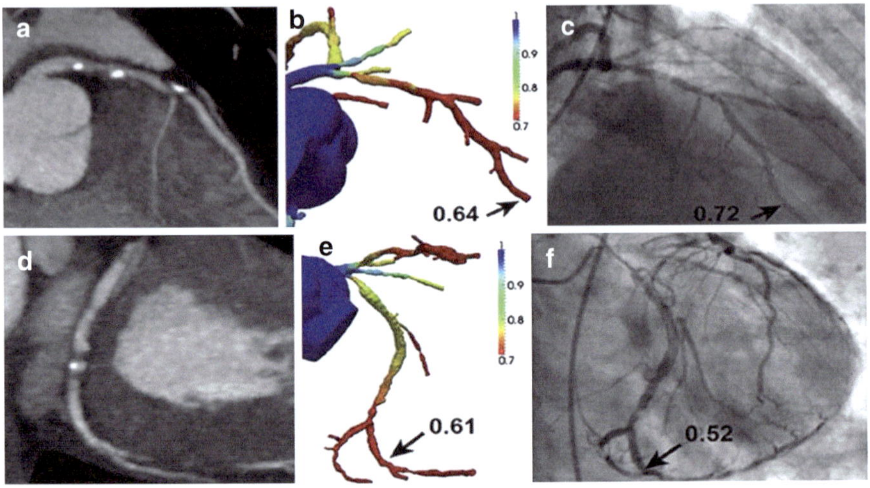

Fig. 9.4 (**a**) CTA demonstrating stenosis in the LAD. (**b**) FFRCTA demonstrates ischemia in the LAD, with a computed value of 0.64. (**c**) ICA with FFR also demonstrates ischemia in the LAD, with a measured value of 0.72. (**d**) CTA demonstrating stenosis in the LCx. (**e**) FFRCTA demonstrates ischemia in the LCx, with a computed value of 0.61. (**f**) ICA with FFR also demonstrates ischemia in the LCx, with a measured value of 0.52 (Adapted with permission from Taylor et al. [13])

to SPECT (0.85) and CCTA (0.90) alone [50]. Another study integrating SPECT and CTA stated PPV of 77 % compared to 31 % for CTA alone in detecting myocardial ischemia [51]. Sato and colleagues [52] reported augmentation of PPV from 69 to 85 % by combining SPECT information to non-evaluable coronary arteries on CCTA.

In a study of 107 patients, $H_2{}^{15}O$ PET/64-slice CTA had a diagnostic accuracy of 98 % with significant improvement in PPV of 96 % for hybrid imaging compared to 76 % for CTA alone [53]. The reference standard was ICA with FFR $\leq$0.80 when feasible. Another study confirmed these findings with reported sensitivity and specificity of 98 % and 91 %, respectively [54]. Danad et al. [55] attested the "gatekeeper" role of hybrid imaging for downstream revascularization and referral for ICA. Of 5 % of the patients with "normal" CTA that were referred for invasive angiography, none had significant CAD. Among the patients that had an equivocal CTA result, 18 % with normal PET-MPI were referred for ICA compared to 71 % in abnormal MPI group, though no coronary revascularization was done in the normal PET-MPI group. Similarly, 72 % patients underwent revascularization for concurrent CTA stenosis and abnormal perfusion versus 26 % with obstructive stenosis ($\geq$50 %) on CTA but normal PET imaging. Hybrid imaging had incremental diagnostic utility in 29 % of the patients, particularly influencing individuals with multivessel disease and/or intermediate-grade stenosis. Thus, combined anatomic-physiologic information derived from hybrid imaging, particularly in the setting of equivocal functional imaging, has been of clinical significance leading to the proportionate decline in false-positive testing. This improved accuracy was most relevant in the segments perfused by the left circumflex and right coronary artery, affirming the inconsistencies that exist among the myocardial segments perfused by respective coronary vessel [56].

9.3.2 Myocardial CT Perfusion

Numerous single-center studies initially established the diagnostic efficacy of CTP in assessing the flow-limiting stenosis. Using 64-row and 256-row MDCT scanner systems and defining the gold standard as a combination of quantitative coronary angiography and concurrent perfusion abnormalities by SPECT, George et al. on per-patient basis reported the sensitivity, specificity, PPV, and NPV of 86 %, 92 %, 92 %, and 85 % for combined CTA and CTP, respectively. For per-vessel/territory analysis, these corresponding values to detect obstructive stenosis were 79 %, 91 %, 75 %, and 92 %, respectively [30]. Blankstein et al. showed that CTP alone had a sensitivity of 93 % and a specificity of 74 % for the detection of vessels with at least 50 % stenosis and a corresponding SPECT perfusion abnormality [31]. Myocardial CTP has also been compared to invasive FFR in the single-center study by Bettencourt et al. [57] This study enrolled 101 symptomatic patients at intermediate to high risk for CAD. When compared to invasive FFR, myocardial CTP has a diagnostic accuracy of 85 % and a sensitivity, specificity, PPV, and NPV of 89, 83, 80, and 90 %, respectively. Radiation dose was quite low at 5.0 ± 0.96 mSv for the CTA and CTP study combined. Another single-center study examined the added value of CTP over CTA in the diagnosis of in-stent restenosis. Studying 91 patients with suspected in-stent restenosis, Rief et al. [58] tested the diagnostic performance of CTA alone and in combination with CTP. Compared to CTA alone, nondiagnostic rates dropped from 20 to 0 %. There were significant improvements in accuracy, sensitivity, and specificity. Overall diagnostic performance measured by the AUC of the receiver-operator characteristic curve was 0.76 for CTA alone and 0.90 for CTA + CTP ($p < 0.001$).

Following the encouraging results from the single-center experiences, the coronary artery evaluation using 320-row multidetector computed tomography angiography and myocardial perfusion study (CORE320) was an international, multicenter study aimed to establish the incremental diagnostic utility of CTP over CTA against the reference standard of invasive coronary angiography and a corresponding perfusion deficit on SPECT-MPI. The study included patients with prior intracoronary stents and prior myocardial infarction. The study enrolled 381 patients and demonstrated a sensitivity of 94 % and specificity of 64 % for the presence of ≥50 % stenosis by CTA alone to predict the reference standard of combined ICA-SPECT with an AUC (0.84, 95 % CI: 0.79–0.88). The study confirmed significant increase in the patient-based diagnostic accuracy when CTP was added to the CTA (AUC 0.87, 95 % CI: 0.84–0.91). The AUCs for combined CTA-CTP imaging continued to rise to 0.90 for patients without prior myocardial infarction and 0.93 for patients without prior CAD. For the combination of a CTA stenosis ≥50 % stenosis and a CTP perfusion deficit, the sensitivity, specificity, PPV, and NPV values were 80 %, 74 %, 65 %, and 86 %, respectively [12]. A subsequent multicenter study verified that

CTP had a good agreement with SPECT (87 %) imaging and the diagnostic accuracy of CTA (0.69) for detecting a reversible perfusion defect on SPECT improved to 0.85 with the combination of CTP [59]. This study demonstrated that myocardial CTP is non-inferior to SPECT myocardial perfusion imaging for the detection of ≥2 segmental reversible perfusion deficits. Interestingly, CTP has been noted to have a higher sensitivity than SPECT-MPI for detecting of multivessel disease [60].

9.3.3 CT-FFR

CT-FFR derived using rest CTA images has been shown to have improved diagnostic accuracy in predicting lesion-specific ischemia, as determined by invasive FFR. In the Discover-Flow study, Koo et al. [61] in a per-vessel analyses reported better diagnostic accuracy of CT-FFR (AUC, 0.84) compared to CTA stenosis of ≥50 % (AUC, 0.59). On a per-patient basis, CT-FFR had an AUC of 0.87 with stated sensitivity of 94 %, specificity of 82 %, NPV of 0.91, and PPV of 0.85, respectively. In follow-up to the Discover-Flow trial, DEFACTO studied 252 patients with CT-FFR compared to the reference standard invasive FFR. CT-FFR did improve diagnostic accuracy from 64 to 73 %, but overall the trial did not meet its non-inferiority margin. More recently, the Analysis of Coronary Blood Flow Using CT Angiography: Next Steps (NXT) trial evaluated the diagnostic performance of updated iteration of CT-FFR utilizing invasive FFR as a reference standard [14]. In this study, a rigorous quality control mechanism was put in place for CTA and invasive FFR. Of the 365 subjects enrolled with a clinical indication for ICA, 251 subjects made it into the final analysis with 103 studies rejected due to CTA or FFR quality issues. In this study, CT-FFR – on per-patient basis – had an improved diagnostic accuracy with AUC of 0.81 versus 0.53 of CTA alone for detecting flow-limiting stenosis by invasive FFR. CT-FFR had better per-patient sensitivity of 86 %, specificity of 79 %, PPV of 65 %, and NPV of 93 % compared to CTA with corresponding values of 94 %, 34 %, 40 %, and 92 %, respectively. In a meta-analyses to assess the diagnostic performance of CT-FFR, Li and coauthors [62], in a per-patient analysis, reported pooled sensitivity of 89 %, specificity of 71 %, PPV of 70 %, and NPV of 90 % to predict the gold standard of invasive FFR ≤ 0.8. At the vessel level, there was improvement in diagnostic performance of CT-FFR with pooled specificity of 78 % and a comparable sensitivity of 83 %, respectively [62]. Overall, CT-FFR appears to be a robust method to improve the accuracy of CTA to predict the hemodynamic significance. However, CT-FFR has not been extensively tested in patients with prior revascularization or prior infarcts.

9.4 Limitations

Hybrid imaging has significant implications in terms of additional cost, contrast, and radiation exposure. An additional scan may also confer diagnostic delays and logistic challenges that significantly add to patient anxiety and inconvenience.

Therefore, concerted efforts are being made to minimize these problems. Recent years have witnessed significant advances in imaging technology to decrease radiation dose. For SPECT-MPI, introduction of novel small-footprint cardiac scanners armed with solid-state detectors [63] and performance of half-dose perfusion imaging [64] have led to significant reduction in radiation exposure. Optimizing diagnostic yield by using high-efficiency cameras and employing stress-first protocols in individuals with predefined low-intermediate CAD risk have pushed the radiation doses for SPECT imaging to as low as 2.2 mSV [65]. The PET perfusion tracers (i.e., $H_2\ ^{15}O$, $^{13}NH_3$, and ^{82} Rb) construe low radiation doses (1–2 mSv) and may be advantageous for hybrid imaging [66]. Recent advances in CT technology with emphasis on dose reduction techniques like limiting scan length, ECG-gated dose modulation, prospective ECG-triggering, and high-pitch scanning protocols have resulted in significant reductions in effective radiation dose [67]. Additionally, post-processing methods such as iterative reconstruction [68] and availability of next-generation scanners with faster gantry rotation time and wide volume coverage have implied substantial reduction in the amount of radiation during diagnostic testing. With current strategies, a hybrid stress-only SPECT/CTA or PET/CTA studies could be performed with radiation exposure less than or equivalent to invasive diagnostic angiography [69]. Availability of PET perfusion tracers limited by on-site cyclotron is a significant hindrance for performance of PET/CTA hybrid imaging. Although [81] Rb is a generator-based tracer, it requires large patient flow for its commercial viability. Industrial delivery of perfusion tracers with longer half-lives similar to fluorodeoxyglucose (^{18}F) may help alleviate this problem.

MDCT imaging may be influenced by problems arising from image artifacts, lower contrast resolution, contrast dose, and optimal contrast timing. Imaging artifacts are an inherent limitation to CT technology with particular references to artifacts arising out of cardiac motion, beam-hardening, and reconstruction artifacts [70, 71]. Motion artifacts can be further incited by vasodilator stress agents that increase the average heart rate by 20–25 beats/min. These motion artifacts could be avoided by using β-blocker medications and improving the temporal resolution of the scan by using multicycle reconstruction or dual-source CT. Availability of wide-area multi-detector scanner that allows coverage of entire cardiac volume in a single gantry rotation has considerably mitigated this problem [30, 32]. Beam-hardening artifacts are similar to attenuation artifacts in SPECT and arise from the high-attenuation structures (bones and contrast filled ventricular cavity and vessels) that absorb low-energy photons in proximity with the myocardium resulting in low-attenuation streaks. This can be negated by using corrections built into the reconstruction algorithms and by accounting for these artifacts during interpretation of the scan [71, 72].

Strict adherence to imaging protocols to ensure optimum image quality is critical for CT-FFR assessment. CT-FFR requires accurate anatomic framework derived using the image segmentation algorithms that can be influenced by image quality. Hence, the artifacts may have an amplified effect on the calculation of CT-FFR. The presence of coronary calcification and/or stents may result in misrepresentation of CT-FFR. Additional limitations of CT-FFR relate to physiological assumption models that include population as well as patient-specific data. Deduced relationships relating myocardial mass to total coronary flow, the relative coronary microvascular resistance calculated based on vessel size, or reduction in vascular resistance in response to adenosine-mediated hyperemia will not be consistent among all individuals. Extrapolation of these assumptions to calculate lesion-specific ischemia involves certain degree of variation.

While the results of integrated imaging modalities in assessing lesion-specific or patient-specific ischemia are promising, the data from the published studies are limited and lack uniform reference standard. The applicability and usefulness of combined imaging modalities have not yet been tested beyond clinical trials in the real-world clinical scenario. Currently, there are no data on the cost-effectiveness and improvements in patient outcomes as well as which patient subset will benefit from integrated imaging accounting for cost and radiation dose.

9.5 Prognostic Value

The presence of obstructive CAD and corresponding perfusion defect has a synergistic effect on incidence of adverse cardiovascular events; however, the presence of either conveys an independent prognostic risk. Consistent with this principle, a number of studies have documented improved efficiency of hybrid imaging in predicting adverse cardiovascular risk [11]. In a single-center study of 335 consecutively enrolled patients, Pazhenkottil and coauthors [11] stratified the patients based on CTA stenosis and the presence or absence of matching SPECT perfusion deficit. Combination of abnormal CTA-SPECT translated into worst prognosis with annual major adverse cardiovascular event rate of 21.0 and 6.0 % incidence of death/myocardial infarction. Normal dual-modality scan had lowest major event rate of 2.2 % with 1.3 % risk of death or coronary events. Patient with CTA stenosis and discordant result on MPI had intermediate major adverse event rate of 7.8 % and hard event rate of 2.8 %, respectively. Van Werkhoven et al. [73] had similar findings with annual event rate of 1.0 % (death/MI 0.6 %) in patients with normal CTA (<50 % stenosis) and a normal SPECT-MPI, whereas adverse event rate in patients with obstructive CAD (≥50 %) and corresponding SPECT perfusion abnormality was 9.0 % (death/infarction = 6.0 %). These findings are currently limited to single-center data with relatively smaller cohort size.

Given recent emergence of CTP and CT-FFR technology, outcomes data to assess the prognostic utility is currently in an early stage. Nevertheless, dissociating from the concept of hemodynamically significant stenosis and prognosis, CTA had focused our attention on the significance of total atherosclerotic plaque burden, plaque characteristics, and remodeling status [74]. Studies have projected total atherosclerotic burden as a reliable prognostic marker compared to inducible myocardial ischemia [75, 76]. Integration of these results in improving the risk prediction models in combination with coronary flow reserve and myocardial blood flow and perfusion currently awaits more evidence and data.

9.6 Clinical Perspective

Sequential imaging to obtain anatomic and hemodynamic information can be challenging, particularly in view of establishing "diagnostic yield" of second scan over the first. In a usual clinical setup, additional scan is performed if the result of initial modality is equivocal or if adjunct information is required to define therapeutic strategies. In this regard, individual's pretest likelihood of CAD can help determine the order of the scans. Given the excellent NPV of CTA, anatomic assessment should be performed first in the patients with low to intermediate likelihood of CAD, followed by perfusion imaging in those with obstructive CAD on CTA. Conversely, if the pretest likelihood of CAD is high indicating higher prevalence of obstructive CAD, starting with perfusion imaging may be a better approach, with anatomic imaging being triggered after an abnormal, equivocal, or suboptimal perfusion testing.

Hybrid imaging may be clinically useful in coronary stenosis of moderate severity (30–90 %) where quantitative stenosis may not be a reliable indicator of physiologic significance of a lesion. For such cases, perfusion imaging or CT-FFR can be added to CTA to assess the flow-limiting stenosis. This may be beneficial in a patient with multivessel disease where culprit lesion/s can be identified in the setting of "balanced ischemia." Left main stenosis can also be diagnostically challenging for radionuclide perfusion imaging. The presence of stenosis on CTA and a corresponding large anterior perfusion deficit permit accurate detection of flow-obstructing left main stenosis. In a patient with heavily calcified coronary arteries and uninterpretable coronary segments, perfusion imaging provides useful information about downstream hemodynamic effects, increasing the diagnostic certainty of an obstructive CAD. Quantitative perfusion imaging can also identify microvascular dysfunction, represented by reduced myocardial blood flow in the absence of obstructive epicardial CAD. Finally, dual-modality imaging provides quantitative estimation of the "myocardium at risk" and helps differentiate patient with extensive scar versus significant myocardial ischemia. This is clinically vital so as to guide revascularization approach in those with viable myocardium while avoiding coronary intervention in individuals with no potential for myocardial recovery [77].

9.7 Future Advancement

Rapid evolution of CT technology led by the improvement in temporal and spatial resolution along with post-processing techniques has allowed faster scan acquisition at higher heart rates [78–80]. The role of cardiac MDCT imaging as a comprehensive CAD assessment tool using solo imaging platform, aided by automated and semiautomated analysis software, is currently in sight. It will soon be feasible to obtain enhanced information about coronary morphology and lesion-specific ischemia and/or downstream hemodynamic effects based on single-scan acquisition.

Cardiovascular molecular imaging provides important insights into the biological and vascular processes at the cellular levels. PET-CT imaging has emerged as a powerful imaging tool designed to decipher pathophysiological and metabolic mechanisms of plaque progression and rupture that has led to better understanding of the concept of vulnerable plaque [81–83]. Recent preclinical evidences suggest that macrophage-specific iodine-based contrast agents such as N1177 can noninvasively identify high-risk atherosclerotic features and localize and quantify inflammation in the atherosclerotic plaque [84]. Translation of these promising molecular imaging techniques into the clinical practice remains to be seen.

References

1. Miller JM, Rochitte CE, Dewey M, et al. Diagnostic performance of coronary angiography by 64-row CT. N Engl J Med. 2008;359:2324–36.
2. Arbab-Zadeh A, Miller JM, Rochitte CE, et al. Diagnostic accuracy of computed tomography coronary angiography according to pre-test probability of coronary artery disease and severity of coronary arterial calcification. The CORE-64 (Coronary Artery Evaluation Using 64-Row Multidetector Computed Tomography Angiography) International Multicenter Study. J Am Coll Cardiol. 2012;59:379–87.
3. Uren NG, Melin JA, De Bruyne B, Wijns W, Baudhuin T, Camici PG. Relation between myocardial blood flow and the severity of coronary-artery stenosis. N Engl J Med. 1994;330:1782–8.
4. Di Carli M, Czernin J, Hoh CK, et al. Relation among stenosis severity, myocardial blood flow, and flow reserve in patients with coronary artery disease. Circulation. 1995;91:1944–51.
5. Levine GN, Bates ER, Blankenship JC, et al. 2011 ACCF/AHA/SCAI Guideline for Percutaneous Coronary Intervention. A report of the American College of Cardiology Foundation/American Heart Association Task Force on Practice Guidelines and the Society for Cardiovascular Angiography and Interventions. J Am Coll Cardiol. 2011;58:e44–122.
6. Weiner DA, Ryan TJ, McCabe CH, Chaitman BR, et al. The role of exercise testing in identifying patients with improved survival after coronary artery bypass surgery. J Am Coll Cardiol. 1986;8:741–8.
7. Shaw LJ, Berman DS, Maron DJ, et al. Optimal medical therapy with or without percutaneous coronary intervention to reduce ischemic burden: results from the Clinical Outcomes Utilizing Revascularization and Aggressive Drug Evaluation (COURAGE) trial nuclear substudy. Circulation. 2008;117:1283–91.
8. Tonino PA, De Bruyne B, Pijls NH, et al. Fractional flow reserve versus angiography for guiding percutaneous coronary intervention. N Engl J Med. 2009;360:213–24.
9. Czernin J, Muller P, Chan S, et al. Influence of age and hemodynamics on myocardial blood flow and flow reserve. Circulation. 1993;88:62–9.
10. Schelbert HR. Anatomy and physiology of coronary blood flow. J Nucl Cardiol. 2010;17:545–54.
11. Pazhenkottil AP, Nkoulou RN, Ghadri JR, et al. Prognostic value of cardiac hybrid imaging integrating single-photon emission computed tomography with coronary computed tomography angiography. Eur Heart J. 2011;32:1465–71.
12. Rochitte CE, George RT, Chen MY, et al. Computed tomography angiography and perfusion to assess coronary artery stenosis causing perfusion defects by single photon emission computed tomography: the CORE320 study. Eur Heart J. 2014;35(17):1120–30.
13. Taylor CA, Fonte TA, Min JK. Computational fluid dynamics applied to cardiac computed tomography for noninvasive quantification of fractional flow reserve: scientific basis. J Am Coll Cardiol. 2013;61:2233–41.

14. Norgaard BL, Leipsic J, Gaur S, et al. Diagnostic performance of noninvasive fractional flow reserve derived from coronary computed tomography angiography in suspected coronary artery disease: the NXT trial (Analysis of Coronary Blood Flow Using CT Angiography: Next Steps). J Am Coll Cardiol. 2014;63:1145–55.
15. Nakazato R, Park HB, Berman DS, et al. Noninvasive fractional flow reserve derived from computed tomography angiography for coronary lesions of intermediate stenosis severity: results from the DeFACTO study. Circ Cardiovasc Imaging. 2013;6:881–9.
16. Dilsizian V. SPECT and PET myocardial perfusion imaging: tracers and techniques. In: Dilsizian V, Narula J, editors. Atlas of nuclear cardiology. 4th ed. New York/Heidelberg/Dordrecht/London: Springer; 2013. p. 55–94.
17. Di Carli MF, Dorbala S, Meserve J, El Fakhri G, Sitek A, Moore SC. Clinical myocardial perfusion PET/CT. J Nucl Med. 2007;48:783–93.
18. Klocke FJ, Baird MG, Lorell BH, et al. ACC/AHA/ASNC guidelines for the clinical use of cardiac radionuclide imaging–executive summary: a report of the American College of Cardiology/American Heart Association Task Force on Practice Guidelines (ACC/AHA/ASNC Committee to Revise the 1995 Guidelines for the Clinical Use of Cardiac Radionuclide Imaging). J Am Coll Cardiol. 2003;42:1318–33.
19. Bergmann SR, Fox KA, Rand AL, et al. Quantification of regional myocardial blood flow in vivo with H215O. Circulation. 1984;70:724–33.
20. Hutchins GD, Schwaiger M, Rosenspire KC, Krivokapich J, Schelbert H, Kuhl DE. Noninvasive quantification of regional blood flow in the human heart using N-13 ammonia and dynamic positron emission tomographic imaging. J Am Coll Cardiol. 1990;15:1032–42.
21. Knuuti J, Kajander S, Maki M, Ukkonen H. Quantification of myocardial blood flow will reform the detection of CAD. J Nucl Cardiol. 2009;16:497–506.
22. Kajander SA, Joutsiniemi E, Saraste M, et al. Clinical value of absolute quantification of myocardial perfusion with (15)O-water in coronary artery disease. Circ Cardiovasc Imaging. 2011;4:678–84.
23. Parkash R, deKemp RA, Ruddy TD, et al. Potential utility of rubidium 82 PET quantification in patients with 3-vessel coronary artery disease. J Nucl Cardiol. 2004;11:440–9.
24. Yoshinaga K, Katoh C, Noriyasu K, et al. Reduction of coronary flow reserve in areas with and without ischemia on stress perfusion imaging in patients with coronary artery disease: a study using oxygen 15-labeled water PET. J Nucl Cardiol. 2003;10:275–83.
25. Di Carli MF, Hachamovitch R. New technology for noninvasive evaluation of coronary artery disease. Circulation. 2007;115:1464–80.
26. Javadi MS, Lautamaki R, Merrill J, et al. Definition of vascular territories on myocardial perfusion images by integration with true coronary anatomy: a hybrid PET/CT analysis. J Nucl Cardiol. 2010;51:198–203.
27. Di Carli MF. Hybrid imaging: integration of nuclear imaging and cardiac CT. Cardiol Clin. 2009;27:257–63.
28. Mahnken AH, Bruners P, Katoh M, Wildberger JE, Gunther RW, Buecker A. Dynamic multisection CT imaging in acute myocardial infarction: preliminary animal experience. Eur Radiol. 2006;16:746–52.
29. Garcia MJ, Lessick J, Hoffmann MH. Accuracy of 16-row multidetector computed tomography for the assessment of coronary artery stenosis. JAMA. 2006;296:403–11.
30. George RT, Arbab-Zadeh A, Miller JM, et al. Adenosine stress 64- and 256-row detector computed tomography angiography and perfusion imaging: a pilot study evaluating the transmural extent of perfusion abnormalities to predict atherosclerosis causing myocardial ischemia. Circ Cardiovasc Imaging. 2009;2:174–82.
31. Blankstein R, Shturman LD, Rogers IS, et al. Adenosine-induced stress myocardial perfusion imaging using dual-source cardiac computed tomography. J Am Coll Cardiol. 2009;54:1072–84.
32. George RT, Silva C, Cordeiro MA, et al. Multidetector computed tomography myocardial perfusion imaging during adenosine stress. J Am Coll Cardiol. 2006;48:153–60.
33. Cury RC, Magalhaes TA, Borges AC, et al. Dipyridamole stress and rest myocardial perfusion by 64-detector row computed tomography in patients with suspected coronary artery disease. Am J Cardiol. 2010;106:310–5.

34. George RT, Jerosch-Herold M, Silva C, et al. Quantification of myocardial perfusion using dynamic 64-detector computed tomography. Invest Radiol. 2007;42:815–22.
35. Ho KT, Chua KC, Klotz E, Panknin C. Stress and rest dynamic myocardial perfusion imaging by evaluation of complete time-attenuation curves with dual-source CT. JACC Cardiovasc Imaging. 2010;3:811–20.
36. Hein PA, May J, Rogalla P, Butler C, Hamm B, Lembcke A. Feasibility of contrast material volume reduction in coronary artery imaging using 320-slice volume CT. Eur Radiol. 2010;20:1337–43.
37. Ichihara T, George RT, Silva C, Lima JAC, Lardo AC. Quantitative analysis of first-pass contrast-enhanced myocardial perfusion multidetector CT using a Patlak plot method and extraction fraction correction during adenosine stress. Nucl Sci IEEE Trans. 2011;58:133–8.
38. Schuleri KH, Centola M, George RT, et al. Characterization of peri-infarct zone heterogeneity by contrast-enhanced multidetector computed tomography: a comparison with magnetic resonance imaging. J Am Coll Cardiol. 2009;53:1699–707.
39. Senra T, Shiozaki AA, Salemi VM, Rochitte CE. Delayed enhancement by multidetector computed tomography in endomyocardial fibrosis. Eur Heart J. 2008;29:347.
40. Lardo AC, Cordeiro MA, Silva C, et al. Contrast-enhanced multidetector computed tomography viability imaging after myocardial infarction: characterization of myocyte death, microvascular obstruction, and chronic scar. Circulation. 2006;113:394–404.
41. Mahnken AH, Koos R, Katoh M, et al. Assessment of myocardial viability in reperfused acute myocardial infarction using 16-slice computed tomography in comparison to magnetic resonance imaging. J Am Coll Cardiol. 2005;45:2042–7.
42. Gerber BL, Belge B, Legros GJ, et al. Characterization of acute and chronic myocardial infarcts by multidetector computed tomography: comparison with contrast-enhanced magnetic resonance. Circulation. 2006;113:823–33.
43. Cerqueira MD, Verani MS, Schwaiger M, Heo J, Iskandrian AS. Safety profile of adenosine stress perfusion imaging: results from the Adenoscan Multicenter Trial Registry. J Am Coll Cardiol. 1994;23:384–9.
44. Iskandrian AE, Bateman TM, Belardinelli L, et al. Adenosine versus regadenoson comparative evaluation in myocardial perfusion imaging: results of the ADVANCE phase 3 multicenter international trial. J Nucl Cardiol. 2007;14:645–58.
45. Patel AR, Lodato JA, Chandra S, et al. Detection of myocardial perfusion abnormalities using ultra-low radiation dose regadenoson stress multidetector computed tomography. J Cardiovasc Comput Tomogr. 2011;5:247–54.
46. Christian TF, Frankish ML, Sisemoore JH, et al. Myocardial perfusion imaging with first-pass computed tomographic imaging: measurement of coronary flow reserve in an animal model of regional hyperemia. J Nucl Cardiol. 2010;17:625–30.
47. West GB, Brown JH, Enquist BJ. A general model for the origin of allometric scaling laws in biology. Science (New York, NY). 1997;276:122–6.
48. Wilson RF, Wyche K, Christensen BV, Zimmer S, Laxson DD. Effects of adenosine on human coronary arterial circulation. Circulation. 1990;82:1595–606.
49. Schaap J, Kauling RM, Boekholdt SM, et al. Incremental diagnostic accuracy of hybrid SPECT/CT coronary angiography in a population with an intermediate to high pre-test likelihood of coronary artery disease. Eur Heart J Cardiovasc Imaging. 2013;14:642–9.
50. Schaap J, de Groot JA, Nieman K, et al. Added value of hybrid myocardial perfusion SPECT and CT coronary angiography in the diagnosis of coronary artery disease. Eur Heart J Cardiovasc Imaging. 2014;15:1281–8.
51. Hacker M, Jakobs T, Matthiesen F, et al. Comparison of spiral multidetector CT angiography and myocardial perfusion imaging in the noninvasive detection of functionally relevant coronary artery lesions: first clinical experiences. J Nucl Med. 2005;46:1294–300.
52. Sato A, Nozato T, Hikita H, Miyazaki S, et al. Incremental value of combining 64-slice computed tomography angiography with stress nuclear myocardial perfusion imaging to improve noninvasive detection of coronary artery disease. J Nucl Cardiol. 2010;17:19–26.
53. Gaemperli O, Schepis T, Valenta I, et al. Cardiac image fusion from stand-alone SPECT and CT: clinical experience. J Nucl Med. 2007;48:696–703.

54. Danad I, Raijmakers PG, Appelman YE, et al. Hybrid imaging using quantitative H215O PET and CT-based coronary angiography for the detection of coronary artery disease. J Nucl Med. 2013;54:55–63.
55. Danad I, Raijmakers PG, Harms HJ, et al. Effect of cardiac hybrid 15O-water PET/CT imaging on downstream referral for invasive coronary angiography and revascularization rate. Eur Heart J Cardiovasc Imaging. 2013;15:170–9.
56. Slomka PJ, Cheng VY, Dey D, et al. Quantitative analysis of myocardial perfusion SPECT anatomically guided by coregistered 64-slice coronary CT angiography. J Nucl Med. 2009; 50:1621–30.
57. Bettencourt N, Chiribiri A, Schuster A, et al. Direct comparison of cardiac magnetic resonance and multidetector computed tomography stress-rest perfusion imaging for detection of coronary artery disease. J Am Coll Cardiol. 2013;61:1099–107.
58. Rief M, Zimmermann E, Stenzel F, et al. Computed tomography angiography and myocardial computed tomography perfusion in patients with coronary stents: prospective intraindividual comparison with conventional coronary angiography. J Am Coll Cardiol. 2013;62:1476–85.
59. Cury RC, Kitt TM, Feaheny K, et al. A randomized, multicenter, multivendor study of myocardial perfusion imaging with regadenoson CT perfusion vs single photon emission CT. J Cardiovasc Comput Tomogr. 2015;9(2):103–12.
60. George RT, Mehra VC, Chen MY, et al. Myocardial CT perfusion imaging and SPECT for the diagnosis of coronary artery disease: a head-to-head comparison from the CORE320 multicenter diagnostic performance study. Radiology. 2014;272:407–16.
61. Koo BK, Erglis A, Doh JH, et al. Diagnosis of ischemia-causing coronary stenoses by noninvasive fractional flow reserve computed from coronary computed tomographic angiograms. Results from the prospective multicenter DISCOVER-FLOW (Diagnosis of Ischemia-Causing Stenoses Obtained Via Noninvasive Fractional Flow Reserve) study. J Am Coll Cardiol. 2011;58:1989–97.
62. Li S, Tang X, Peng L, Luo Y, Dong R, Liu J. The diagnostic performance of CT-derived fractional flow reserve for evaluation of myocardial ischaemia confirmed by invasive fractional flow reserve: a meta-analysis. Clin Radiol. 2015;70(5):476–86.
63. Duvall WL, Croft LB, Ginsberg ES, et al. Reduced isotope dose and imaging time with a high-efficiency CZT SPECT camera. J Nucl Cardiol. 2011;18:847–57.
64. Gaemperli O, Kaufmann PA. Lower dose and shorter acquisition: pushing the boundaries of myocardial perfusion SPECT. J Nucl Cardiol. 2011;18:830–2.
65. Einstein AJ, Johnson LL, DeLuca A, et al. Radiation dose and prognosis of ultra-low dose stress-first myocardial perfusion SPECT in patients with chest pain using a high-efficiency camera. J Nucl Med. 2015;56(4):545–51.
66. Namdar M, Hany TF, Koepfli P, et al. Integrated PET/CT for the assessment of coronary artery disease: a feasibility study. J Nucl Med. 2005;46:930–5.
67. Halliburton SS, Abbara S, Chen MY, et al. SCCT guidelines on radiation dose and dose-optimization strategies in cardiovascular CT. J Cardiovasc Comput Tomogr. 2011;5:198–224.
68. Chen MY, Steigner ML, Leung SW, et al. Simulated 50 % radiation dose reduction in coronary CT angiography using adaptive iterative dose reduction in three-dimensions (AIDR3D). Int J Cardiovasc Imaging. 2013;29:1167–75.
69. Husmann L, Herzog BA, Gaemperli O, et al. Diagnostic accuracy of computed tomography coronary angiography and evaluation of stress-only single-photon emission computed tomography/computed tomography hybrid imaging: comparison of prospective electrocardiogram-triggering vs. retrospective gating. Eur Heart J. 2009;30:600–7.
70. Mehra VC, Ambrose M, Valdiviezo-Schlomp C, et al. CT-based myocardial perfusion imaging-practical considerations: acquisition, image analysis, interpretation, and challenges. J Cardiovasc Transl Res. 2011;4:437–48.
71. Mehra VC, Valdiviezo C, Arbab-Zadeh A, et al. A stepwise approach to the visual interpretation of CT-based myocardial perfusion. J Cardiovasc Comput Tomogr. 2011;5:357–69.
72. Kitagawa K, George RT, Arbab-Zadeh A, Lima JA, Lardo AC. Characterization and correction of beam-hardening artifacts during dynamic volume CT assessment of myocardial perfusion. Radiology. 2010;256:111–8.

73. van Werkhoven JM, Schuijf JD, Gaemperli O, et al. Prognostic value of multislice computed tomography and gated single-photon emission computed tomography in patients with suspected coronary artery disease. J Am Coll Cardiol. 2009;53:623–32.
74. Arbab-Zadeh A, Fuster V. The Myth of the "Vulnerable Plaque": transitioning from a focus on individual lesions to atherosclerotic disease burden for coronary artery disease risk assessment. J Am Coll Cardiol. 2015;65:846–55.
75. Mancini GB, Hartigan PM, Shaw LJ, et al. Predicting outcome in the COURAGE trial (Clinical Outcomes Utilizing Revascularization and Aggressive Drug Evaluation): coronary anatomy versus ischemia. JACC Cardiovasc Interv. 2014;7:195–201.
76. Arbab-Zadeh A. Fractional flow reserve-guided percutaneous coronary intervention is not a valid concept. Circulation. 2014;129:1871–8; discussion 1878.
77. Shaw LJ, Hachamovitch R, Berman DS, et al. The economic consequences of available diagnostic and prognostic strategies for the evaluation of stable angina patients: an observational assessment of the value of precatheterization ischemia. Economics of Noninvasive Diagnosis (END) Multicenter Study Group. J Am Coll Cardiol. 1999;33:661–9.
78. Cho I, Elmore K, OH B, Schulman-Marcus J, et al. Heart-rate dependent improvement in image quality and diagnostic accuracy of coronary computed tomographic angiography by novel intracycle motion correction algorithm. Clin Imaging. 2015;39:421–6. doi:10.1016/j.clinimag.2014.11.020. ec 9. pii: S0899-7071(14)00305-2.
79. Tomizawa N, Maeda E, Akahane M, et al. Coronary CT angiography using the second-generation 320-detector row CT: assessment of image quality and radiation dose in various heart rates compared with the first-generation scanner. Int J Cardiovasc Imaging. 2013;29:1613–8.
80. Gassenmaier T, Petri N, Allmendinger T, et al. Next generation coronary CT angiography: in vitro evaluation of 27 coronary stents. Eur Radiol. 2014;24:2953–61.
81. Saraste A, Nekolla SG, Schwaiger M. Cardiovascular molecular imaging: an overview. Cardiovasc Res. 2009;83:643–52.
82. Nahrendorf M, Sosnovik DE, French BA, et al. Multimodality cardiovascular molecular imaging, part II. Circ Cardiovasc Imaging. 2009;2:56–70.
83. Knuuti J, Bengel FM. Positron emission tomography and molecular imaging. Heart. 2008;94:360–7.
84. Hyafil F, Cornily JC, Rudd JH, Machac J, Feldman LJ, Fayad ZA. Quantification of inflammation within rabbit atherosclerotic plaques using the macrophage-specific CT contrast agent N1177: a comparison with 18F-FDG PET/CT and histology. J Nucl Med. 2009;50:959–65.
85. Naya M, et al. Quantitative relationship between the extent and morphology of coronary atherosclerotic plaque and down-stream myocardial perfusion. J Am Coll Cardiol. 2011;58:1807–16.

Three-Dimensional Fusion Display of CT Coronary Angiography and Myocardial Perfusion

10

Oliver Gaemperli, Philipp A. Kaufmann, and Aju P. Pazhenkottil

10.1 Introduction

10.1.1 Definition of Fusion Display

The term fusion display or fusion imaging refers to the assessment of two imaging data sets by spatial superposition (usually in a 3D hybrid display) and where both modalities contribute equally to the image information. Fusion imaging has faced increasing clinical acceptance as it provides anatomical information on the presence of coronary artery lesions combined with functional information on its pathophysiologic consequences with regard to myocardial perfusion or metabolism.

10.1.2 Clinical Background

Despite major advances in diagnosis and treatment, coronary artery disease (CAD) remains a leading cause of morbidity and mortality in Western countries. Invasive coronary angiography (ICA) using x-ray is still seen as the gold standard for the assessment of CAD. However, a major drawback of this technique is its invasive nature which is associated with a non negligible rate of morbidity and mortality. Moreover,

O. Gaemperli (✉)
Department of Nuclear Medicine, University Hospital Zurich, Zurich, Switzerland
e-mail: Oliver.Gaemperli@usz.ch

P.A. Kaufmann
Department of Nuclear Medicine, University Hospital Zurich, Zurich, Switzerland

A.P. Pazhenkottil
Department of Nuclear Medicine, University Hospital Zurich, Zurich, Switzerland
e-mail: Aju.pazhenkottil@usz.ch

T.H. Schindler et al. (eds.), *Molecular and Multimodality Imaging in Cardiovascular Disease*, DOI 10.1007/978-3-319-19611-4_10

angiography alone does not allow to assess the functional impact of a given lesion on myocardial perfusion and metabolism [1–3]. It has been shown that only 30–50 % of stenoses with a luminal narrowing of ≥50 % assessed by coronary computed tomography angiography (CCTA) are associated with reversible perfusion defects on MPI [4–6]. The latter, however, has important implications for the prognosis and treatment of stable CAD patients: two large randomized trials including patients with known CAD assessed by ICA have failed to demonstrate a prognostic benefit of revascularization compared with optimal medical treatment if patients were not stratified by prior ischemia testing [7, 8]. The randomized FAME I trial, however, has shown that ischemia-guided revascularization is associated with better outcomes than angiography-guided revascularization [9], while the prospective randomized FAME II trial demonstrated superiority of revascularization over optimal medical treatment for patients with flow-limiting coronary stenosis (FFR <0.8) [10]. Consequently, current guidelines recommend testing for myocardial ischemia, beyond the assessment of coronary morphology alone, prior to any revascularization procedure [11]. Therefore, a tool for the noninvasive integration of coronary anatomy, which is assessed by multislice CCTA, and of myocardial perfusion or viability assessed by single-photon emission computed tomography (SPECT) or positron emission tomography (PET) is helpful for the detection of CAD and for establishing appropriate treatment decisions. Especially with the latest advances and technological improvement using dedicated fusion scanners, the scan duration as well as the radiation burden could be lowered, leading to an increasing acceptance of fusion imaging in clinical routine.

10.2 Technical Considerations

10.2.1 Hardware

CCTA allows an accurate noninvasive visualization of coronary arteries. No other noninvasive technique has yet matched CCTA in terms of resolution, accuracy, and clinical robustness with regard to coronary artery visualization. Tremendous advances have been seen in the recent years with regard to resolution, speed, and accuracy in the field of cardiac CT, which paved the way for the first attempts in cardiac fusion imaging. Two main factors are the reason why fusion imaging was accepted in clinical practice and is now a routine technique in many specialized imaging centers: the excellent image quality and high diagnostic accuracy of state-of-the-art multislice CT devices and the low radiation exposure of modern cardiac CT acquisition protocols. However, while novel techniques such as CT perfusion, CT-derived fractional flow reserve, as well as CT transluminal attenuation gradient offer physiological information on myocardial perfusion, these techniques remain still under clinical investigation. Therefore, a technique assessing the functional significance of a luminal narrowing, such as SPECT or PET, is an important complementary tool.

The principle of hybrid devices originated from the great success of hybrid PET/CT imaging in oncologic patients for the purpose of staging neoplastic diseases. Similar hybrid systems combining SPECT or PET cameras with dedicated CT scanners have been introduced widening the application of hybrid devices for cardiac indications with the latest advances in hybrid imaging combining PET with MR (see Chap. 2).

Initially, the main purpose of a CT acquisition in a hybrid scanner was to provide a fast transmission scan for attenuation correction, avoiding the long exposure times from linear sources. However, the purpose nowadays is shifting toward high-end diagnostic assessment of coronary arteries. There are several manufacturers producing commercially available hybrid SPECT/CT scanners [12].

10.2.2 Post-Processing and Image Analysis Software

It is essential to have dedicated software packages for the accurate coregistration of hybrid images by fusion of CCTA and radionuclide imaging datasets. Different manufacturers now offer dedicated image fusion software that run on standard workstations and allow 3D reconstruction from datasets obtained on different devices and even with stand-alone systems from different manufacturers. Therefore, it is not necessary to have a dedicated hybrid device to obtain fused images.

Furthermore, most of the recent cardiac SPECT/CT devices allow improved image reconstruction algorithms for SPECT analysis, modeling the specific geometry of the detectors and the collimator to improve count sensitivity and reduce image noise. These iterative reconstruction algorithms have increased the image quality considerably, particularly in obese patients. In contrast to the hybrid imaging of other organs, the assessment of fusion images of the heart is challenging for several reasons, particularly because of respiratory-based changes as well as cardiac motion throughout the cardiac cycle. Moreover, the intrinsic disagreement in size and shape of the left ventricle in nongated SPECT images and diastole-gated CCTA has to be considered during image coregistration. Therefore, the manual superposition and correction of dataset misalignment are crucial. The next step after correcting for misalignment includes the tracking of the coronary arteries, which is performed similar as in standard CCTA image reconstruction software, as well as the modeling of the perfusion data into a 3D volume rendering of the left ventricle. Finally, both images will be integrated to 3D images. Modern software packages offer fusion of image datasets from different modalities and even different manufacturers. With datasets of acceptable quality, the process of image fusion takes no longer than 5 min per patient in experienced hands.

10.3 Clinical Value of Fusion CT Angiography and Myocardial Perfusion Imaging

10.3.1 Diagnostic Value for Assessment of CAD

Cardiac fusion imaging combining SPECT or PET with CCTA was first introduced in 2005 [13]. Sincc its introduction, cardiac fusion imaging has immensely gained importance in daily clinical routine. A number of trials have assessed the diagnostic accuracy of cardiac fusion imaging, summarized in Table 10.1.

Table 10.1 Summary of available diagnostic studies in cardiac fusion imaging

First author	Publication year	Hybrid system	*N*	Reference standard for definition of significant CAD	Sens	Spec	PPV	NPV
Namdar	2005	$^{13}N\text{-}NH_3$ PET/4-slice CCTA	25	Flow-limiting coronary stenoses requiring revascularization (ICA + PET)	90	98	82	99
Rispler	2007	SPECT/16-slice CCTA	56	Flow-limiting coronary stenoses (>50 % stenosis on ICA + SPECT pos.)	96	95	77	99
Groves	2009	^{82}Rb PET/64-slice CCTA	33	>50 % stenosis on ICA	88	100	97	99
Sato	2010	SPECT/64-slice CCTA[a]	130	>50 % stenosis on ICA	94	92	85	97
Kajander	2010	$^{15}O\text{-}H_2O$ PET/64-slice CCTA	107	Flow-limiting coronary stenosis (>50 % stenosis of ICA + FFR)	93	99	96	99
Schaap	2013	SPECT/64-slice CCTA	98	Flow-limiting coronary stenosis (>50 % stenosis of ICA + FFR)	96	95	96	95
Danad	2013	$^{15}O\text{-}H_2O$ PET/64-slice CCTA[b]	120	Flow-limiting coronary stenosis (>50 % stenosis of ICA + FFR)	76	92	86	84
Thomassen	2013	$^{15}O\text{-}H_2O$ PET/64-slice CCTA	44	>50 % stenosis on ICA (QCA)	91	100	100	92

[a]Hybrid SPECT/CCTA only applied for non-evaluable arteries on CCTA (14 %)
[b]Non-fused images

Overall, the diagnostic accuracy of fusion imaging is very high with a sensitivity, specificity, positive predictive value and negative predictive value of 76–96 %, 92–100 %, 77–100 %, and 84–99 %, respectively. The incremental value of fusion cardiac imaging lies in the accurate spatial co-localization of myocardial perfusion defects assessed by SPECT or PET and subtending coronary arteries (Fig. 10.1). However, there are some limitations which apply to these early clinical studies such as the difference in hybrid systems, the variable reference standard (either invasive coronary angiography alone or in combination with SPECT or FFR), the single-center design, as well as the small sample size.

In the first clinical study documenting the feasibility and clinical robustness of noninvasive fusion imaging after fusion of $^{13}N\text{-}NH_3$ PET with four-slice CCTA in 25 patients with CAD, the hybrid PET/CCTA images allowed identifying

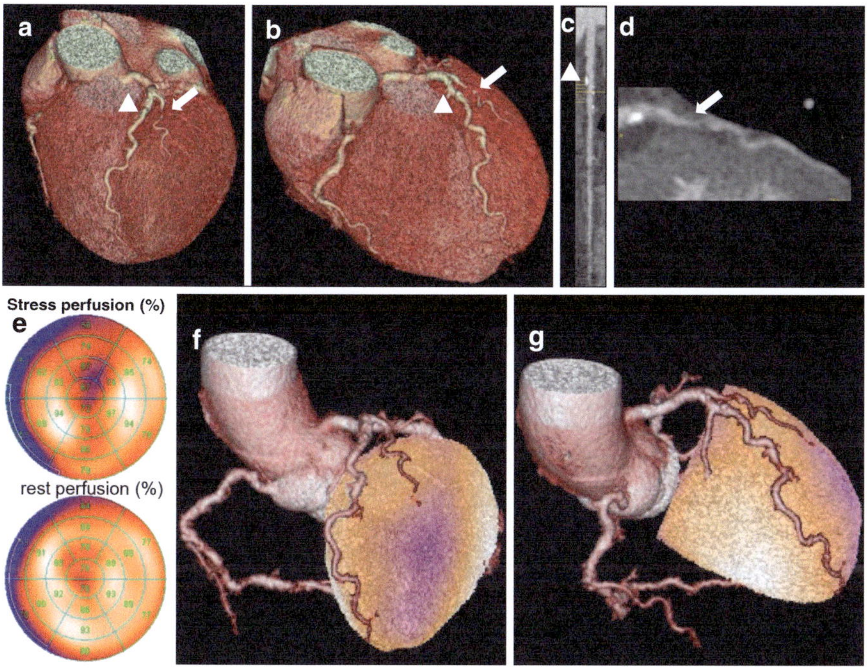

Fig. 10.1 Panel (**a**, **b**) show different views of a cardiac 3D CCTA reconstruction documenting an intermediate stenosis in the proximal LAD (*arrowhead*) as well as an intermediate stenosis without calcification (soft plaque) in the first diagonal branch (*DA*, *arrow*). Curved multiplanar reformation of the LAD and the first DA are seen in Panels **c** and **d**, respectively. SPECT MPI (Panel **e**) reveals a reversible anteroapical perfusion defect, which can be accurately attributed to the corresponding territory of the first DA by fused SPECT/CCTA images (Panel **f**, **g**)

flow-limiting coronary lesions requiring a revascularization procedure (as defined by ICA and PET) with a sensitivity, specificity, positive predictive value (PPV), and negative predictive value (NPV) of 90 %, 98 %, 82 %, and 99 %, respectively (Table 10.1) [13]. Similar results were documented in a study by Rispler and coworkers, who were able to show an increase in specificity (from 63 to 95 %) and PPV (from 31 to 77 %) with SPECT/CCTA compared to CCTA alone [14]. Another study by Sato and coworkers demonstrated a particular improvement in specificity and PPV by adding SPECT information in non-evaluable arteries on CCTA (from 80 to 92 % and from 69 to 85 %, respectively) [15]. Kajender and coworkers demonstrated in a study of 107 patients who underwent $^{15}O\text{-}H_2O$ PET/64-slice CCTA that hybrid images increased the PPV significantly from 76 to 96 % compared to CCTA alone [16]. Moreover, in that study, the hemodynamic significance of ICA stenoses was confirmed by fractional flow reserve (FFR) in 18 of 40 patients providing a more comprehensive reference standard. Similarly, Schaap and coworkers showed an improvement of specificity from 62 and 79 % when using CCTA alone and SPECT alone, respectively, to a specificity of 95 % in a combined approach [17]. In a study using $^{15}O\text{-}H_2O$ PET/64-slice CCTA on

120 patients with an intermediate likelihood for CAD, the diagnostic accuracy of quantitative $^{15}O\text{-}H_2O$ PET/64-slice CCTA was superior to either $^{15}O\text{-}H_2O$ PET or CCTA alone [18]. Finally, in a study by Thomassen and coworkers, the quantitative hybrid PET/CCTA imaging yielded an excellent sensitivity, specificity, positive predictive value, and negative predictive value of 91, 100, 100, and 92 % pointing out the benefit especially in increasing the positive predictive value, which was 71 % for CCTA alone and 87 % for SPECT alone [19].

These studies have documented the incremental diagnostic value of fusion imaging compared to one imaging modality alone. Furthermore, so far, there have been three studies which have specifically evaluated the additional value of fusion cardiac imaging over the side-by-side analysis of CCTA and myocardial perfusion images. In the first study, the number of lesions with equivocal hemodynamic relevance could be significantly reduced using SPECT/CCTA fusion compared with the side-by-side analysis in 38 patients with perfusion defects on SPECT [20]. In another study conducted by Santana and coworkers, a higher diagnostic performance for fused SPECT/CCTA imaging compared to the side-by-side analysis of SPECT and CCTA ($p = 0.007$) for the diagnosis of obstructive CAD on ICA could be demonstrated [21]. This was mainly true in patients with multivessel disease. Finally, Slomka and coworkers demonstrated an improved diagnostic value of cardiac fusion imaging mainly in the territories of the circumflex artery and the right coronary artery in a study implementing motion-frozen SPECT data and CCTA-guided SPECT contour and territory adjustments [22].

In summary, cardiac fusion imaging combining the anatomic information from CCTA with the functional information from myocardial perfusion imaging offers an incremental diagnostic value in the identification of hemodynamically significant coronary artery stenoses and thereby in guiding clinicians on the appropriate treatment (medical versus revascularization). The added value has not only been proven when comparing to one imaging modality alone, but also when comparing to the side-by-side analysis.

10.3.2 Clinical Indication for Fusion Imaging

As the combined hybrid approach is associated with increased radiation burden as well as higher costs, it is of great importance to select patients carefully. It is still an open question which patients do truly benefit from such an integrated approach. For the vast majority of patients referred for noninvasive testing, a single imaging method (either CCTA or myocardial perfusion imaging depending on the clinical situation) is sufficient. In the following clinical scenarios, the hybrid approach might be helpful.

10.3.2.1 Intermediate Pretest Likelihood

It is essential to assess the pretest likelihood in every patients presenting with symptoms of CAD. The main determinants of likelihood are age, gender, characteristics of chest pain, and ECG changes during exercise test. In patients with an intermediate pretest likelihood, the probability of an inconclusive or intermediate result in either of the imaging method is higher. Thus, in such situations, a combined approach is helpful to determine the relevance of a given lesion. For example, in a patient with an intermediate stenosis in CCTA, the subsequent assessment of the functional significance by myocardial perfusion imaging is needed to decide whether the patient can be treated medically or should undergo invasive revascularization. There are several centers with hybrid imaging facilities performing such an integrated approach sequentially.

10.3.2.2 Significant Side-Branch Disease

Although side branches (diagonal and posterolateral branches) of main coronary arteries are often seen as clinically irrelevant, patients may still suffer from symptoms such as angina as these side branches may induce ischemia. In such situations, fusion images provide an accurate method to assess the hemodynamic significance of such lesions, especially as the coregistration allows to exactly determine the vessel causing the ischemia.

10.3.2.3 Multivessel Disease

It is well known that patients with multivessel disease (MVD) are at increased risk for future adverse cardiac events. Although angiographically suspected, a large number of patients with MVD do not have any perfusion abnormality. Studies have shown that fusion imaging has an incremental diagnostic value compared to perfusion imaging alone, particularly in patients with MVD. Moreover, fusion imaging allows to accurately detect the culprit lesion, so that fusion imaging can been seen as a “gatekeeper” for ICA and revascularization.

10.3.2.4 Chronic Total Occlusion

In patients with chronic total occlusion (CTO), fusion imaging may be very helpful as it gives on one hand anatomic information such as the morphology of the vessel, the presence and the course of collateral vessels, the presence and amount of calcifications, and the length of occlusion and on the other hand allows to assess perfusion defects in the area of the CTO (Fig. 10.2). This information is especially needed, since revascularization procedures in CTO are associated with higher rates of complications, higher radiation burden, as well as larger amounts of contrast media used. Hence, it is of utmost importance to first evaluate the anatomic and functional information gained from fusion imaging before planning any potentially harmful interventions.

10.3.3 Prognostic Value of Fusion Imaging

Several studies have so far documented the incremental diagnostic value of fusion imaging (see above). However, only a few studies have assessed the prognostic value of fusion imaging. In a study including more than 500 patients, Van Werkhoven and coworkers showed on one hand that the anatomic information

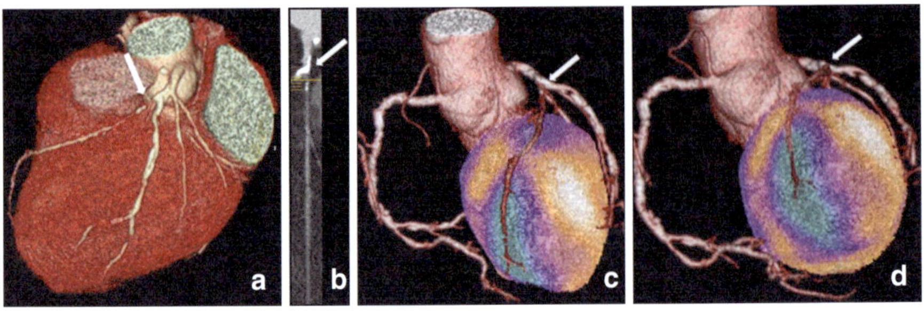

Fig. 10.2 Panel (**a**) is a 3D CCTA reconstruction of a patient with a chronic total occlusion (*arrow*) of the proximal LAD (documented by multiplanar reformation of the LAD in Panel **b**). Panels (**c**, **d**) are different views of a 3D-fused SPECT/CCTA reconstruction revealing a large perfusion defect in the territory of the LAD

from CCTA has incremental prognostic information over baseline clinical variables and MPI, particularly in patients with a normal MPI. Consequently, there is a higher risk in patients with an abnormal CCTA despite a normal SPECT scan, which may justify aggressive risk factor modification [23]. The first study documenting the prognostic value of fused SPECT/CCTA images included 324 consecutive patients which were subdivided into three groups: (1) stenosis by CCTA and a matching reversible SPECT defect (i.e., the perfusion defect was exactly at the area provided by the stenotic coronary artery on the 3D fusion display), (2) unmatched CCTA and SPECT finding, and (3) normal finding by CCTA and SPECT [24]. There was a significantly higher event rate (death or myocardial infarction) on follow-up (median of 2.8 years) in patients with a corresponding matched hybrid finding. A matched finding on fusion imaging proved to be an independent predictor for major adverse cardiovascular events. The annual death/MI rate was 6.0, 2.8, and 1.3 % for patients with matched, unmatched, and normal findings (Fig. 10.3).

In addition, a few studies have proven that fusion imaging has an impact on downstream resource utilization and most notably on revascularization rates. The first report demonstrated that revascularization rates within 60 days were 41 %, 11 %, and 0 % for matched, unmatched, and normal findings, respectively ($p<0.001$) [25]. In a similar study by Schaap and colleagues, revascularization rates were even higher with 90 %, 31 %, and 0 % for matched, unmatched, and normal findings, respectively ($p<0.001$) [26]. Fiechter and coworkers documented a revascularization rate of 91 and 8 % in patients with matched and unmatched hybrid findings, respectively [27]. Finally, a recent study by Danad and coworkers documented the revascularization rates per invasive coronary angiogram were 65 and 26 % in patients who displayed obstructive CAD on CTCA in combination with abnormal and normal MPI, respectively [28].

In conclusion, although prognostic information is still limited to a number of small single-center studies, the 3D fusion display of CCTA and myocardial

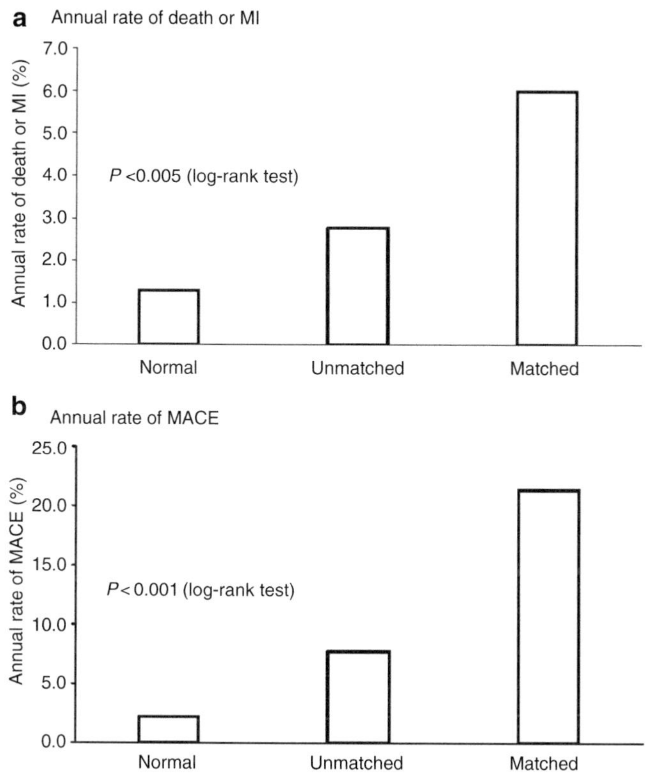

Fig. 10.3 The prognostic value of cardiac fusion imaging shown by the annual event rate. (**a**) A matched hybrid finding predicts a higher annual rate of all-cause death or nonfatal myocardial infarction (*MI*) as well as (**b**) major adverse cardiac events (death, MI, unstable angina requiring hospitalization, and coronary revascularization) (Reprinted with permission from Oxford University Press from Pazhenkottil et al. [24])

perfusion allowing anatomical and functional assessment of CAD may gain importance in the near future in cardiovascular imaging.

10.4 Future Perspective of Fusion Imaging

So far, the main focus of fusion imaging by combining CT with nuclear imaging methods was in assessing patients with suspected or known coronary artery disease. However, recently, fusion imaging is increasingly widening its application possibilities, going beyond the assessment of myocardial perfusion alone. Furthermore, the use of other modalities (e.g., cardiac MR) may expand existing indications for fusion imaging. A number of novel fusion imaging approaches hold promise to make their way into clinical practice or are used already in very specialized centers.

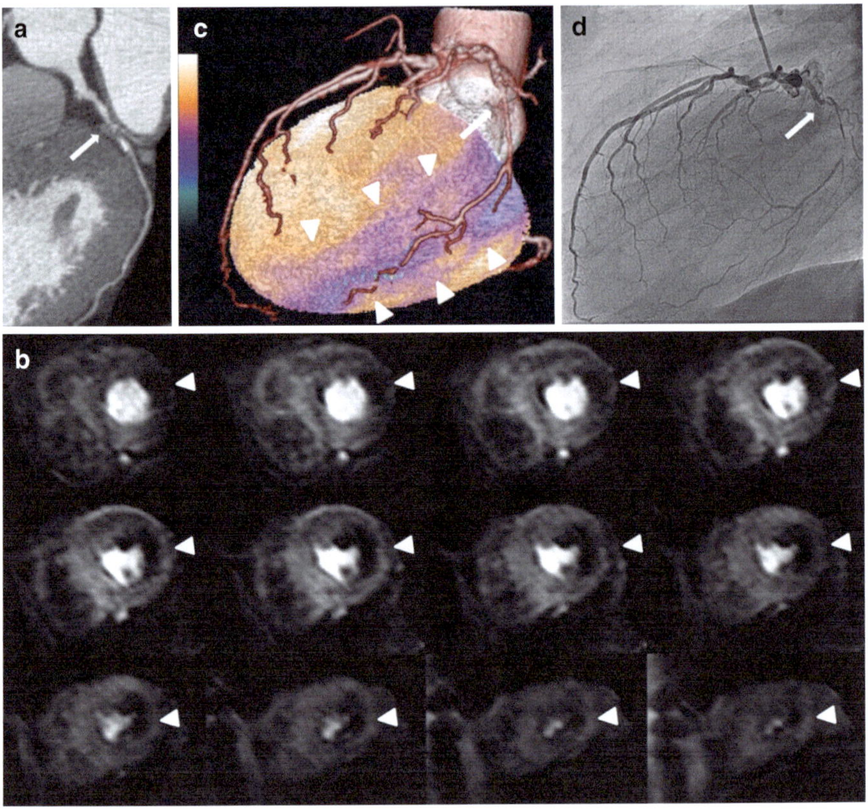

Fig. 10.4 First fusion of 3D CMR with CCTA. Panel (**a**) shows a curved multiplanar reformation of the left circumflex artery with a high-grade stenosis (*arrow*) in the large first obtuse marginal branch (OM1) leading to a lateral perfusion defect on CMR (Panel **b**: *arrowheads*). Panel (**c**) documents a perfect match of perfusion defect by 3D fusion imaging combining CMR and CCTA (*white arrowheads*). Invasive coronary angiography confirmed a subtotal occlusion of the OM1 (*white arrow*), which was successfully revascularized (Panel **d**) (Reprinted by permission from Oxford University Press from Manka et al. [29])

10.4.1 Hybrid CCTA/MR

Recently, feasibility of fusion of CCTA with 3D cardiac magnetic resonance (CMR) has been documented (Fig. 10.4) [29]. The use of stress MR instead of SPECT or PET for fusion imaging has the advantage of a higher spatial resolution and the avoidance of ionizing radiation. This development has been made possible by dedicated faster kt SENSE perfusion sequences which allow to obtain a full-coverage volumetric 3D dataset of CMR perfusion in the left ventricle (instead of the standard first-pass perfusion MR acquiring only three distinct short axes of the left ventricle, which was not enough to extrapolate onto a volumetric perfusion dataset).

10.4.2 Cardiac Resynchronization Therapy

Patients with severe symptomatic heart failure, particularly those with ischemic heart disease, are considered for cardiac resynchronization therapy (CRT) which is now an accepted therapeutic option improving symptoms and prognosis in such patients. Unfortunately, around 30 % of all patients receiving a CRT device are nonresponders. Therefore, dedicated methods to predict CRT response are warranted. It has been shown that an accurate assessment of mechanical dyssynchrony is feasible by phase analysis of gated perfusion SPECT scans [30]. By the combined assessment of viability by SPECT/PET and venous anatomy by CCTA, a better long-term result in CRT patients may be achieved. Particularly the fusion imaging approach allows visualization of venous morphology and identifying suitable veins for percutaneous lead insertion as well as assessing viability in this territory at the same time [31].

References

1. White CW, Wright CB, Doty DB, et al. Does visual interpretation of the coronary arteriogram predict the physiologic importance of a coronary stenosis? N Engl J Med. 1984;310:819–24.
2. Tonino PA, Fearon WF, De Bruyne B, et al. Angiographic versus functional severity of coronary artery stenoses in the FAME study fractional flow reserve versus angiography in multivessel evaluation. J Am Coll Cardiol. 2010;55:2816–21.
3. Uren NG, Melin JA, De Bruyne B, Wijns W, Baudhuin T, Camici PG. Relation between myocardial blood flow and the severity of coronary-artery stenosis. N Engl J Med. 1994;330: 1782–8.
4. Hacker M, Jakobs T, Hack N, et al. Sixty-four slice spiral CT angiography does not predict the functional relevance of coronary artery stenoses in patients with stable angina. Eur J Nucl Med Mol Imaging. 2007;34:4–10.
5. Gaemperli O, Schepis T, Valenta I, et al. Functionally relevant coronary artery disease: comparison of 64-section CT angiography with myocardial perfusion SPECT. Radiology. 2008; 248:414–23.
6. Schuijf JD, Wijns W, Jukema JW, et al. Relationship between noninvasive coronary angiography with multi-slice computed tomography and myocardial perfusion imaging. J Am Coll Cardiol. 2006;48:2508–14.
7. Boden WE, O'Rourke RA, Teo KK, et al. Optimal medical therapy with or without PCI for stable coronary disease. N Engl J Med. 2007;356:1503–16.
8. Frye RL, August P, Brooks MM, et al. A randomized trial of therapies for type 2 diabetes and coronary artery disease. N Engl J Med. 2009;360:2503–15.
9. Tonino PA, De Bruyne B, Pijls NH, et al. Fractional flow reserve versus angiography for guiding percutaneous coronary intervention. N Engl J Med. 2009;360:213–24.
10. De Bruyne B, Pijls NH, Kalesan B, et al. Fractional flow reserve-guided PCI versus medical therapy in stable coronary disease. N Engl J Med. 2012;367:991–1001.
11. Task Force M, Montalescot G, Sechtem U, et al. 2013 ESC guidelines on the management of stable coronary artery disease: the Task Force on the management of stable coronary artery disease of the European Society of Cardiology. Eur Heart J. 2013;34:2949–3003.
12. Gaemperli O, Kaufmann PA, Alkadhi H. Cardiac hybrid imaging. Eur J Nucl Med Mol Imaging. 2014;41 Suppl 1:S91–103.
13. Namdar M, Hany TF, Koepfli P, et al. Integrated PET/CT for the assessment of coronary artery disease: a feasibility study. J Nucl Med. 2005;46:930–5.

14. Rispler S, Keidar Z, Ghersin E, et al. Integrated single-photon emission computed tomography and computed tomography coronary angiography for the assessment of hemodynamically significant coronary artery lesions. J Am Coll Cardiol. 2007;49:1059–67.
15. Sato A, Nozato T, Hikita H, et al. Incremental value of combining 64-slice computed tomography angiography with stress nuclear myocardial perfusion imaging to improve noninvasive detection of coronary artery disease. J Nucl Cardiol. 2010;17:19–26.
16. Kajander S, Joutsiniemi E, Saraste M, et al. Cardiac positron emission tomography/computed tomography imaging accurately detects anatomically and functionally significant coronary artery disease. Circulation. 2010;122:603–13.
17. Schaap J, Kauling RM, Boekholdt SM, et al. Incremental diagnostic accuracy of hybrid SPECT/CT coronary angiography in a population with an intermediate to high pre-test likelihood of coronary artery disease. Eur Heart J Cardiovasc Imaging. 2013;14:642–9.
18. Danad I, Raijmakers PG, Appelman YE, et al. Hybrid imaging using quantitative H215O PET and CT-based coronary angiography for the detection of coronary artery disease. J Nucl Med. 2013;54:55–63.
19. Thomassen A, Petersen H, Diederichsen AC, et al. Hybrid CT angiography and quantitative 15O-water PET for assessment of coronary artery disease: comparison with quantitative coronary angiography. Eur J Nucl Med Mol Imaging. 2013;40:1894–904.
20. Gaemperli O, Schepis T, Valenta I, et al. Cardiac image fusion from stand-alone SPECT and CT: clinical experience. J Nucl Med. 2007;48:696–703.
21. Santana CA, Garcia EV, Faber TL, et al. Diagnostic performance of fusion of myocardial perfusion imaging (MPI) and computed tomography coronary angiography. J Nucl Cardiol. 2009;16:201–11.
22. Slomka PJ, Cheng VY, Dey D, et al. Quantitative analysis of myocardial perfusion SPECT anatomically guided by coregistered 64-slice coronary CT angiography. J Nucl Med. 2009;50:1621–30.
23. van Werkhoven JM, Schuijf JD, Gaemperli O, et al. Prognostic value of multislice computed tomography and gated single-photon emission computed tomography in patients with suspected coronary artery disease. J Am Coll Cardiol. 2009;53:623–32.
24. Pazhenkottil AP, Nkoulou RN, Ghadri JR, et al. Prognostic value of cardiac hybrid imaging integrating single-photon emission computed tomography with coronary computed tomography angiography. Eur Heart J. 2011;32:1465–71.
25. Pazhenkottil AP, Nkoulou RN, Ghadri JR, et al. Impact of cardiac hybrid single-photon emission computed tomography/computed tomography imaging on choice of treatment strategy in coronary artery disease. Eur Heart J. 2011;32(22):2824–9.
26. Schaap J, de Groot JA, Nieman K, et al. Hybrid myocardial perfusion SPECT/CT coronary angiography and invasive coronary angiography in patients with stable angina pectoris lead to similar treatment decisions. Heart. 2013;99:188–94.
27. Fiechter M, Ghadri JR, Wolfrum M, et al. Downstream resource utilization following hybrid cardiac imaging with an integrated cadmium-zinc-telluride/64-slice CT device. Eur J Nucl Med Mol Imaging. 2012;39:430–6.
28. Danad I, Raijmakers PG, Harms HJ, et al. Effect of cardiac hybrid (1)(5)O-water PET/CT imaging on downstream referral for invasive coronary angiography and revascularization rate. Eur Heart J Cardiovasc Imaging. 2014;15:170–9.
29. Manka R, Kuhn FP, Kuest SM, Gaemperli O, Kozerke S, Kaufmann PA. Hybrid cardiac magnetic resonance/computed tomographic imaging: first fusion of three-dimensional magnetic resonance perfusion and low-dose coronary computed tomographic angiography. Eur Heart J. 2011;32(21):2625.
30. Chen J, Garcia EV, Folks RD, Cooke CD, Faber TL, Tauxe EL, et al. Onset of left ventricular mechanical contraction as determined by phase analysis of ECG-gated myocardial perfusion SPECT imaging: development of a diagnostic tool for assessment of cardiac mechanical dyssynchrony. J Nucl Cardiol. 2005;12:687–95.
31. van der Hoeven BL, Schalij MJ, Delgado V. Multimodality imaging in interventional cardiology. Nat Rev Cardiol. 2012;9:333–46.

Combining CT Coronary Angiography and Myocardial Flow Reserve: Is It the Future?

11

Paul Knaapen

11.1 Introduction

Coronary artery disease (CAD) is the leading cause of death in the Western world. An accurate and early diagnosis is therefore warranted to determine the presence and extent of disease to guide clinical management. Invasive coronary angiography (ICA), in conjunction with intracoronary pressure measurements for intermediate coronary lesions, is considered the reference standard for this purpose [1]. With supreme temporal and spatial resolution, ICA provides reliable and accurate information on coronary luminal abnormalities. Furthermore, simultaneous assessment of fractional flow reserve (FFR) identifies patients who are eligible for revascularization, and FFR-driven percutaneous coronary intervention (PCI) improves outcome [2–4]. The invasive nature and high costs, however, warrant noninvasive screening to act as gatekeeper for conventional angiography and select those patients in whom obstructive CAD is most likely [5].

Coronary computed tomography angiography (CCTA) has recently emerged as a noninvasive alternative for its invasive counterpart to evaluate coronary anatomy [6]. The widespread availability of CT technology and ease of implementation in daily clinical practice has resulted in an exponential utilization of this imaging modality [7]. CCTA has proven particularly useful to exclude CAD due to its excellent sensitivity. Much like ICA, however, CCTA is a purely anatomical imaging technique, and hemodynamic consequences for a given epicardial cannot be determined, emphasizing the role of myocardial perfusion imaging (MPI) in the noninvasive evaluation of CAD [8]. Although several imaging modalities are available to assess myocardial perfusion, positron emission tomography (PET) has shown to possess the highest diagnostic accuracy to diagnose CAD [9–11]. Moreover,

P. Knaapen, MD
Department of Cardiology, VU University Medical Center of Amsterdam, Amsterdam, The Netherlands
e-mail: p.knaapen@vumc.nl

T.H. Schindler et al. (eds.), *Molecular and Multimodality Imaging in Cardiovascular Disease*, DOI 10.1007/978-3-319-19611-4_11

PEt allows to quantify myocardial blood flow (MBF) and flow reserve (MFR) in absolute terms, which adds important diagnostic and prognostic value in the evaluation of patients with (suspected) CAD. Due to its limited availability, methodological complexity, and high cost, cardiac PET has long been considered to be a research tool only. With the introduction of hybrid PET/CT, predominantly driven by its success in clinical oncology, cardiac PET is becoming increasingly available. This growth in hardware has been paralleled by improvements in radiotracer availability and advances in post-processing software. Consequently, cardiac PET has witnessed more widespread use and routine implementation in the clinical arena. Moreover, these hybrid devices now allow to acquire anatomical and functional information of the coronary tree in a single imaging session [12]. This chapter will discuss the advantages of hybrid imaging with PET/CT and quantification of flow over each modality separately in patients suspected of CAD.

11.2 Coronary Computed Tomography Angiography

Over the last decade, CCTA has developed as a valuable noninvasive alternative for the visualization of coronary anatomy. Current multislice CT scanners in combination with modern acquisition protocols enable robust and reproducible assessment of coronary artery morphology with relatively high temporal and spatial resolution accomplished at acceptable radiation dose [13]. The diagnostic accuracy of CCTA has been extensively studied, and pooled analysis of the literature demonstrates a consistent and unequaled high sensitivity (96 %) and negative predictive value (NPV, 94 %), positioning CCTA as a perfect tool to rule out CAD [14]. This holds particularly true in patients with a low pretest likelihood of disease. In contrast, specificity (76 %) and positive predictive value (PPV, 84 %) are generally moderate [14]. Lesion assessment is less accurate in comparison with ICA owing to the lower spatial and temporal resolution. Image quality is further affected by several additional factors such as heart rate and rhythm, body size, motion artifacts, quality of contrast opacification, and coronary calcifications. Although proper patient selection, preparation, and tailored imaging protocols can optimize image quality, coronary calcification is unamendable. The latter causes blooming artifacts and systemic overestimation of lesion severity [15]. Dual-energy CT acquisitions may reduce this issue, yet both invasive and noninvasive coronary imaging of a stenosis will continuously fail to accurately predict its functional aspects [16]. Hybrid imaging studies have shown that of CCTA deemed positive scans, approximately only half are actually associated with perfusion defects as documented with nuclear MPI [8, 17, 18]. Therefore, functional assessment is mandatory in the presence of an apparent obstructive stenosis to discern its hemodynamic relevance. Of interest, studies have unequivocally demonstrated that CCTA as an initial diagnostic test conveys increased downstream test utilization, costs, as well as revascularization procedures without a clear benefit in outcome [19–21].

The prognostic value of CCTA beyond traditional risk factors has been well documented, whereby adverse cardiac events are extremely rare in case of normal findings, and risk gradually increases in line with the extent of CAD [22–24]. An additional advantage of CT-based angiography is the fact that plaque morphology can be assessed. Noncalcified plaques are shown to bear an unfavorable prognosis. Noncalcified lesions, although not necessarily of obstructive nature impeding myocardial perfusion, are associated with plaque vulnerability and the occurrence of acute coronary syndromes due to plaque rupture [25–27]. The clinical implications of these observations are under investigation, and the impact of preventive medical strategies instigated by the detection of CT-graded nonobstructive CAD on outcome remains to be elucidated.

11.3 Positron Emission Tomography

Positron emission tomography (PET) is widely accepted as the reference technique to assess myocardial perfusion noninvasively in vivo [28]. For this purpose, four tracers in particular have been validated. Of the available tracers, ^{82}Rb, $^{13}NH_3$, and $H_2{}^{15}O$ are the most commonly used for the assessment of myocardial perfusion [29]. ^{18}F-flurpiridaz is an emerging perfusion tracer not yet available for clinical use, but holds great potential and is currently being tested in phase three trials [30]. Each of these tracers possesses unique characteristics with their individual pros and cons pertaining (costs of) radionuclide production, physical half-life, image quality, radiation exposure, compatibility with exercise acquisition protocols, and tracer kinetics for quantification (Table. 11.1). None of the perfusion tracers excels on all of these features. Choice of tracer is therefore multifactorial and frequently depends on practical and logistical considerations.

11.3.1 Perfusion Tracer Characteristics

$H_2{}^{15}O$ is characterized by fundamentally different properties as compared with ^{82}Rb, $^{13}NH_3$, and ^{18}F-flurpiridaz [28, 31, 32]. ^{82}Rb is a potassium analog that is rapidly and actively taken up by myocardial cells via the Na/K ATP transporter [33], whereas $^{13}NH_3$ is incorporated into the glutamine pool by active transport and passive diffusion processes [34]. ^{18}F-flurpiridaz is a pyridazinone derivative that avidly binds to mitochondrial complex-1 [35]. The latter tracers are transported across the cell membrane and effectively become metabolically trapped while cleared from the intravascular compartment, yielding excellent qualitative gradable imaging due to high tissue-to-background ratios. In contrast, $H_2{}^{15}O$ is a freely diffusible, metabolically inert tracer that promptly reaches equilibrium between blood and tissue and is not accumulated in the myocardium. As a consequence, radiotracer distribution images of $H_2{}^{15}O$ are of little diagnostic value. The lack of diagnostic images has long prohibited the use of $H_2{}^{15}O$ for diagnostic imaging of CAD and virtually all studies on qualitative imaging for CAD have been conducted with ^{82}Rb or $^{13}NH_3$ [36]. In recent years, however, digital subtraction techniques and parametric imaging by automated software packages now generate qualitative gradable $H_2{}^{15}O$

Table 11.1 Characteristics of cardiac perfusion tracers

	$H_2{}^{15}O$	$^{13}NH_3$	^{82}Rb	^{18}F-flurpiridaz
Half-life	123 s	9.97 min	76 s	110 min
Production	Cyclotron	Cyclotron	Generator	Cyclotron
Kinetics	Freely diffusible, metabolically inert	Metabolically trapped in the myocardium	Metabolically trapped in the myocardium	Metabolically trapped in the myocardium
Mean positron range in tissue	1.1 mm	0.4 mm	2.8 mm	0.2 mm
Scan duration Gating/LV function	6 min –	20 min +	6 min +	20 min +
Radiation dose (3D) according to protocol in references	~0.4 mSv/370 MBq	~1 mSv/550 MBq	~0.7 mSv/555 MBq (2D: ~2.3 mSv/1,850 MBq)	~2.1 mSv/111 MBq (rest) ~4.6 mSv/244 MBq (stress)
Exercise protocol compatible	–	–	–	+
Quantification	Excellent	Good	Moderate	Very good
Image quality	Good (parametric images)	Very good	Good	Excellent

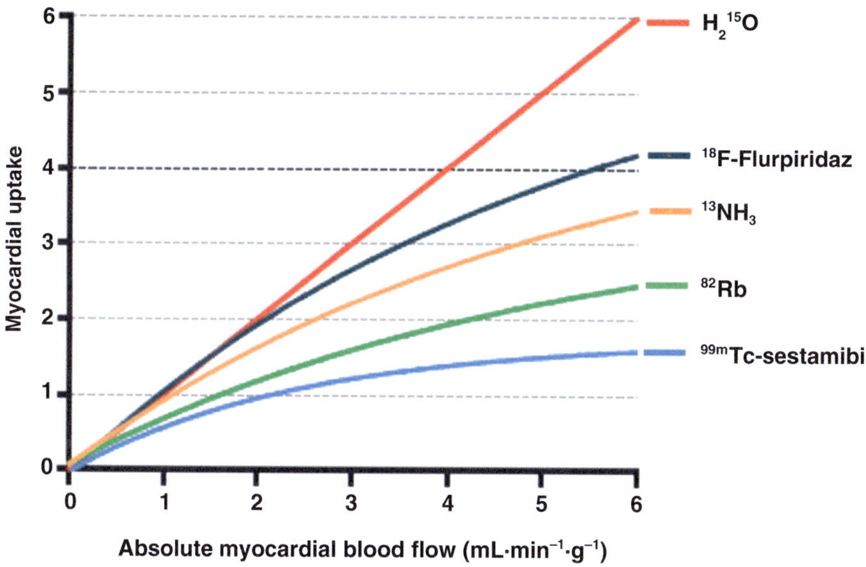

Fig. 11.1 Kinetics of myocardial perfusion tracers; graphical presentation of the relationship between absolute myocardial blood flow of PET radiotracers and actual tracer uptake. 18F-flurpiridaz is not yet available for clinical use

perfusion images comparable to the aforementioned tracers [37–39]. These developments have enabled $H_2{}^{15}O$ to be utilized in clinical practice [40–42].

Next to relative uptake images, PET measures absolute levels of tracer concentration. Acquisition of PET in a dynamic fashion (i.e., multiple frames initiated upon administration of the tracer) generates time-activity curves of tracer flux between arterial blood and tissues [28]. This information allows to mathematically compute MBF in absolute terms (in units of mL · min^{-1} · g^{-1}) and calculate myocardial flow reserve (MFR). The ideal tracer accumulates in/or clears from the myocardium proportionally linear to perfusion, irrespective of flow rate or metabolic state [43]. $H_2{}^{15}O$ is the only tracer that meets these criteria and is therefore considered the gold standard for quantification of MBF [44]. An important limitation of the other aforementioned tracers is that myocardial extraction from arterial blood is incomplete and curvilinear with increasing flow rates, frequently referred to as the "roll-off" phenomenon (Fig. 11.1) [45].

This results in progressive underestimation of MBF measurements as actual flow increases. Correction models based on animal experiments can be employed yet induce noise, particularly when large correction factors are required with severely blunted extraction at high perfusion levels. Nonetheless, each of these tracers has been tested in animal experiments against microsphere-quantified perfusion, the invasive reference standard. $H_2{}^{15}O$ and $^{13}NH_3$ in particular have been well validated and display close agreement with microsphere flow and demonstrate low test-retest variability (10–15 %) [31, 44, 46–48]. Quantification of ^{82}Rb is less reliable as this tracer harbors intrinsic limitations (ultrashort physical half-life, long positron range, and low extraction fraction). Nonetheless, recent studies have shown MBF measurements of ^{82}Rb to be feasible [49]. Limited data are available pertaining the quantification of ^{18}F-flurpiridaz, but its characteristics and kinetics should allow for highly reliable perfusion measurements [30, 43, 50].

11.3.2 Tracer Production and Availability

A pivotal issue that has proven to be the major obstacle for cardiac PET perfusion imaging is the necessity to produce the utilized tracers on-site. Of the currently available tracers, $H_2{}^{15}O$ and $^{13}NH_3$ require a cyclotron in the near proximity of the scanning facilities. ^{82}Rb is produced by a ^{82}Sr/^{82}Rb generator obviating the need for a cyclotron and is therefore more convenient to implement in clinical practice. The parent isotope ^{82}Sr, however, needs to be replenished every 28 days at relatively high costs ($20.000). Therefore, high volume patient throughput is needed to be cost-effective. These issues of local tracer production have clearly limited the widespread use of cardiac perfusion PET. This may soon be overcome by the dawning perspective of fluorine-labeled tracers such as ^{18}F-flurpiridaz [30]. Its longer physical half-life of 110 min allows for off-site production and could be as successful for cardiology as ^{18}F-FDG PET has been for clinical oncology. Another advantage of ^{18}F-labeled flow tracers is the fact that they allow to be used in physical exercise protocols whereby the radioisotope is administered during maximal exertion. ^{82}Rb, $H_2{}^{15}O$, and $^{13}NH_3$ require injection while the patient is lying within the scanner, as tracer decay is too rapid to transport the patient from the treadmill or stationary bike to the scanner. These tracers can therefore only be utilized in conjunction with pharmacological stressor agents.

11.4 Diagnostic Accuracy and Prognosis

The vast majority of the studies on the diagnostic accuracy have been conducted with static uptake images of ^{82}Rb and $^{13}NH_3$ [51]. Pooled analysis of these studies displays weighted sensitivity, specificity, NPV, and PPV which were 91, 86, 81, and 93 %, respectively, although it must be acknowledged that virtually all of these studies were compared with invasive coronary angiography without FFR and therefore lack an appropriate reference standard [14]. In comparison with single-photon emission computed tomography (SPECT) and cardiovascular magnetic resonance imaging (CMR), MPI with PET consistently yields the highest diagnostic accuracy [9–11]. Traditionally, these images (regardless of the utilized technique like SPECT, PET, CMR, or CT) are graded in a qualitative manner whereby perfusion defects are identified based on the relative distribution of the tracer. Unfortunately, conditions that are accompanied by lack of normal myocardium to act as reference limit such a qualitative approach and may yield false-negative results or underestimation of the extent of disease (e.g., in the case of multivessel disease and/or microvascular

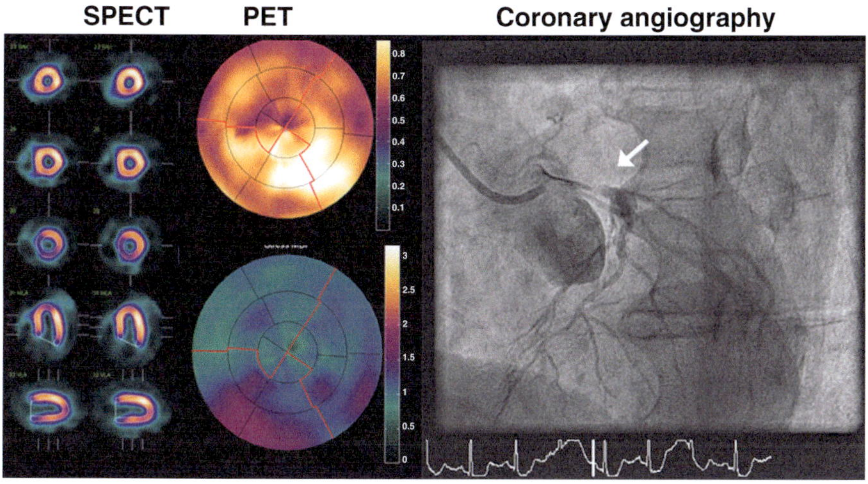

Fig. 11.2 A 73-year-old male with atypical angina without cardiovascular risk factors, and no prior cardiac history was evaluated for coronary artery disease with 99mTc-sestamibi SPECT (*left panel rest* and *right panel stress*) and PET (*upper panel rest, lower panel stress*). Tracer distribution was homogenous during rest and stress on the SPECT images, and the visual and automated grading yielded a normal test result. Polar maps of PET displayed normal resting perfusion but diffusely blunted hyperemic MBF. Coronary angiography revealed a subtotal occlusion of the left main coronary artery (*white arrow*). SPECT imaging was false negative due to balanced ischemia, which was unmasked by the quantitative nature of the PET imaging

dysfunction). As already mentioned, PET offers the possibility to routinely quantify MBF and thus overcome these limitations (Fig. 11.2).

Indeed, there is mounting evidence that quantitative analysis with PET is superior to static uptake image grading [52–55]. Also compelling are the recent observations that hyperemic MBF quantification outperforms MFR to diagnose obstructive CAD, highlighting the potential of stress-only protocols [40, 42, 56, 57]. Reported thresholds of what should be considered pathological hyperemic MBF or MFR are unfortunately not uniform [51]. It appears that cutoff values are, at least in part, related to tracer kinetics and these should not be considered interchangeable [58]. Next to these technical issues, the detection of hemodynamically significant CAD is based on the presence of a flow-limiting epicardial coronary lesion, whereas PET measurements reflect the composite of perfusion throughout the entire coronary artery tree (roughly divided into the epicardial coronary compartment and the microvasculature) (see Fig. 11.3).

Definition of a single threshold will therefore remain elusive given its dependency on microvascular vasomotor function. The latter is related to age, gender, and cardiovascular risk profile [59, 60]. Nonetheless, recently, Danad et al. have explored optimal values for hyperemic MBF and MFR in a large multicenter trial using $H_2^{15}O$ PET whereby each patient was referred for invasive coronary angiography and FFR when appropriate [57]. Optimal thresholds were set at 2.3 $mL \cdot min^{-1} \cdot g^{-1}$ and 2.5 for hyperemic MBF and MFR, respectively. For hyperemic MBF, sensitivity,

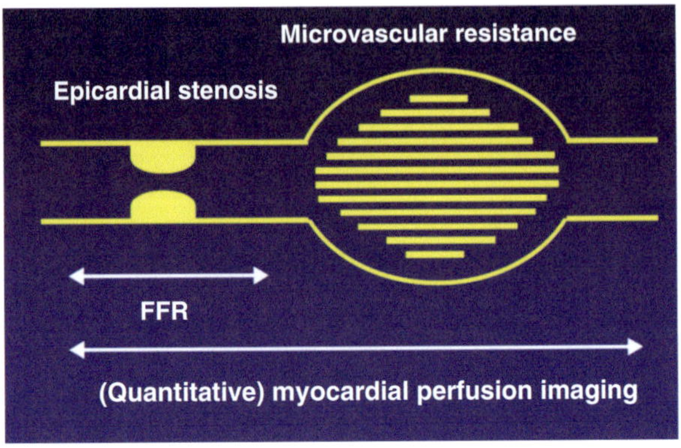

Fig. 11.3 Graphical representation of the coronary vascular bed, divided into the epicardial conduit arteries and the microvasculature. The detection of coronary artery disease is based on the functional evaluation of an epicardial stenosis. Quantitative myocardial perfusion imaging provides an integrated measurement of perfusion of the entire coronary vascular bed, whereas, for example, fractional flow reserve (*FFR*) solely measures the pressure gradient across the coronary lesion. FFR and perfusion imaging therefore provide different information on coronary vascular health and are not necessarily concordant [51, 59]

specificity, and accuracy of hyperemic MBF for the detection of functionally relevant CAD were 87, 84, and 85 %, respectively. Of notice, these values were superior to MFR (84, 73, and 77 % for MFR, respectively) (Fig. 11.4). These data now pave the way for quantitative perfusion imaging, potentially with stress-only protocols, to be utilized in clinical practice.

In terms of prognosis, there is analogy to large-scale SPECT databases [61]. The extent and severity of (reversible) perfusion defects documented with PET hold strong prognostic information beyond traditional cardiovascular risk factors [51]. The quantitative nature of PET has shown incremental value. Of particular interest is the fact that apparent normal perfusion images with a homogenous tracer distribution can be reclassified based on diffusely blunted hyperemic MBF or MFR. Several studies have revealed that this subset of patients is at increased risk for future cardiac events [62–65].

11.5 Hybrid Cardiac PET/CT

Either an anatomical or functional approach in the evaluation of CAD has its limitations. Atherosclerosis is a gradual process that develops over decades. The advancing stages of CAD have been described by Glagov et al. [66]. Fig. 11.5 displays that noninvasive MPI with PET is particularly useful to document myocardial ischemia in advanced disease when coronary lesions become so tight that flow is hampered. In case of a normal scan, however, MPI PET cannot distinguish the different stages prior to the development of ischemia.

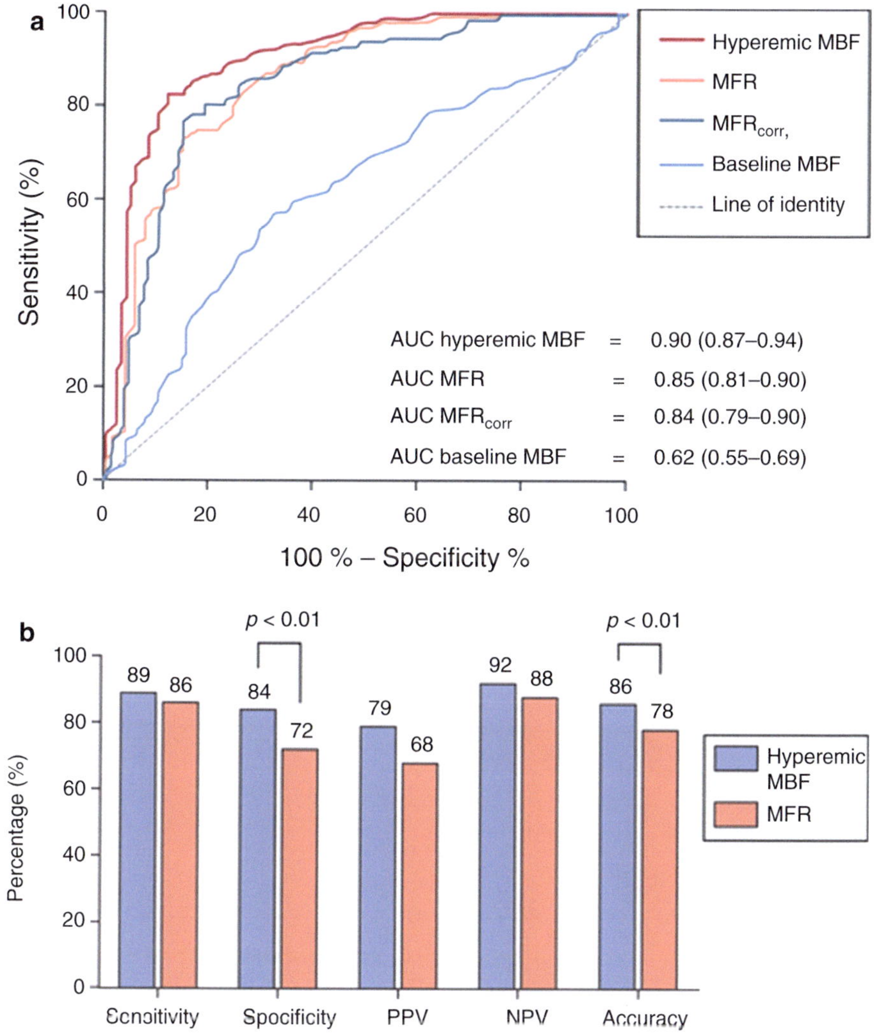

Fig. 11.4 *Upper panel*: ROC curve analysis with corresponding AUCs and 95 % CI displaying the diagnostic performance of hyperemic MBF, MFR, MFRcorr, and baseline MBF for the detection of hemodynamically significant CAD as indicated by FFR per patient. *Lower panel*: sensitivity, specificity, PPV, NPV, and accuracy on a per-patient basis of quantitative PET MPI using hyperemic MBF and MFR, respectively, as a perfusion parameter (Adapted from Danad et al. [59])

Conversely, CCTA can accurately document the very early stages of coronary disease but does not have the ability to predict the hemodynamic consequences in more advanced stage of disease. Therefore, a hybrid assessment provides complementary rather than overlapping information. In recent years, CT technology has been fused with PET. These hybrid devices are now available up to 128-slice CT and state-of-the-art PET equipment, enabling the near simultaneous evaluation of

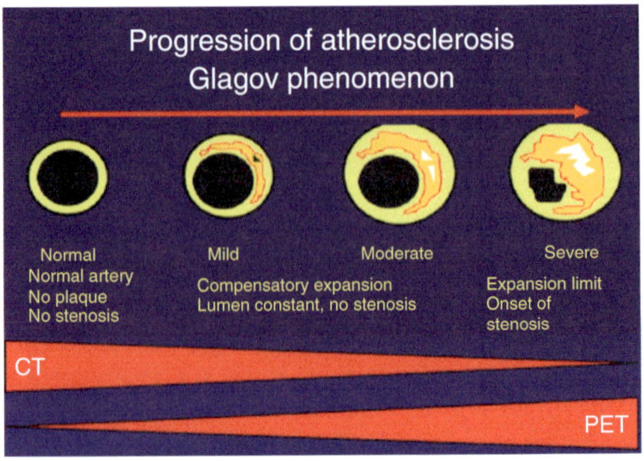

Fig. 11.5 The gradual stages of coronary artery disease. CT-based angiography is particularly useful to document the early stages of disease, whereas PET perfusion only displays abnormalities in the later stages of disease. The combination of CT and PET therefore acts complimentary

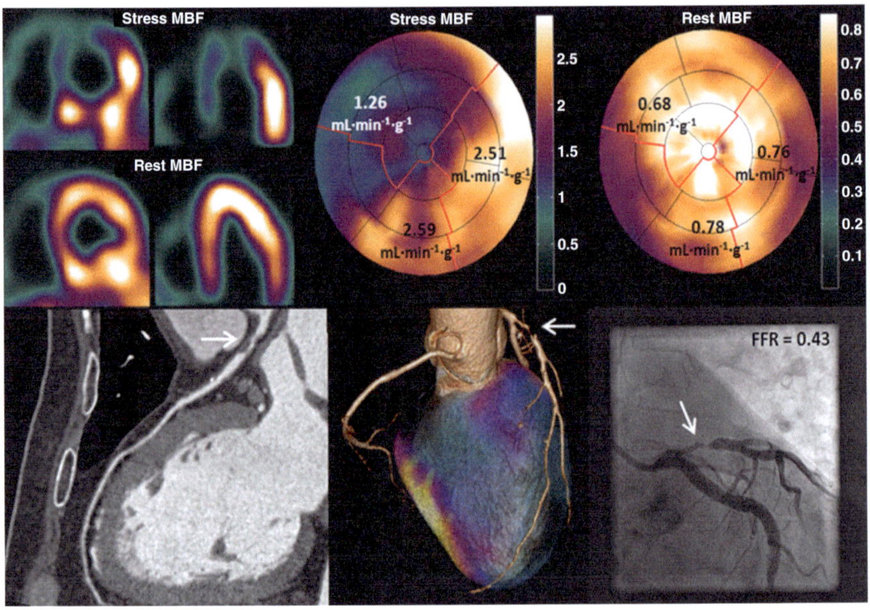

Fig. 11.6 A 52-year-old male with atypical angina. Hybrid 15O-water PET/CTCA imaging reveals a severely reduced hyperemic perfusion (1.26 ml · min^{-1} · g^{-1}) in the area supplied by the LAD artery with single-vessel disease documented with CCTA. Invasive coronary angiography can be planned with ad hoc percutaneous coronary intervention

coronary anatomy and quantitative myocardial perfusion in a single scanning session, which can be as short as 30 min (Fig. 11.6).

The number of studies on the diagnostic value of PET/CCTA for CAD is small yet convincingly demonstrates enhanced accuracy as compared with either modality alone (Table. 11.2) [40, 41, 67, 68]. Similar observations have been made in protocols of CCTA in conjunction with SPECT or CMR [69–73]. Hybrid imaging

Table 11.2 Diagnostic performance of cardiac hybrid PET/CCTA imaging (results shown on a per-patient basis)

Author	Hybrid PET/CT system	*N*	Reference standard for definition of obstructive CAD	Sensitivity CCTA/PET/hybrid (%)	Specificity CCTA/PET/hybrid (%)	NPV CCTA/PET/hybrid (%)	PPV CCTA/PET/hybrid (%)
Groves et al. [67]	^{82}Rb PET/64-slice CCTA	33	ICA > 50 %	100/92/96	82/89/100	100/80/91	92/96/100
Kajander et al. [41]	[^{15}O]H_2O PET/64-slice CCTA	107	ICA > 50 % + FFR ≤ 0.80	95/95/95	87/91/100	97/97/98	81/86/100
Danad et al. [40]	[^{15}O]H_2O PET/64-slice CCTA	120	ICA > 50 % + FFR ≤ 0.80	100/76/76	34/82/92	100/83/84	51/76/86
Thomassen et al. [68]	[^{15}O]H_2O PET/64-slice CCTA	44	ICA > 50 %	91/91/91	64/86/100	88/90/92	71/87/100
Weighted summary		304		97/89/90	67/87/98	96/88/91	74/86/97

CCTA, coronary computed tomography angiography, *CAD* coronary artery disease, *NPV* negative predictive value, *PPV* positive predictive value

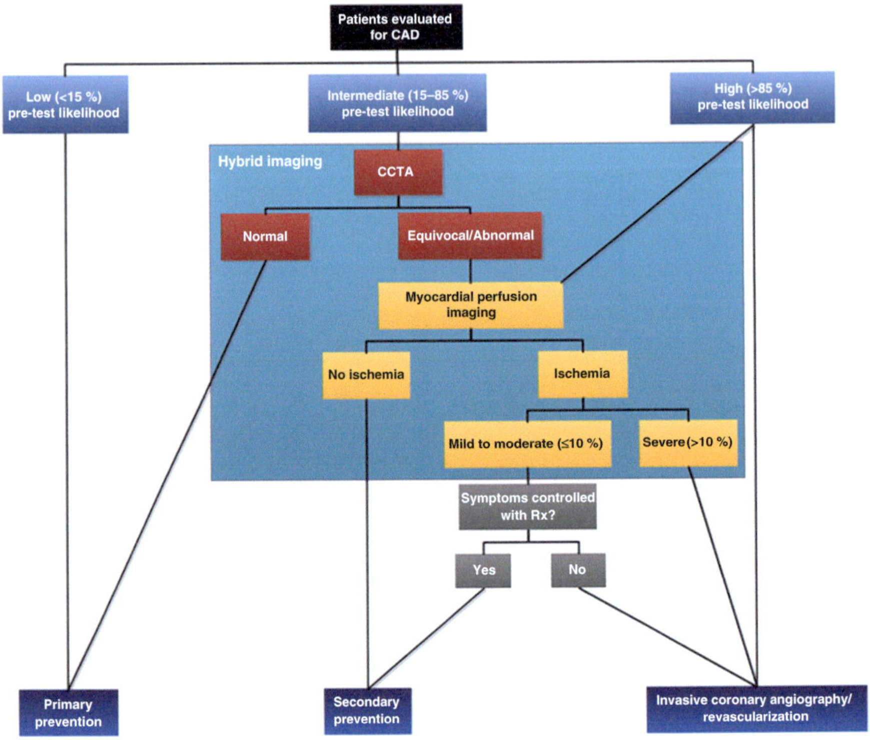

Fig. 11.7 Proposed diagnostic algorithm for diagnosing CAD using CCTA and myocardial perfusion imaging

is shown to be particularly useful for enhancing the moderate specificity and PPV of CCTA.

Besides enhanced diagnostic value, profiling the anatomical and functional status of the coronary tree additionally yields incremental prognostic data. Combining coronary calcium scoring (CAC) with MPI adds prognostic value in patients with and without myocardial ischemia, although ischemia appears to be a more potent predictor of future cardiac events than coronary calcification [74, 75]. To date, studies on the prognostic relevance of PET combined with CCTA are lacking. Nevertheless, data obtained from hybrid SPECT/CCTA studies reveal a more accurate risk stratification of the combined anatomical and functional approach [76, 77]. The hybrid approach provides particular additional value to risk stratify patients when either functional or anatomical evaluation displays ambiguous results. In a large cohort of patients ($n=1,295$), Kim et al. recently highlighted that sequential imaging with SPECT and CCTA was of limited incremental prognostic value when either SPECT MPS or CCTA was clearly abnormal (i.e., SSS ≥ 4 or CT-graded diameter stenosis ≥90 %, respectively) [78]. Figure 11.7 displays a proposed algorithm for the diagnostic work-up for patients suspected of CAD. CCTA should be the initial test and be complemented with MPI in case of a documented coronary lesion or poor interpretable CT scan. MPI should subsequently act as gatekeeper for ICA. Adding routine quantitative MBF and MFR with PET appears to provide the most comprehensive diagnostic evaluation in this category of patients.

Even though steadily increasing, the availability of hybrid PET/CCTA is still limited. Therefore, latest efforts have been directed toward deriving physiological information from CT technology directly. Three methodological avenues are currently being explored. First, as adopted from well-defined CMR protocols, CT perfusion (CTP) by acquisition of a dynamic first pass (stress) sequence has demonstrated to be feasible. Although CTP is in its early development and still faces many technical issues, a recent multicenter trial utilizing 320-slice CT scanners demonstrated that CTP enhanced the diagnostic accuracy over CCTA alone [79]. Second, noninvasive estimation of FFR through computational fluid dynamics analysis solely based on the anatomical features of the coronary arteries obtained with CCTA has recently emerged [80]. Multicenter trials have shown that FFR-CT may indeed raise diagnostic accuracy of CCTA [81–83]. The model, however, is based on numerous assumptions and the overall incremental value appears to be limited [82]. Moreover, the tremendous computational complexity requires hours of off-line analysis hampering its implementation in clinical practice for the time being. Hence, a much simpler approach of this principle was proposed as a third option whereby contrast opacification along the course of a coronary artery is documented by linear regression. The rationale behind this so-called transluminal attenuation gradient (TAG) is that contrast opacification may in theory fall off more rapidly in the presence of a functionally significant stenosis than in the absence of stenosis [84]. Although elegant in its simplicity, the fundamental concept of these approaches whereby hyperemic functional consequences of a coronary lesion are attempted to be disclosed at baseline conditions is questionable and lacks additional diagnostic value over CCTA alone [85]. Clearly, deriving functional data from cardiac CT is work in progress.

11.6 Summary

Hybrid cardiac PET/CCTA allows for a comprehensive evaluation of patients suspected of coronary artery disease. Within a single session, complementary diagnostic information on anatomy and physiology is obtained to guide patient management in an optimal fashion. The added diagnostic and prognostic value of routine quantification of MBF and MFR is a feature that is unique for this type of advanced imaging. Although current evidence supports its use in clinical practice for appropriately selected patients, studies in larger cohorts and in multicenter setting are needed to further clarify unresolved issues like incremental value over alternative (hybrid) approaches, cost-effectiveness, and impact on patient outcome.

References

1. Bashore TM, Bates ER, Berger PB, et al. American College of Cardiology/Society for Cardiac Angiography and Interventions Clinical Expert Consensus Document on cardiac catheterization laboratory standards. A report of the American College of Cardiology Task Force on Clinical Expert Consensus Documents. J Am Coll Cardiol. 2001;37(8):2170–214.
2. Pijls NH, De Bruyne B, Peels K, et al. Measurement of fractional flow reserve to assess the functional severity of coronary-artery stenoses. N Engl J Med. 1996;334:1703–8.

3. Tonino PAL, De Bruyne B, Pijls NHJ, et al. Fractional flow reserve versus angiography for guiding percutaneous coronary intervention. N Engl J Med. 2009;360:213–24.
4. De Bruyne B, Pijls NHJ, Kalesan B, et al. Fractional flow reserve-guided PCI versus medical therapy in stable coronary disease. N Engl J Med. 2012;367:991–1001.
5. Task Force Members, Montalescot G, Sechtem U, Achenbach S, et al. 2013 ESC guidelines on the management of stable coronary artery disease: the Task Force on the management of stable coronary artery disease of the European Society of Cardiology. Eur Heart J. 2013;34:2949–3003.
6. Schroeder S, Achenbach S, Bengel F, et al. Cardiac computed tomography: indications, applications, limitations, and training requirements: report of a Writing Group deployed by the Working Group Nuclear Cardiology and Cardiac CT of the European Society of Cardiology and the European Council of Nuclear Cardiology. Eur Heart J. 2008;29:531–56.
7. Shaw LJ, Marwick TH, Zoghbi WA, et al. Why all the focus on cardiac imaging? JACC Cardiovasc Imaging. 2010;3:789–94.
8. Danad I, Raijmakers PG, Harms HJ, et al. Effect of cardiac hybrid 15O-water PET/CT imaging on downstream referral for invasive coronary angiography and revascularization rate. Eur Heart J Cardiovasc Imaging. 2014;15:170–9.
9. Jaarsma C, Leiner T, Bekkers SC, et al. Diagnostic performance of noninvasive myocardial perfusion imaging using single-photon emission computed tomography, cardiac magnetic resonance, and positron emission tomography imaging for the detection of obstructive coronary artery disease: a meta-analysis. J Am Coll Cardiol. 2012;59:1719–28.
10. Parker MW, Iskandar A, Limone B, et al. Diagnostic accuracy of cardiac positron emission tomography versus single photon emission computed tomography for coronary artery disease: a bivariate meta-analysis. Circ Cardiovasc Imaging. 2012;5:700–7.
11. Mc Ardle BA, Dowsley TF, DeKemp RA, Wells GA, Beanlands RS. Does rubidium-82 PET have superior accuracy to SPECT perfusion imaging for the diagnosis of obstructive coronary disease? A systematic review and meta-analysis. J Am Coll Cardiol. 2012;60:1828–37.
12. Knaapen P, de Haan S, Hoekstra OS, et al. Cardiac PET-CT: advanced hybrid imaging for the detection of coronary artery disease. Neth Heart J. 2010;18:90–8.
13. Bogaard K, van der Zant FM, Knol RJJ, et al. High-pitch prospective ECG-triggered helical coronary computed tomography angiography in clinical practice: image quality and radiation dose. Int J Cardiovasc Imaging. 2014;31:1–9.
14. Danad I, Raijmakers PG, Knaapen P. Diagnosing coronary artery disease with hybrid PET/CT: it takes two to tango. J Nucl Cardiol. 2013;20:874–90.
15. Leber AW, Knez A, von Ziegler F, et al. Quantification of obstructive and nonobstructive coronary lesions by 64-slice computed tomography: a comparative study with quantitative coronary angiography and intravascular ultrasound. J Am Coll Cardiol. 2005;46:147–54.
16. Tonino PAL, Fearon WF, De Bruyne B, et al. Angiographic versus functional severity of coronary artery stenoses in the FAME study fractional flow reserve versus angiography in multivessel evaluation. J Am Coll Cardiol. 2010;55:2816–21.
17. Gaemperli O, Schepis T, Valenta I, et al. Functionally relevant coronary artery disease: comparison of 64-section CT angiography with myocardial perfusion SPECT. Radiology. 2008; 248:414–23.
18. Schuijf JD, Wijns W, Jukema JW, et al. Relationship between noninvasive coronary angiography with multi-slice computed tomography and myocardial perfusion imaging. J Am Coll Cardiol. 2006;48:2508–14.
19. Shreibati JB, Baker LC, Hlatky MA. Association of coronary CT angiography or stress testing with subsequent utilization and spending among Medicare beneficiaries. JAMA. 2011;306:2128–36.
20. Hachamovitch R, Nutter B, Hlatky MA, et al. Patient management after noninvasive cardiac imaging results from SPARC (Study of myocardial perfusion and coronary anatomy imaging roles in coronary artery disease). J Am Coll Cardiol. 2012;59:462–74.
21. Nielsen LH, Ortner N, Nørgaard BL, Achenbach S, Leipsic J, Abdulla J. The diagnostic accuracy and outcomes after coronary computed tomography angiography vs. conventional functional testing in patients with stable angina pectoris: a systematic review and meta-analysis. Eur Heart J Cardiovasc Imaging. 2014;15:961–71.

22. Hulten EA, Carbonaro S, Petrillo SP, Mitchell JD, Villines TC. Prognostic value of cardiac computed tomography angiography: a systematic review and meta-analysis. J Am Coll Cardiol. 2011;57:1237–47.
23. Min JK, Dunning A, Lin FY, et al. Age- and sex-related differences in all-cause mortality risk based on coronary computed tomography angiography findings results from the International Multicenter CONFIRM (Coronary CT Angiography Evaluation for Clinical Outcomes: An International Multicenter Registry) of 23,854 patients without known coronary artery disease. J Am Coll Cardiol. 2011;58:849–60.
24. Hadamitzky M, Täubert S, Deseive S, et al. Prognostic value of coronary computed tomography angiography during 5 years of follow-up in patients with suspected coronary artery disease. Eur Heart J. 2013;34:3277–85.
25. Blankstein R, Ferencik M. The vulnerable plaque: can it be detected with Cardiac CT? Atherosclerosis. 2010;211:386–9.
26. Versteylen MO, Kietselaer BL, Dagnelie PC, et al. Additive value of semiautomated quantification of coronary artery disease using cardiac computed tomographic angiography to predict future acute coronary syndrome. J Am Coll Cardiol. 2013;61:2296–305.
27. Motoyama S, Sarai M, Harigaya H, et al. Computed tomographic angiography characteristics of atherosclerotic plaques subsequently resulting in acute coronary syndrome. J Am Coll Cardiol. 2009;54:49–57.
28. Knaapen P, Camici PG, Marques KM, et al. Coronary microvascular resistance: methods for its quantification in humans. Basic Res Cardiol. 2009;104:485–98.
29. Knaapen P, Lubberink M. Cardiac positron emission tomography: myocardial perfusion and metabolism in clinical practice. Clin Res Cardiol. 2008;97:791–6.
30. Rischpler C, Park M-J, Fung GSK, Javadi M, Tsui BMW, Higuchi T. Advances in PET myocardial perfusion imaging: F-18 labeled tracers. Ann Nucl Med. 2012;26:1–6.
31. Iida H, Kanno I, Takahashi A, et al. Measurement of absolute myocardial blood flow with H215O and dynamic positron-emission tomography. Strategy for quantification in relation to the partial-volume effect. Circulation. 1988;78:104–15.
32. Schindler TH, Schelbert HR, Quercioli A, Dilsizian V. Cardiac PET imaging for the detection and monitoring of coronary artery disease and microvascular health. JACC Cardiovasc Imaging. 2010;3:623–40.
33. Huang SC, Williams BA, Krivokapich J, Araujo L, Phelps ME, Schelbert HR. Rabbit myocardial 82Rb kinetics and a compartmental model for blood flow estimation. Am J Physiol. 1989;256:H1156–64.
34. Schelbert HR, Phelps ME, Huang SC, et al. N-13 ammonia as an indicator of myocardial blood flow. Circulation. 1981;63:1259–72.
35. Yalamanchili P, Wexler E, Hayes M, et al. Mechanism of uptake and retention of F-18 BMS-747158-02 in cardiomyocytes: a novel PET myocardial imaging agent. J Nucl Cardiol. 2007;14:782–8.
36. Di Carli MF, Hachamovitch R. New technology for noninvasive evaluation of coronary artery disease. Circulation. 2007;115:1464–80.
37. Nesterov SV, Han C, Mäki M, et al. Myocardial perfusion quantitation with 15O-labelled water PET: high reproducibility of the new cardiac analysis software (Carimas). Eur J Nucl Med Mol Imaging. 2009;36:1594–602.
38. Harms HJ, Knaapen P, de Haan S, Halbmeijer R, Lammertsma AA, Lubberink M. Automatic generation of absolute myocardial blood flow images using [15O]H2O and a clinical PET/CT scanner. Eur J Nucl Med Mol Imaging. 2011;38:930–9.
39. Harms HJ, Nesterov SV, Han C, et al. Comparison of clinical non-commercial tools for automated quantification of myocardial blood flow using oxygen-15-labelled water PET/CT. Eur Heart J Cardiovasc Imaging. 2013;15(4):431–41.
40. Danad I, Raijmakers PG, Appelman YE, et al. Hybrid imaging using quantitative H215O PET and CT-based coronary angiography for the detection of coronary artery disease. J Nucl Med. 2013;54:55–63.
41. Kajander S, Joutsiniemi E, Saraste M, et al. Cardiac positron emission tomography/computed tomography imaging accurately detects anatomically and functionally significant coronary artery disease. Circulation. 2010;122:603–13.

42. Danad I, Raijmakers PG, Harms HJ, et al. Impact of anatomical and functional severity of coronary atherosclerotic plaques on the transmural perfusion gradient: a [15O]H2O PET study. Eur Heart J. 2014;35:2094–105.
43. Maddahi J. Properties of an ideal PET perfusion tracer: new PET tracer cases and data. J Nucl Cardiol. 2012;19 Suppl 1:S30–7.
44. Bergmann SR, Fox KA, Rand AL, et al. Quantification of regional myocardial blood flow in vivo with H215O. Circulation. 1984;70:724–33.
45. Saraste A, Kajander S, Han C, Nesterov SV, Knuuti J. PET: is myocardial flow quantification a clinical reality? J Nucl Cardiol. 2012;19:1044–59.
46. Bol A, Melin JA, Vanoverschelde JL, et al. Direct comparison of [13N]ammonia and [15O] water estimates of perfusion with quantification of regional myocardial blood flow by microspheres. Circulation. 1993;87:512–25.
47. Kaufmann PA, Gnecchi-Ruscone T, Yap JT, Rimoldi O, Camici PG. Assessment of the reproducibility of baseline and hyperemic myocardial blood flow measurements with 15O-labeled water and PET. J Nucl Med. 1999;40:1848–56.
48. Hutchins GD, Schwaiger M, Rosenspire KC, Krivokapich J, Schelbert H, Kuhl DE. Noninvasive quantification of regional blood flow in the human heart using N-13 ammonia and dynamic positron emission tomographic imaging. J Am Coll Cardiol. 1990;15:1032–42.
49. Lautamäki R, George RT, Kitagawa K, et al. Rubidium-82 PET-CT for quantitative assessment of myocardial blood flow: validation in a canine model of coronary artery stenosis. Eur J Nucl Med Mol Imaging. 2009;36:576–86.
50. Nekolla SG, Reder S, Saraste A, et al. Evaluation of the novel myocardial perfusion positron-emission tomography tracer 18F-BMS-747158-02: comparison to 13N-ammonia and validation with microspheres in a pig model. Circulation. 2009;119:2333–42.
51. Gould KL, Johnson NP, Bateman TM, et al. Anatomic versus physiologic assessment of coronary artery disease. Role of coronary flow reserve, fractional flow reserve, and positron emission tomography imaging in revascularization decision-making. J Am Coll Cardiol. 2013;62:1639–53.
52. Muzik O, Duvernoy C, Beanlands RS, et al. Assessment of diagnostic performance of quantitative flow measurements in normal subjects and patients with angiographically documented coronary artery disease by means of nitrogen-13 ammonia and positron emission tomography. J Am Coll Cardiol. 1998;31:534–40.
53. Kajander SA, Joutsiniemi E, Saraste M, et al. Clinical value of absolute quantification of myocardial perfusion with (15)O-water in coronary artery disease. Circ Cardiovasc Imaging. 2011;4:678–84.
54. Hajjiri MM, Leavitt MB, Zheng H, Spooner AE, Fischman AJ, Gewirtz H. Comparison of positron emission tomography measurement of adenosine-stimulated absolute myocardial blood flow versus relative myocardial tracer content for physiological assessment of coronary artery stenosis severity and location. JACC Cardiovasc Imaging. 2009;2:751–8.
55. Fiechter M, Ghadri JR, Gebhard C, et al. Diagnostic value of 13N-ammonia myocardial perfusion PET: added value of myocardial flow reserve. J Nucl Med. 2012;53:1230–4.
56. Joutsiniemi E, Saraste A, Pietilä M, et al. Absolute flow or myocardial flow reserve for the detection of significant coronary artery disease? Eur Heart J Cardiovasc Imaging. 2014;15:659–65.
57. Danad I, Uusitalo V, Kero T, et al. Quantitative assessment of myocardial perfusion in the detection of significant coronary artery disease: cutoff values and diagnostic accuracy of quantitative [(15)O]H2O PET imaging. J Am Coll Cardiol. 2014;64:1464–75.
58. Knaapen P. Quantitative myocardial blood flow imaging: not all flow is equal. Eur J Nucl Med Mol Imaging. 2014;41:116–8.
59. Danad I, Raijmakers PG, Appelman YE, et al. Coronary risk factors and myocardial blood flow in patients evaluated for coronary artery disease: a quantitative [15O]H2O PET/CT study. Eur J Nucl Med Mol Imaging. 2012;39:102–12.
60. Liga R, Rovai D, Sampietro T, et al. Insulin resistance is a major determinant of myocardial blood flow impairment in anginal patients. Eur J Nucl Med Mol Imaging. 2013;40:1905–13.

61. Shaw LJ, Iskandrian AE. Prognostic value of gated myocardial perfusion SPECT. J Nucl Cardiol. 2004;11:171–85.
62. Ziadi MC, DeKemp RA, Williams KA, et al. Impaired myocardial flow reserve on rubidium-82 positron emission tomography imaging predicts adverse outcomes in patients assessed for myocardial ischemia. J Am Coll Cardiol. 2011;58:740–8.
63. Herzog BA, Husmann L, Valenta I, et al. Long-term prognostic value of 13N-ammonia myocardial perfusion positron emission tomography added value of coronary flow reserve. J Am Coll Cardiol. 2009;54:150–6.
64. Farhad H, Dunet V, Bachelard K, et al. Added prognostic value of myocardial blood flow quantitation in rubidium-82 positron emission tomography imaging. Eur Heart J Cardiovasc Imaging. 2013;14:1203–10.
65. Fukushima K, Javadi MS, Higuchi T, et al. Prediction of short-term cardiovascular events using quantification of global myocardial flow reserve in patients referred for clinical 82Rb PET perfusion imaging. J Nucl Med. 2011;52:726–32.
66. Glagov S, Weisenberg E, Zarins CK, Stankunavicius R, Kolettis GJ. Compensatory enlargement of human atherosclerotic coronary arteries. N Engl J Med. 1987;316:1371–5.
67. Groves AM, Speechly-Dick M-E, Kayani I, et al. First experience of combined cardiac PET/64-detector CT angiography with invasive angiographic validation. Eur J Nucl Med Mol Imaging. 2009;36:2027–33.
68. Thomassen A, Petersen H, Diederichsen ACP, Mickley H, Jensen LO, Johansen A, et al. Hybrid CT angiography and quantitative 15O-water PET for assessment of coronary artery disease: comparison with quantitative coronary angiography. Eur J Nucl Med Mol Imaging. 2013;40:1894–904.
69. Rispler S, Keidar Z, Ghersin E, et al. Integrated single-photon emission computed tomography and computed tomography coronary angiography for the assessment of hemodynamically significant coronary artery lesions. J Am Coll Cardiol. 2007;49:1059–67.
70. Sato A, Nozato T, Hikita H, et al. Incremental value of combining 64-slice computed tomography angiography with stress nuclear myocardial perfusion imaging to improve noninvasive detection of coronary artery disease. J Nucl Cardiol. 2010;17:19–26.
71. Schaap J, Kauling RM, Boekholdt SM, et al. Incremental diagnostic accuracy of hybrid SPECT/CT coronary angiography in a population with an intermediate to high pre-test likelihood of coronary artery disease. Eur Heart J Cardiovasc Imaging. 2013;14:642–9.
72. Schaap J, de Groot JAH, Nieman K, et al. Added value of hybrid myocardial perfusion SPECT and CT coronary angiography in the diagnosis of coronary artery disease. Eur Heart J Cardiovasc Imaging. 2014;15(11):1281–8.
73. Groothuis JGJ, Beek AM, Brinckman SL, et al. Combined non-invasive functional and anatomical diagnostic work-up in clinical practice: the magnetic resonance and computed tomography in suspected coronary artery disease (MARCC) study. Eur Heart J. 2013;34:1990–8.
74. Schenker MP, Dorbala S, et al. Interrelation of coronary calcification, myocardial ischemia, and outcomes in patients with intermediate likelihood of coronary artery disease: a combined positron emission tomography/computed tomography study. Circulation. 2008;117:1693–700.
75. Naya M, Murthy VL, Foster CR, et al. Prognostic interplay of coronary artery calcification and underlying vascular dysfunction in patients with suspected coronary artery disease. J Am Coll Cardiol. 2013;61:2098–106.
76. van Werkhoven JM, Schuijf JD, Gaemperli O, et al. Prognostic value of multislice computed tomography and gated single-photon emission computed tomography in patients with suspected coronary artery disease. J Am Coll Cardiol. 2009,53.623–32.
77. Pazhenkottil AP, Nkoulou RN, Ghadri J-R, et al. Prognostic value of cardiac hybrid imaging integrating single-photon emission computed tomography with coronary computed tomography angiography. Eur Heart J. 2011;32:1465–71.
78. Kim H-L, Kim Y-J, Lee S-P, et al. Incremental prognostic value of sequential imaging of single-photon emission computed tomography and coronary computed tomography angiography in patients with suspected coronary artery disease. Eur Heart J Cardiovasc Imaging. 2014;15:878–85.

79. Rochitte CE, George RT, Chen MY, et al. Computed tomography angiography and perfusion to assess coronary artery stenosis causing perfusion defects by single photon emission computed tomography: the CORE320 study. Eur Heart J. 2014;35:1120–30.
80. Taylor CA, Fonte TA, Min JK. Computational fluid dynamics applied to cardiac computed tomography for noninvasive quantification of fractional flow reserve: scientific basis. J Am Coll Cardiol. 2013;61:2233–41.
81. Koo B-K, Erglis A, Doh J-H, et al. Diagnosis of ischemia-causing coronary stenoses by noninvasive fractional flow reserve computed from coronary computed tomographic angiograms. Results from the prospective multicenter DISCOVER-FLOW (Diagnosis of Ischemia-Causing Stenoses Obtained Via Noninvasive Fractional Flow Reserve) study. J Am Coll Cardiol. 2011;58:1989–97.
82. Min JK, Leipsic J, Pencina MJ, et al. Diagnostic accuracy of fractional flow reserve from anatomic CT angiography. JAMA. 2012;308:1237–45.
83. Nørgaard BL, Leipsic J, Gaur S, et al. Diagnostic performance of noninvasive fractional flow reserve derived from coronary computed tomography angiography in suspected coronary artery disease: the NXT trial (Analysis of Coronary Blood Flow Using CT Angiography: Next Steps). J Am Coll Cardiol. 2014;63:1145–55.
84. Wong DTL, Ko BS, Cameron JD, et al. Transluminal attenuation gradient in coronary computed tomography angiography is a novel noninvasive approach to the identification of functionally significant coronary artery stenosis: a comparison with fractional flow reserve. J Am Coll Cardiol. 2013;61:1271–9.
85. Stuijfzand WJ, Danad I, Raijmakers PG, et al. Additional value of transluminal attenuation gradient in CT angiography to predict hemodynamic significance of coronary artery stenosis. JACC Cardiovasc Imaging. 2014;7:374–86.

12 Adding CT Measurements of Coronary Artery Calcification to Nuclear Myocardial Perfusion Imaging for Risk Stratification

Mouaz H. Al-Mallah

12.1 Introduction

Coronary artery disease remains one of the main causes of mutuality and morbidity in the current century [1]. Multiple tools are used in the diagnosis and assessment of suspected patients with CAD. Despite that, establishing the diagnosis of CAD remains a challenge in certain cases. In this chapter, we will review one of the most commonly used tools in the workup of patients with suspected CAD, nuclear myocardial perfusion imaging (MPI). Then we will discuss the incremental role of coronary artery calcium (CAC) scoring among patients undergoing MPI.

12.2 Nuclear Myocardial Perfusion Imaging

Nuclear MPI is a commonly used test and a practical choice in the evaluation of patients known or suspected to have CAD. The most commonly used tests include SPECT MPI and less often positron emission tomography (PET MPI). Both exercise and vasodilator stress MPI can be performed with SPECT and can be performed with acceptable diagnostic accuracy [2]. Among the various available imaging agents with SPECT, technetium-labeled tracers are predominantly used due to technetium higher energy and short half-life [3]. Given its wide use and long-standing history, there is significant data to support MPI routine use in the assessment and prognostication of suspected CAD as well as assessment of response to therapy [4–7]. Combining MPI with exercise stress testing provides important estimation of the cardiorespiratory fitness and adds significant prognostic value [8]. Pooled data

M.H. Al-Mallah, MD, MSc, FACC, FAHA, FESC
Cardiac Imaging, King Abdul-Aziz Cardiac Center,
King Abdul-Aziz Medical Center,
National Guard Health Affairs, Riyadh, Kingdom of Saudi Arabia
e-mail: mouaz74@gmail.com

T.H. Schindler et al. (eds.), *Molecular and Multimodality Imaging in Cardiovascular Disease*, DOI 10.1007/978-3-319-19611-4_12

of the various stress protocols revealed a sensitivity of 90 % and specificity of nearly 80 % [9]. The addition of gated imaging allows for evaluation of left ventricular wall motion and ejection fraction and further improves the diagnostic accuracy [10, 11]. Moreover, the advent of hybrid scanners allows for CT-based attenuation correction and improves the diagnostic accuracy by reducing artifacts and improving the study specificity [12].

In the recent years, cardiac PET emerged as a robust tool for evaluation of myocardial ischemia [13–15]. PET MPI is almost exclusively performed via pharmacological stress testing. It provides a better diagnostic accuracy compared to SPECT owing its better spatial resolution and image quality as well as superior specificity [15, 16]. In a pooled analysis of 15 studies and 1344 patients, PET was superior to SPECT in detecting CAD with a sensitivity and specificity of 90 % and 88 %, respectively [16]. The ability to evaluate left ventricular wall motion abnormalities during maximum hyperemia at peak stress with PET significantly improves detection of significant ischemia [17]. Moreover, noninvasive measurement of myocardial blood flow (MBF) and myocardial flow reserve can be performed with PET improving detection of multivessel epicedial CAD [18] and allowing for evaluation of the functional significance of intermediate anatomical lesions [19, 20].

However, considerable discrepancy has been shown between the extent of the anatomical stenosis and inducible ischemia on MPI [21, 22]. While this is seen with PET and SPECT, it is most pronounced with SPECT MPI. In a study of 101 patients with angiographic left main CAD (> or=50 % stenosis) and no prior myocardial infarction or coronary revascularization, gated exercise or adenosine stress technetium SPECT MPI identified high-risk ischemic features in 56 % of patients visually and 59 % quantitatively [23]. More importantly, 13 % of the patients had no evidence of significant perfusion defects. Thus, further tools may be needed to improve the overall accuracy of MPI and provide a comprehensive evaluation of the different pathophysiological processes in CAD as well as aid in the decision making of equivocal MPI tests as well as optimization of medical therapy.

12.3 Coronary Artery Calcium Score

On the other hand, the relationship between CAC and CAD has been established for over a decade. Several studies indicated a strong positive correlation between CAC and significant CAD by angiography or histology [24–26]. Although CAC can be evaluated by many imaging modalities including plain chest radiographs and fluoroscopy, the use of multislice computed tomography (MSCT) systems is the most reproducible technique used to detect CAC [27]. CAC scoring has several advantages. It is a fast test that takes less than ten seconds of breath hold to acquire. There is no need for any patient preparation and no intravenous contrast injection. In addition, CAC scoring can be performed on any MSCT system that has gating capabilities and can be routinely performed with very low radiation doses (less than millisievert) [28, 29].

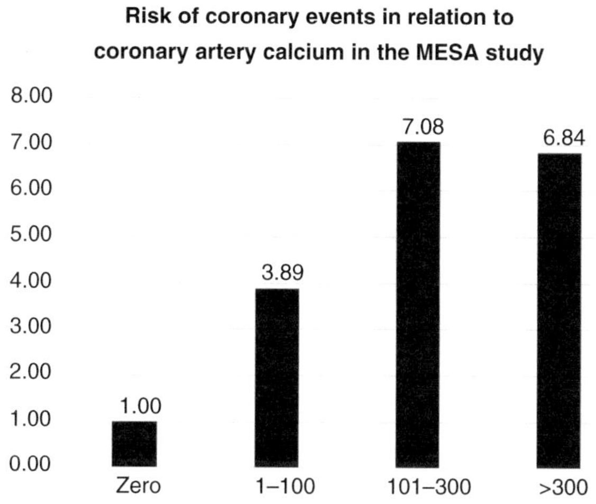

Fig. 12.1 Risk of coronary events in relation to coronary artery calcium in the MESA study. The increase in coronary calcium score more than 100 was associated with more than sixfold increase in coronary events [39]

Calcium detected on these non-contrast CT scans is scored using the Agatston technique that was first described in 1990 [30]. This score takes into account both the density and the volume of the arterial calcification. The presence of a nonzero CAC score has been associated with a high likelihood of significant CAD (sensitivity of 94–100 %, specificity 44–66 %) [31–33]. More importantly, the absence of CAC is associated with a very low probability (<2 %) of significant coronary stenosis (≥50 %) even among symptomatic patients [34, 35]. However, CAC score is significantly affected by gender and race. Data from the Multi-Ethnic Study of Atherosclerosis (MESA) demonstrated that the CAC increases with age and is higher in Caucasian males in comparison to other ethnicities [36, 37]. For the same CAC score, African Americans, for example, tend to have more diffuse CAD compared to Caucasians.

The prognostic value of CAC scoring performed as a single test has also been proven in both asymptomatic and symptomatic cohorts [38]. The Multi-Ethnic Study of Atherosclerosis (MESA) clearly demonstrated the increased cardiac events with increasing CAC score over a follow-up duration of 5 years (Fig. 12.1) [39].

A meta-analysis by Pletcher et al. demonstrated that in comparison to CAC score of zero Agatston unit (AU), CAC score of (1–100 AU) has 2.1 relative risk for cardiac event including cardiac death, nonfatal myocardial infarction (MI), or stroke, while CAC score > 400AU has a much higher risk of cardiac event (relative risk 4.3) [40]. In another analysis, a CAC score of zero was associated with a very low risk of cardiac death or MI (annual event rate less than 0.4 %) [41]. In addition, many studies have shown that CAC provides incremental prognostic value over traditional risk factors [42] or biomarkers such as high sensitivity C-reactive protein [43]. However, the most important role of CAC remains its ability to reclassify patients within different risk categories as determined by the Framingham Risk Score (FRS) or even the newly described American College of Cardiology/American Heart Association risk estimator equation. Greenland et al. have showed that in the MESA cohort, the addition of CAC score to a prediction model based on traditional risk factors significantly improved the classification of risk and placed more individuals in the most extreme risk categories [44]. A total of 23 % of those who experienced events were reclassified to high risk, and an additional 13 % without events were reclassified to low risk. In the Heinz Nixdorf Recall study, CAC scoring reclassified 21.7 % and 30.6 % of the intermediate-risk group into the low- and high-risk groups, respectively, using CAC <100 and CAC >400 as cutoff values [45]. Recently, data from the MESA showed that nearly all risk score estimators overestimate the risk of patients by 25–115 % compared to calcium score using cardiac events as the endpoint [46].

CAC scoring has also an important role in the evaluation of patients with diabetes, a condition that is highly prevalent among patients referred to the nuclear labs. Several studies demonstrated that diabetic patients have a higher prevalence of CAC and a higher score compared to nondiabetic [47–49]. In a review of 10,377 asymptomatic individuals referred for CAC evaluation with a mean follow-up of 5 years, Raggi et al. found that CAC predicted all-cause mortality in diabetics [50]. In this cohort, the overall mortality was proportionate to the degree of calcification and at any given CAC score, the mortality was higher in diabetic compared to nondiabetic at any CAC score. In the same context, the absence of CAC was associated with low mortality irrespective of the presence of DM (Fig. 12.2).

However, the inherent difference between CAC and MPI should be kept in mind while utilizing both tests. While CAC is a measure of subclinical atherosclerotic burden, MPI evaluates the functional significance of coronary artery lesions. Looking at the same disease condition from different angles may provide more accurate diagnosis and assessment of the outcome. In the second part of this chapter, we will review the complimentary role of nuclear MPI and calcium score in patients referred to nuclear laboratories.

12.4 CAC Incremental Diagnostic Value

The addition of calcium score to nuclear MPI appears to add significant diagnostic value. CAC score could unmask significant CAD in patients with otherwise normal or low-risk MPI. Berman and colleagues evaluated 1195 subjects (51 % symptomatic) with both single-photon emission computed tomography (SPECT) and CAC scoring. Inducible ischemia was highly prevalent with high CAC and rarely seen when CAC <100 AU (<2 %) [51]. However, as shown in Fig. 12.3, many patients with normal SPECT MPI may have significant atherosclerosis which could be detected by CAC scoring [51].

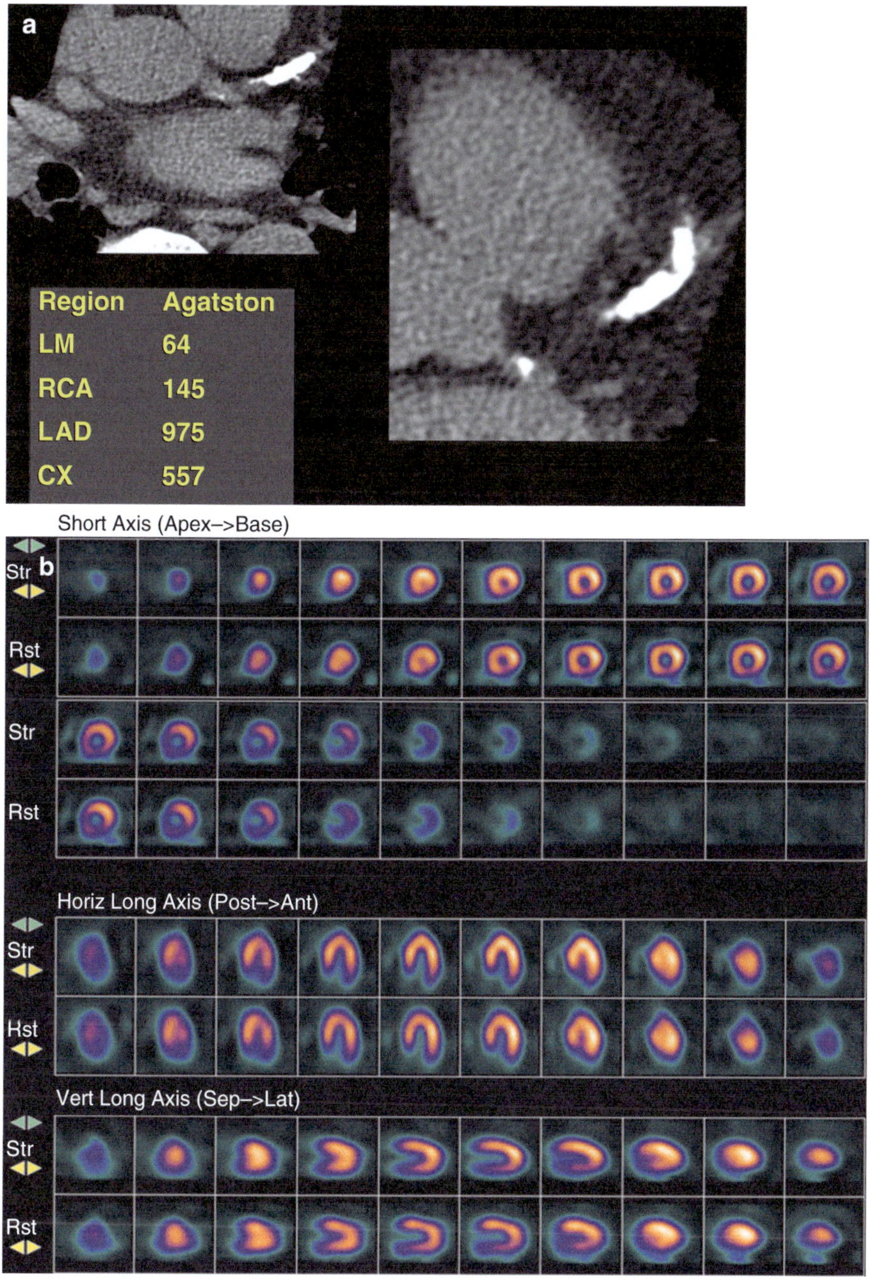

Fig. 12.2 (**a**) Coronary calcium score in a 71-year-old ex-smoker patient with chest pain and normal ECG. It shows severe coronary calcification in all three vessels with very high score of 1741 AU. (**b**) SPECT myocardial perfusion imaging: No significant perfusion defects are seen (other than diaphragmatic attenuation). The patient had severe three-vessel disease on coronary angiography and underwent coronary artery bypass surgery

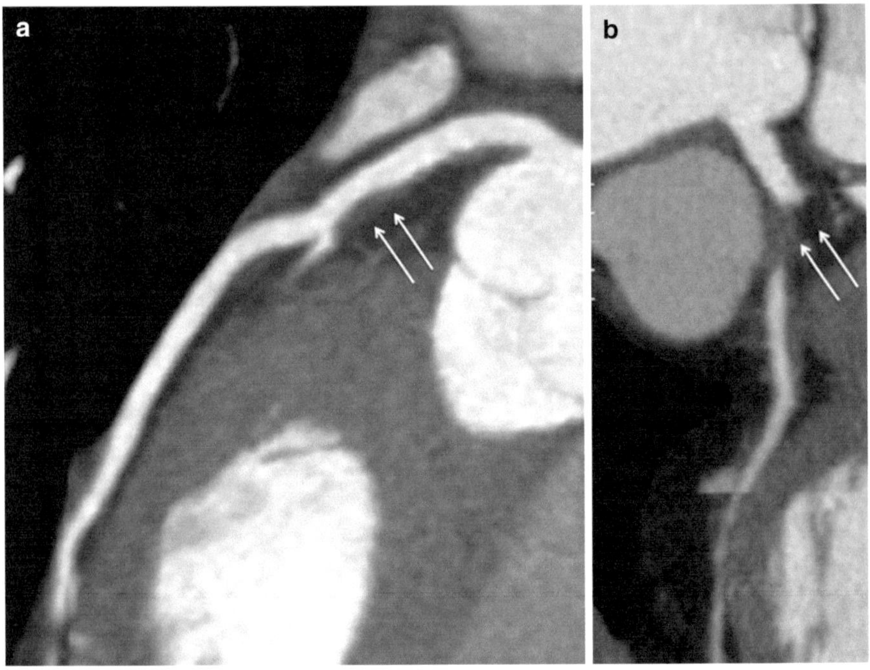

Fig. 12.3 Coronary CT angiography in a 70-year-old female with chest pain and normal ECG and cardiac markers. Coronary calcium score was zero. The patient has a non obstructive noncalcified plaque CAD in the LAD (**a**). The mid-RCA artery has a total occlusion with noncalcified plaque (**b**). *Arrow* indicates the location of the stenosis (**a**, **b**)

In a study of 77 intermediate-risk subjects referred for invasive angiography, CAC scoring and SPECT MPI were done [52]. A CAC score of 709 AU had high accuracy to detect significant CAD missed by SPECT MPI. This was also confirmed in another cohort of 864 asymptomatic patients [53] where a CAC score >1000 AU was able to detect significant coronary stenosis (≥50 %) on invasive angiography despite normal myocardial perfusion on SPECT [54]. This increased diagnostic accuracy is mostly related to the fact that a combined MPI-CAC study evaluates both anatomical and physiological aspects of the disease; thus allowing overcoming the limitations of physiological testing in patients where the anatomical burden of the disease is very significant.

12.5 Impact of Medical Therapy and Compliance

The identification of subclinical atherosclerosis by CAC can also help optimize the clinicians to optimize the medical therapy of patients with normal perfusion on MPI but higher atherosclerotic burden on CAC scoring. Nasir et al. found that only 59 % of subjects with CAC >400 AU and 65 % of subjects with CAC 100–399 AU did not qualify for pharmacotherapy by National Cholesterol Education Program

(NCEP) Panel III guidelines leaving a significant number of patients with atherosclerosis without potentially lifesaving therapies [35]. Bybee et al. found that substantial number of patients with subclinical atherosclerosis and normal perfusion on PET were not receiving adequate therapy [55]. Only 41.5 % of patients with CAC 100–399 AU and 47.7 % of patients with CAC >400 AU were receiving statin with similar proportion of patients receiving aspirin. Increasing CAC score was associated with a higher chance of optimizing the medical therapy after PET result; the increasing CAC score was independently associated with initiation and optimization of medical therapy [55]. However, the prognostic value of this practice (adding intensive medical therapy to patients with normal perfusion and high CAC score) needs further evaluation and testing in a randomized controlled setting. Despite the proven utility of CAC in the diagnosis and prognosis of CAD, the exact score at which secondary preventive therapy should start is not well defined. The St. Francis Heart Study showed that asymptomatic patient with CAC >80th percentile did not benefit of daily atorvastatin therapy [56]. However, benefit with statin therapy was shown in a post hoc analysis of the same study in patients with CAC >80th percentiles and family history of CAD [57]. In an analysis of the MESA population who fulfilled the JUPITAR trial inclusion criteria, Blaha et al. reported that 5-year NNT was 24 and 19 for coronary heart disease and cardiovascular disease, respectively, when CAC >100 AU [58]. Therefore, although the exact CAC score to start statin therapy is not precisely defined, it is fair to say that statin therapy is reasonable to be started when CAC >100 AU [59]. Furthermore, it is important to note that the current guidelines recommend stress testing for asymptomatic patients with CAC >400 AU [60, 54].

12.6 Incremental Prognostic Value

The prognostic value of nuclear MPI has been extensively studied both with SPECT and PET imaging. While a normal exercise SPECT is associated with <1 % annual event rate of future cardiac event, an abnormal SPECT is associated with higher all-cause and cardiac mortality and cardiac events that are proportionate to the extent of abnormalities [61–63]. In addition, registry data suggested that nuclear MPI can be used to guide medical decisions. A reversible perfusion defect less than 10 % of the left ventricle would best be treated with medical therapy, while significant ischemia would best be treated with revascularization when feasible [64]. This approach is being tested in a large-scale National Institute of Health (NIH)-funded trial [65].

Several large-scale studies have examined the prognostic value of CAC over myocardial perfusion with SPECT. In 1126 patients (10 % diabetic) who underwent both CAC and SPECT MPI, Chang et al. found that all-cause mortality and nonfatal MI increased significantly with the severity of CAC [66]. CAC score >400 AU was associated with a 2.75-fold increase in all-cause mortality and nonfatal MI despite normal SPECT after a median follow-up duration of 7 years. Additionally, all-cause mortality and nonfatal MI exponentially increased with increasing severity of CAC in both normal and abnormal SPECT groups. Although the extent of ischemia on SPECT predicted hard cardiac event, adding CAC to the SPECT findings (normal/abnormal) further reclassified patients irrespective of the degree of ischemia on SPECT. Multiple smaller studies reported confirmed the above finding of the incremental prognostic value of CAC score over SPECT MPI [67, 68]. However, this added prognostic value may not be seen in short follow-up durations. A study of 1153 with a mean follow-up of 32 months showed that high CAC score failed to add incremental prognostic value in patients with normal perfusion on SPECT [69].

12.7 Addition of CAC to Positron Emission Tomography (PET)

The prognostic value of PET MPI has been demonstrated in several recent studies [70]. In a multicenter registry of 7061 patients referred for rubidium-82 stress PET, the extent and severity of perfusion abnormality were independent predictors of cardiac and all-cause mortalities [71]. Severely abnormal PET was associated with fivefold increase in cardiac mortality, and perfusion PET was able to reclassify nearly 12 % of patients. In addition, noninvasive coronary flow reserve adds incremental prognostic value to perfusion abnormalities on PET [72, 73].

In concordance with SPECT literature, a study of 695 intermediate-risk patients who underwent rubidium-82 PET imaging showed that an abnormal PET scan was seen more often with increasing CAC score [74]. The frequency of abnormal scans among patients with a CAC score > or = 400 was higher than that in patients with a CAC score of 1–399 (48.5 % versus 21.7 %, P <0.001). However, the frequency of ischemia among patients with no CAC was 16.0 %, and its absence only afforded a negative predictive value of 84.0 %. Among patients with normal PET myocardial perfusion imaging, the annualized event rate in patients with no CAC was lower than in those with a CAC score > or = 1000 (2.6 % versus 12.3 %, respectively). Likewise, in patients with ischemia on PET myocardial perfusion imaging, the annualized event rate in those with no CAC was lower than among patients with a CAC score > or = 1000 (8.2 % versus 22.1 %) (Fig. 12.4).

This was also seen in patients referred to our laboratory. With very high prevalence of diabetes mellitus (55 %), hypercholesterolemia (90 %), and hypertension (87 %), the prevalence of perfusion defects increased with increasing CAC score. While nearly 54 % of patients with CAC >400 AU had an abnormal scan [75], the absence of CAC excluded ischemia in 206 intermediate-risk subjects with a negative predictive value (NPV) of 99 % (Fig. 12.5) [76]. These findings support the notion that CAC is predictive of abnormal myocardial perfusion on PET and thus may be used to improve the diagnostic accuracy of PET MPI.

Since most PET systems are hybrid machines including both PET and CT used primarily for attenuation correction, CAC score can be easily performed in the same setting. The interplay between CAC and coronary flow reserve (CFR) measured on PET was investigated in 901 patients with a mean follow-up of 1.53 years. The annual major adverse cardiac event (MACE), including cardiac death, nonfatal MI,

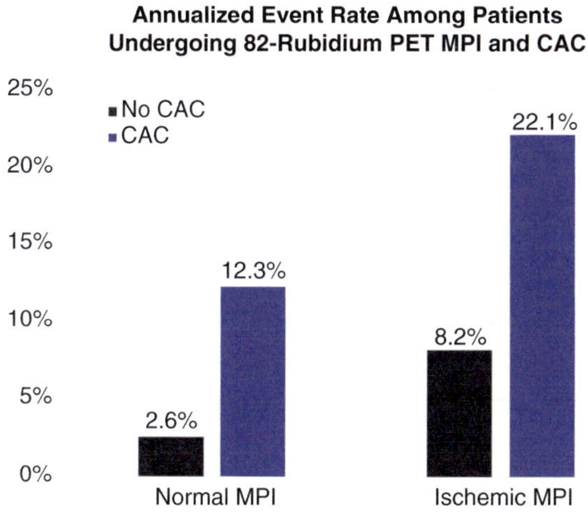

Fig. 12.4 Event rate among patients undergoing both 82-rubidium PET MPI and CAC. Among patients with normal PET myocardial perfusion imaging, the annualized event rate in patients with no CAC was lower than in those with a CAC score ≥ 1,000 (2.6 % versus 12.3 %, respectively). Likewise, in patients with ischemia on PET myocardial perfusion imaging, the annualized event rate in those with no CAC was lower than among patients with a CAC score ≥ 1,000 (8.2 % versus 22.1 %)

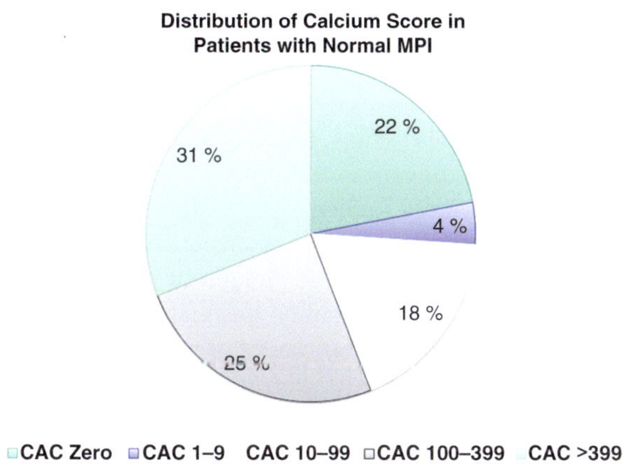

Fig. 12.5 Distribution of coronary calcium score in a patients with normal myocardial perfusion imaging. Patients with normal myocardial perfusion imaging have a wide range of coronary calcium. Nearly one third of the patients have high calcium score of more than 400 [51]

revascularization, and admission for heart failure, increased with CFR <2 [77]. Although there was no direct association between CAC and short-term MACE in this study, CFR <2 occurred at higher frequency with increasing CAC score. Moreover, there was a significant association between low CFR (<2) and annual MACE across all levels of CAC [77]. The findings of this study may suggest that

CAC although reflective of overall atherosclerotic burden is likely to represent a late manifestation of atherosclerosis than reflecting the activity of the disease. CAC may be predicative of late events, while CFR and myocardial ischemia could be predictive of short-term events.

Finally, evaluating CAC allows for measurement of other potential high-risk markers. There is some data to suggest that epicardial fat is associated with presence and outcome of CAD [78, 79]. It can be easily measured on the gated non-contrast CT used for CAC scoring. It has been associated with ischemia on SPECT MPI with odd ratio of 2.68 in patients without known CAD [80]. Measurement of pericardial fat may help in the decision making of obscure cases of SPECT and may help further in stratification of the patients in general. In addition, other vascular and cardiac nonvascular calcifications can be measured, many of which add independent prognostic value. However, further data is needed to confirm the added role of epicardial fat and noncoronary cardiac calcifications.

12.8 Practical Considerations

Despite the clearly demonstrated incremental diagnostic and prognostic value of coronary calcium score in different patient populations, some practical considerations need to be taken into account. Given the fact that CAC and perfusion imaging study are two different distinct processes, it would be expected to have clinical scenarios where the two tests yield discrepant results. The impact of these discrepant results on the patient acute management is not well studied. Management decision should take into account the patients' baseline risk and symptomatic status as well as baseline coronary disease status. Since coronary calcium score has limited role in patients with known coronary disease (prior angioplasty or bypass surgery), these patients need to be primarily studied by perfusion imaging. On the other hand, one would expect a very low prevalence of perfusion defects in patients with zero calcium score (<5 %). Artifacts have to be thought of in this patient population of zero calcium score including misregistration artifacts. Untimely revascularization decisions should be made based on the presence of perfusion defects and the extent of myocardial ischemia. Thus, patients with normal perfusion and patients with high calcium score should not be subjected to coronary angiography unless balanced ischemia is suspected. On the other hand, patients with a true perfusion defect should not be deprived from revascularization just because their calcium score is low.

Conclusion

In conclusion, CAC scoring is a robust and effective tool for the detection of anatomical atherosclerosis, while myocardial perfusion imaging is a superb and validated technique to detect myocardial ischemia and prognosticate patients. While CAC and MPI evaluate two deferent aspects of CAD, anatomy versus physiology, it is likely that in a moderate- or high-risk population, adding CAC measurement to myocardial perfusion imaging with PET and SPECT imaging would give an incremental diagnostic and prognostic value. It will also aid in optimizing the medical therapy and risk stratification of subjects. However, revascularization decisions should be solely made based on the ischemic evaluation rather than the anatomic manifestation of atherosclerosis.

References

1. Go AS, Mozaffarian D, Roger VL, et al. American Heart Association Statistics C, Stroke Statistics S. Heart disease and stroke statistics–2014 update: a report from the american heart association. Circulation. 2014;129:e28–e292.
2. Holly TA, Abbott BG, Al-Mallah M, et al. American Society of Nuclear C. Single photon-emission computed tomography. J Nucl Cardiol. 2010;17:941–73.
3. Melon PG, Beanlands RS, DeGrado TR, Nguyen N, Petry NA, Schwaiger M. Comparison of technetium-99m sestamibi and thallium-201 retention characteristics in canine myocardium. J Am Coll Cardiol. 1992;20:1277–83.
4. Beller GA, Zaret BL. Contributions of nuclear cardiology to diagnosis and prognosis of patients with coronary artery disease. Circulation. 2000;101:1465–78.
5. De Lorenzo A, Lima RS, Siqueira-Filho AG, Pantoja MR. Prevalence and prognostic value of perfusion defects detected by stress technetium-99m sestamibi myocardial perfusion single-photon emission computed tomography in asymptomatic patients with diabetes mellitus and no known coronary artery disease. Am J Cardiol. 2002;90:827–32.
6. Hachamovitch R, Berman DS, Kiat H, et al. Exercise myocardial perfusion SPECT in patients without known coronary artery disease: Incremental prognostic value and use in risk stratification. Circulation. 1996;93:905–14.
7. Iskandrian AS, Chae SC, Heo J, Stanberry CD, Wasserleben V, Cave V. Independent and incremental prognostic value of exercise single-photon emission computed tomographic (SPECT) thallium imaging in coronary artery disease. J Am Coll Cardiol. 1993;22:665–70.
8. Kim C, Kwok YS, Heagerty P, Redberg R. Pharmacologic stress testing for coronary disease diagnosis: a meta-analysis. Am Heart J. 2001;142:934–44.
9. Mahmarian JJ, Verani MS. Myocardial perfusion imaging during pharmacologic stress testing. Cardiol Clin. 1994;12:223–45.
10. Bavelaar-Croon CD, Pauwels EK, van der Wall EE. Gated single-photon emission computed tomographic myocardial imaging: a new tool in clinical cardiology. Am Heart J. 2001;141: 383–90.
11. Chua T, Kiat H, Germano G, et al. Gated technetium-99m sestamibi for simultaneous assessment of stress myocardial perfusion, postexercise regional ventricular function and myocardial viability. Correlation with echocardiography and rest thallium-201 scintigraphy. J Am Coll Cardiol. 1994;23:1107–14.
12. Hendel RC, Berman DS, Cullom SJ, et al. Multicenter clinical trial to evaluate the efficacy of correction for photon attenuation and scatter in SPECT myocardial perfusion imaging. Circulation. 1999;99:2742–9.
13. Heller GV, Calnon D, Dorbala S. Recent advances in cardiac pet and pet/ct myocardial perfusion imaging. J Nucl Cardiol. 2009;16:962–9.
14. Di Carli MF. Advances in positron emission tomography. J Nucl Cardiol. 2004;11:719–32.
15. Al-Mallah MH, Sitek A, Moore SC, Di Carli M, Dorbala S. Assessment of myocardial perfusion and function with PET and PET/CT. J Nucl Cardiol. 2010;17:498–513.
16. Mc Ardle BA, Dowsley TF, de Kemp RA, Wells GA, Beanlands RS. Does rubidium-82 pet have superior accuracy to spect perfusion imaging for the diagnosis of obstructive coronary disease?: a systematic review and meta-analysis. J Am Coll Cardiol. 2012;60:1828–37.
17. Dorbala S, Vangala D, Sampson U, Limaye A, Kwong R, Di Carli MF. Value of vasodilator left ventricular ejection fraction reserve in evaluating the magnitude of myocardium at risk and the

extent of angiographic coronary artery disease: a 82rb PET/CT study. J Nucl Med. 2007;48: 349–58.
18. Sampson UK, Dorbala S, Limaye A, Kwong R, Di Carli MF. Diagnostic accuracy of rubidium-82 myocardial perfusion imaging with hybrid positron emission tomography/computed tomography in the detection of coronary artery disease. J Am Coll Cardiol. 2007;49:1052–8.
19. Di Carli M, Czernin J, Hoh CK, et al. Relation among stenosis severity, myocardial blood flow, and flow reserve in patients with coronary artery disease. Circulation. 1995;91:1944–51.
20. Beanlands RS, Muzik O, Melon P, et al. Noninvasive quantification of regional myocardial flow reserve in patients with coronary atherosclerosis using nitrogen-13 ammonia positron emission tomography. Determination of extent of altered vascular reactivity. J Am Coll Cardiol. 1995;26:1465–75.
21. He ZX, Hedrick TD, Pratt CM, et al. Severity of coronary artery calcification by electron beam computed tomography predicts silent myocardial ischemia. Circulation. 2000;101:244–51.
22. Moser KW, O'Keefe Jr JH, Bateman TM, McGhie IA. Coronary calcium screening in asymptomatic patients as a guide to risk factor modification and stress myocardial perfusion imaging. J Nucl Cardiol. 2003;10:590–8.
23. Berman DS, Kang X, Slomka PJ, et al. Underestimation of extent of ischemia by gated spect myocardial perfusion imaging in patients with left main coronary artery disease. J Nucl Cardiol. 2007;14:521–8.
24. Blankenhorn DH, Stern D. Calcification of the coronary arteries. Am J Roentgenol Radium Ther Nucl Med. 1959;81:772–7.
25. Adams DF, Abrams HL, Ruttley M. The roentgen pathology of coronary artery disease. Semin Roentgenol. 1972;7:319–51.
26. Eggen DA, Strong JP, McGill Jr HC. Coronary calcification. Relationship to clinically significant coronary lesions and race, sex, and topographic distribution. Circulation. 1965;32: 948–55.
27. Wexler L, Brundage B, Crouse J, et al. Coronary artery calcification: pathophysiology, epidemiology, imaging methods, and clinical implications. A statement for health professionals from the american heart association. Writing Group. Circulation. 1996;94:1175–92.
28. El-Hayek G, Benjo A, Uretsky S, et al. Meta-analysis of coronary computed tomography angiography versus standard of care strategy for the evaluation of low risk chest pain: are randomized controlled trials and cohort studies showing the same evidence? Int J Cardiol. 2014;177:238–45.
29. Al-Mallah MH, Aljizeeri A, Alharthi M, Alsaileek A. Routine low-radiation-dose coronary computed tomography angiography. J Saudi Heart Assoc. 2014;25:152–3.
30. Agatston AS, Janowitz WR, Hildner FJ, Zusmer NR, Viamonte Jr M, Detrano R. Quantification of coronary artery calcium using ultrafast computed tomography. J Am Coll Cardiol. 1990;15:827–32.
31. Rumberger JA, Sheedy 3rd PF, Breen JF, Schwartz RS. Coronary calcium, as determined by electron beam computed tomography, and coronary disease on arteriogram. Effect of patient's sex on diagnosis. Circulation. 1995;91:1363–7.
32. Budoff MJ, Georgiou D, Brody A, et al. Ultrafast computed tomography as a diagnostic modality in the detection of coronary artery disease: a multicenter study. Circulation. 1996;93:898–904.
33. Nallamothu BK, Saint S, Bielak LF, et al. Electron-beam computed tomography in the diagnosis of coronary artery disease: a meta-analysis. Arch Intern Med. 2001;161:833–8.
34. Haberl R, Becker A, Leber A, et al. Correlation of coronary calcification and angiographically documented stenoses in patients with suspected coronary artery disease: results of 1,764 patients. J Am Coll Cardiol. 2001;37:451–7.
35. Nasir K, Michos ED, Blumenthal RS, Raggi P. Detection of high-risk young adults and women by coronary calcium and national cholesterol education program panel iii guidelines. J Am Coll Cardiol. 2005;46:1931–6.
36. Bild DE, Detrano R, Peterson D, et al. Ethnic differences in coronary calcification: the multi-ethnic study of atherosclerosis (MESA). Circulation. 2005;111:1313–20.

37. McClelland RL, Chung H, Detrano R, Post W, Kronmal RA. Distribution of coronary artery calcium by race, gender, and age: results from the multi-ethnic study of atherosclerosis (MESA). Circulation. 2006;113:30–7.
38. Sarwar A, Shaw LJ, Shapiro MD, et al. Diagnostic and prognostic value of absence of coronary artery calcification. JACC Cardiovasc Imaging. 2009;2:675–88.
39. Detrano R, Guerci AD, Carr JJ, et al. Coronary calcium as a predictor of coronary events in four racial or ethnic groups. N Engl J Med. 2008;358:1336–45.
40. Pletcher MJ, Tice JA, Pignone M, Browner WS. Using the coronary artery calcium score to predict coronary heart disease events: a systematic review and meta-analysis. Arch Intern Med. 2004;164:1285–92.
41. Greenland P, Bonow RO, Brundage BH, et al. ACC/AHA 2007 clinical expert consensus document on coronary artery calcium scoring by computed tomography in global cardiovascular risk assessment and in evaluation of patients with chest pain: a report of the american college of cardiology foundation clinical expert consensus task force (ACC/AHA writing committee to update the 2000 expert consensus document on electron beam computed tomography) developed in collaboration with the society of atherosclerosis imaging and prevention and the society of cardiovascular computed tomography. J Am Coll Cardiol. 2007;49:378–402.
42. Arad Y, Goodman KJ, Roth M, Newstein D, Guerci AD. Coronary calcification, coronary disease risk factors, c-reactive protein, and atherosclerotic cardiovascular disease events: the St. Francis heart study. J Am Coll Cardiol. 2005;46:158–65.
43. Mohlenkamp S, Lehmann N, Moebus S, et al. Quantification of coronary atherosclerosis and inflammation to predict coronary events and all-cause mortality. J Am Coll Cardiol. 2011;57: 1455–64.
44. Greenland P, LaBree L, Azen SP, Doherty TM, Detrano RC. Coronary artery calcium score combined with framingham score for risk prediction in asymptomatic individuals. JAMA. 2004;291:210–5.
45. Erbel R, Mohlenkamp S, Moebus S, et al. Coronary risk stratification, discrimination, and reclassification improvement based on quantification of subclinical coronary atherosclerosis: the Heinz Nixdorf recall study. J Am Coll Cardiol. 2010;56:1397–406.
46. DeFilippis AP, Young R, Carrubba CJ, et al. An analysis of calibration and discrimination among multiple cardiovascular risk scores in a modern multiethnic cohort. Ann Intern Med. 2015;162:266–75.
47. Khaleeli E, Peters SR, Bobrowsky K, Oudiz RJ, Ko JY, Budoff MJ. Diabetes and the associated incidence of subclinical atherosclerosis and coronary artery disease: Implications for management. Am Heart J. 2001;141:637–44.
48. Hoff JA, Quinn L, Sevrukov A, et al. The prevalence of coronary artery calcium among diabetic individuals without known coronary artery disease. J Am Coll Cardiol. 2003;41: 1008–12.
49. Schurgin S, Rich S, Mazzone T. Increased prevalence of significant coronary artery calcification in patients with diabetes. Diabetes Care. 2001;24:335–8.
50. Raggi P, Shaw LJ, Berman DS, Callister TQ. Prognostic value of coronary artery calcium screening in subjects with and without diabetes. J Am Coll Cardiol. 2004;43:1663–9.
51. Berman DS, Wong ND, Gransar H, et al. Relationship between stress-induced myocardial ischemia and atherosclerosis measured by coronary calcium tomography. J Am Coll Cardiol. 2004;44:923–30.
52. Schepis T, Gaemperli O, Koepfli P, et al. Added value of coronary artery calcium score as an adjunct to gated spect for the evaluation of coronary artery disease in an intermediate-risk population. J Nucl Med. 2007;48:1424–30.
53. Anand DV, Lim E, Raval U, Lipkin D, Lahiri A. Prevalence of silent myocardial ischemia in asymptomatic individuals with subclinical atherosclerosis detected by electron beam tomography. J Nucl Cardiol. 2004;11:450–7.
54. Ghadri JR, Pazhenkottil AP, Nkoulou RN, et al. Very high coronary calcium score unmasks obstructive coronary artery disease in patients with normal spect mpi. Heart. 2011;97: 998–1003.

55. Bybee KA, Lee J, Markiewicz R, et al. Diagnostic and clinical benefit of combined coronary calcium and perfusion assessment in patients undergoing pet/ct myocardial perfusion stress imaging. J Nucl Cardiol. 2010;17:188–96.
56. Arad Y, Spadaro LA, Roth M, Newstein D, Guerci AD. Treatment of asymptomatic adults with elevated coronary calcium scores with atorvastatin, vitamin c, and vitamin e: the St. Francis heart study randomized clinical trial. J Am Coll Cardiol. 2005;46:166–72.
57. Mulders TA, Sivapalaratnam S, Stroes ES, Kastelein JJ, Guerci AD, Pinto-Sietsma SJ. Asymptomatic individuals with a positive family history for premature coronary artery disease and elevated coronary calcium scores benefit from statin treatment: a post hoc analysis from the St. Francis heart study. JACC Cardiovasc Imaging. 2012;5:252–60.
58. Blaha MJ, Budoff MJ, DeFilippis AP, et al. Associations between c-reactive protein, coronary artery calcium, and cardiovascular events: implications for the Jupiter population from mesa, a population-based cohort study. Lancet. 2011;378:684–92.
59. Heart Protection Study Collaborative Group. Mrc/bhf heart protection study of cholesterol lowering with simvastatin in 20,536 high-risk individuals: a randomised placebo-controlled trial. Lancet. 2002;360:7–22.
60. Greenland P, Alpert JS, Beller GA, et al. 2010 ACC/AHA guideline for assessment of cardiovascular risk in asymptomatic adults: a report of the american college of cardiology foundation/american heart association task force on practice guidelines. J Am Coll Cardiol. 2010;56:e50–103.
61. Hachamovitch R, Berman DS, Shaw LJ, et al. Incremental prognostic value of myocardial perfusion single photon emission computed tomography for the prediction of cardiac death: differential stratification for risk of cardiac death and myocardial infarction. Circulation. 1998;97:535–43.
62. Cerci MS, Cerci JJ, Cerci RJ, et al. Myocardial perfusion imaging is a strong predictor of death in women. JACC Cardiovasc Imaging. 2011;4:880–8.
63. Hachamovitch R, Berman DS, Kiat H, et al. Incremental prognostic value of adenosine stress myocardial perfusion single-photon emission computed tomography and impact on subsequent management in patients with or suspected of having myocardial ischemia. Am J Cardiol. 1997;80:426–33.
64. Hachamovitch R, Hayes SW, Friedman JD, Cohen I, Berman DS. Comparison of the short-term survival benefit associated with revascularization compared with medical therapy in patients with no prior coronary artery disease undergoing stress myocardial perfusion single photon emission computed tomography. Circulation. 2003;107:2900–7.
65. Phillips LM, Hachamovitch R, Berman DS, et al. Lessons learned from MPI and physiologic testing in randomized trials of stable ischemic heart disease: courage, Bari 2d, fame, and ischemia. J Nucl Cardiol. 2013;20:969–75.
66. Chang SM, Nabi F, Xu J, et al. The coronary artery calcium score and stress myocardial perfusion imaging provide independent and complementary prediction of cardiac risk. J Am Coll Cardiol. 2009;54:1872–82.
67. Anand DV, Lim E, Hopkins D, et al. Risk stratification in uncomplicated type 2 diabetes: prospective evaluation of the combined use of coronary artery calcium imaging and selective myocardial perfusion scintigraphy. Eur Heart J. 2006;27:713–21.
68. Ramakrishna G, Miller TD, Breen JF, Araoz PA, Hodge DO, Gibbons RJ. Relationship and prognostic value of coronary artery calcification by electron beam computed tomography to stress-induced ischemia by single photon emission computed tomography. Am Heart J. 2007;153:807–14.
69. Rozanski A, Gransar H, Wong ND, et al. Clinical outcomes after both coronary calcium scanning and exercise myocardial perfusion scintigraphy. J Am Coll Cardiol. 2007;49:1352–61.
70. Yoshinaga K, Chow BJ, Williams K, et al. What is the prognostic value of myocardial perfusion imaging using rubidium-82 positron emission tomography? J Am Coll Cardiol. 2006;48:1029–39.

71. Dorbala S, Di Carli MF, Beanlands RS, et al. Prognostic value of stress myocardial perfusion positron emission tomography: results from a multicenter observational registry. J Am Coll Cardiol. 2013;61:176–84.
72. Ziadi MC, Dekemp RA, Williams KA, et al. Impaired myocardial flow reserve on rubidium-82 positron emission tomography imaging predicts adverse outcomes in patients assessed for myocardial ischemia. J Am Coll Cardiol. 2011;58:740–8.
73. Murthy VL, Naya M, Foster CR, et al. Association between coronary vascular dysfunction and cardiac mortality in patients with and without diabetes mellitus. Circulation. 2012;126: 1858–68.
74. Schenker MP, Dorbala S, Hong EC, et al. Interrelation of coronary calcification, myocardial ischemia, and outcomes in patients with intermediate likelihood of coronary artery disease: a combined positron emission tomography/computed tomography study. Circulation. 2008;117: 1693–700.
75. Mahmood N, Al-Mallah M. Correlation between coronary calcium score and PET myocardial perfusion abnormalities. Eur Heart J Cardiovasc Imaging. 2014;15(2):ii142–ii144. doi: http://dx.doi.org/10.1093/ehjci/jeu267.
76. Esteves FP, Khan A, Correia LC, et al. Absent coronary artery calcium excludes inducible myocardial ischemia on computed tomography/positron emission tomography. Int J Cardiol. 2011;147:424–7.
77. Naya M, Murthy VL, Foster CR, et al. Prognostic interplay of coronary artery calcification and underlying vascular dysfunction in patients with suspected coronary artery disease. J Am Coll Cardiol. 2013;61:2098–106.
78. Alexopoulos N, McLean DS, Janik M, Arepalli CD, Stillman AE, Raggi P. Epicardial adipose tissue and coronary artery plaque characteristics. Atherosclerosis. 2010;210:150–4.
79. Cheng VY, Dey D, Tamarappoo B, et al. Pericardial fat burden on ecg-gated noncontrast ct in asymptomatic patients who subsequently experience adverse cardiovascular events. JACC Cardiovasc Imaging. 2010;3:352–60.
80. Tamarappoo B, Dey D, Shmilovich H, et al. Increased pericardial fat volume measured from noncontrast ct predicts myocardial ischemia by spect. JACC Cardiovasc Imaging. 2010;3: 1104–12.

Index

T.H. Schindler et al. (eds.), *Molecular and Multimodality Imaging in Cardiovascular Disease*, DOI 10.1007/978-3-319-19611-4

MIX
Papier aus verantwortungsvollen Quellen
Paper from responsible sources
FSC® C105338

If you have any concerns about our products,
you can contact us on
ProductSafety@springernature.com

In case Publisher is established outside the EU,
the EU authorized representative is:
Springer Nature Customer Service Center GmbH
Europaplatz 3, 69115 Heidelberg, Germany

Printed by Libri Plureos GmbH
in Hamburg, Germany